Autism and Child Psychopathology Series

Series Editor
Johnny L. Matson, Department of Psychology
Louisiana State University
Baton Rouge, LA, USA

Brief Overview

The purpose of this series is to advance knowledge in the broad multidisciplinary fields of autism and various forms of psychopathology (e.g., anxiety and depression). Volumes synthesize research on a range of rapidly expanding topics on assessment, treatment, and etiology.

Description

The **Autism and Child Psychopathology Series** explores a wide range of research and professional methods, procedures, and theories used to enhance positive development and outcomes across the lifespan. Developments in education, medicine, psychology, and applied behavior analysis as well as child and adolescent development across home, school, hospital, and community settings are the focus of this series. Series volumes are both authored and edited, and they provide critical reviews of evidence-based methods. As such, these books serve as a critical reference source for researchers and professionals who deal with developmental disorders and disabilities, most notably autism, intellectual disabilities, challenging behaviors, anxiety, depression, ADHD, developmental coordination disorder, communication disorders, and other common childhood problems. The series addresses important mental health and development difficulties that children and youth, their caregivers, and the professionals who treat them must face. Each volume in the series provides an analysis of methods and procedures that may assist in effectively treating these developmental problems.

Nenad Glumbić • Mirjana Đorđević
Branislav Brojčin

Digital Inclusion of Individuals with Autism Spectrum Disorder

Springer

Nenad Glumbić
Faculty of Special Education and Rehabilitation
University of Belgrade
Belgrade, Serbia

Branislav Brojčin
Faculty of Special Education and Rehabilitation
University of Belgrade
Belgrade, Serbia

Mirjana Đorđević
Faculty of Special Education and Rehabilitation
University of Belgrade
Belgrade, Serbia

ISSN 2192-922X ISSN 2192-9238 (electronic)
Autism and Child Psychopathology Series

ISBN 978-3-031-12036-7 ISBN 978-3-031-12037-4 (eBook)
https://doi.org/10.1007/978-3-031-12037-4

This Springer imprint is published by the registered company Springer Nature Switzerland AG
The registered company address is: Gewerbestrasse 11, 6330 Cham, Switzerland

Preface

A long time ago, in a galaxy far, far away, Star Wars premiered on May 25, 1977, accidentally on the same day when the former Socialist Federal Republic of Yugoslavia celebrated the 85th birthday of its communist leader Tito. Ten years earlier, a James Bond movie was not officially approved for cinema release since it showed a British agent who walked around Yugoslavia freely without anyone arresting him. Fortunately, for the first author of this book, Star Wars had a different fate. Sitting in a dark cinema that no longer exists, in a country that also no longer exists, a 7-year-old boy dreamed of getting a toy resembling the cute R2-D2 robot. At the time, he didn't know that it was actually a British musician and actor, Kenny Baker, dressed in a not very comfortable costume.

Only two decades later, the world experienced a digital revolution that, at least in some aspects, surpassed the boldest predictions of science fiction movie makers. It initially seemed that the expansive development of digital technologies would help overcome numerous inequalities of the modern world. However, it was not long before even the most ardent cyber-optimists realized that digital technologies maintain and sometimes even deepen the existing inequalities. Availability and accessibility of devices are only one issue in the complex picture of digital inclusion of certain social groups.

It was believed that certain groups of people could greatly benefit from modern information and communication technologies. A predictable environment, the possibility to limit and delay communication, and a lot of visual content and reinforcers make cyberspace almost an ideal environment for people with autism. And indeed, some people with autism spectrum disorder overcome numerous difficulties with the help of digital technologies. It can often be heard that the Internet is for people with autism what sign language is for the deaf. However, we should always bear in mind that not all people with autism are computer experts, nor is the use of digital technologies alone enough to ensure their social participation.

Thus, we started writing this book with a desire to show the great potential of using information and communication technologies in education, employment, leisure, self-advocacy, treatment, preparation for medical interventions, and all other life aspects of people with autism. At the same time, it was very important for us to indicate the dark side of using the Internet (cyberbullying and cybercrime, development of addictive behavior, etc.). We should point out that certain aspects of using information and communication technologies are limited only to individuals with high-functioning autism and that various forms of the digital divide are still quite present in the modern world.

We are aware that this book presents the current situation in this field and raises certain issues rather than offering solutions. We leave it as a testimony of one period for future readers who would like to know what was happening in terms of the digital inclusion of people with autism a long time ago, in a galaxy far, far away.

Belgrade, Serbia

Nenad Glumbić
Mirjana Đorđević
Branislav Brojčin

Contents

List of Figures

List of Tables

About the Authors

Nenad Glumbić is a full professor at the University of Belgrade, Faculty of Special Education and Rehabilitation. He graduated from the Faculty of Special Education and Rehabilitation, where he also earned his master's degree and PhD (2000), defending the first doctorate in the field of autism in Serbia. He is the author of more than 400 papers and 5 books. His areas of interest include autism spectrum disorder and intellectual disabilities. He has participated in numerous projects and professional and scientific conferences, and is an associate in organizations that provide support to people with autism. In his spare time, he writes short stories and posts for https://www.instagram.com/autism__today/.

Mirjana Đorđević is an associate professor at the University of Belgrade, Faculty of Special Education and Rehabilitation. Her research areas include intellectual disabilities, autism, and support for families and children. She is the founder and manager of the first club for young people with high-functioning autism in Serbia. She is a team member in numerous projects, professional associations, and working groups. In recent years, she has been engaged in developing a national program of family-oriented early interventions.

Branislav Brojčin is a full professor at the University of Belgrade, Faculty of Special Education and Rehabilitation. His areas of interest include inclusive education, development of communication competence, and improvement of attitudes toward people with disabilities. He has collaborated in developing the legal framework of inclusive education in Serbia and training programs for staff, providing additional support for people with disabilities in an educational environment. He cooperates with schools and non-governmental organizations dealing with quality inclusive education.

Chapter 1
Digital Participation and Disability Digital Divide

1.1 Digital Divide

Modern information and communications technology (ICT) and using the Internet have caused significant changes in communication, education, employment, leisure activities, and overall social participation (Grishchenko, 2020). The expansion of digital technologies is considered to be of great importance for further economic development and poverty reduction (United Nations E-Government Survey, 2018). However, it should be kept in mind that ICT development is not a magic wand which will solve all inequalities of the modern world. The initial cyberoptimism of the 1980s started waning with the growing differences in access to digital devices. This was referred to as digital divide (DD).

The origin of this term is associated with Larry Irving, who was the assistant secretary of commerce for communications and information and administrator of the National Telecommunications and Information Administration (NTIA) in Clinton's administration. However, Irving himself denied being the author of this term, claiming, as it usually happens, to "have stolen" it from someone but could not remember whom (according to Gunkel, 2003). The phrase DD first appeared in the mid-1990s, while it became more widely used in 1999 after the publication of the third NTIA's "Falling Through the Net" report in which DD was defined as "the divide between those with access to new technologies and those without" (NTIA, 1999: xiii).

The first research studies on DD focused on the issues of access to digital devices, hardware, software, and Internet connection. Access inequalities were associated with the income and education level of potential users and their age, gender, race, and other sociodemographic characteristics (Van Dijk, 2017). Inequalities in owning digital devices, Internet access possibilities, broadband connection availability, and software accessibility represent first-level DD (Dewan & Riggins, 2005; Robinson et al., 2020).

N. Glumbić et al., *Digital Inclusion of Individuals with Autism Spectrum Disorder*, Autism and Child Psychopathology Series,
https://doi.org/10.1007/978-3-031-12037-4_1

It soon became clear that mere access to digital devices and the Internet did not ensure equality for users due to huge differences in their digital skills and the ways of using the Internet. Thus, research focus shifted from the issue of physical access to the issue of effective use of digital technologies, and the newly determined inequalities in skills and patterns of using digital devices were referred to as second-level DD (Hargittai, 2002). From 2005 to 2015, second-level DD was the main research topic in the field of digital inequalities (Van Dijk, 2017). Such research made it possible to classify the skills needed for using the Internet and types of activities people perform online, as well as to understand their interrelationship (Van Deursen & Helsper, 2015). It was shown that people with similar access level used the Internet in different ways (Brandtzæg et al., 2011). With regard to three criteria (frequency and diversity of Internet use and preference for certain content), these authors divided all users into the following groups: non-users, sporadic users, instrumental users, entertainment users, and advanced users. Significant differences were found in the distribution of certain types of users depending on the country, age, access, and other variables. Further technological development will only increase the existing inequalities between different types of users, confirming the existence of the "rich get richer" effect.

Despite significant progress in bridging first-level DD, inequality in ICT access is still a very relevant issue. Thus, for example, global 4G population coverage was 85% in 2020 (97% in developed world countries and 40.5% in the least developed countries). Over 80% of European urban area population had Internet and computer access, while in rural areas of Africa, only 6% of households had Internet access, and only 2% had computer access (ITU, 2020). This issue of digital inequalities is extremely important since all those without unlimited access to ICTs and the Internet in the future will not be able to use various online resources and will therefore be marginalized in society (Lee et al., 2015). Thus, it is not surprising that Internet access is nowadays being more and more recognized as a human rights issue. The global goal accepted by UNESCO is to achieve Internet access according to "1 for 2" formula, which means that 1GB of mobile broadband data should be available for the maximum of 2% of gross national income per capita (Alliance for Affordable Internet, 2020).

A comprehensive understanding of DD phenomenon is not possible unless research attention focuses on the outcomes of Internet use. Desirable digital outcomes can be achieved in different areas: economic (e.g., finding a well-paid job, purchasing goods and services at reasonable prices), social (e.g., expanding the circle of friends, finding a partner), political (e.g., expressing political views, participating in various political actions), institutional (e.g., making doctor's appointments, calculating taxes), and educational (e.g., acquiring knowledge, skills, formal education) (Van Deursen & Helsper, 2015). Vulnerable social groups which do not have Internet access invest much more energy and effort to exercise their rights and get certain products and services offline. However, as Internet communication develops, some services may not be available at all unless the potential user has access to modern ICTs. Insufficient access to offline services further hinders their participation in digital space, thus completing the digital vicious cycle (Warren, 2007). Nevertheless, even users with virtually unlimited Internet access and with similar Internet use profiles do not necessarily have the same benefits from using it. These differences in outcomes were first referred to as third-level DD in 2011 (Wei et al., 2011). The reason why individuals and certain social groups have difficulties in transferring their Internet use into tangible offline outcomes is the subject of contemporary DD research. In accordance with the modern DD concept, the policy of digital inclusion does not primarily focus on the development of digital infrastructure, but on providing visible benefits of online interactions. Hence, digital inclusion is seen as one aspect of social inclusion in digital society aimed at overcoming the existing inequalities and digital isolation of its members (Plotichkina et al., 2020). Digital inclusion and DD studies are complementary research areas which examine different layers of inequality in the digital world (Carmi & Yates, 2020).

We have seen that the DD concept is very complex and dynamic. The appearance of new forms of digital inequalities has caused changes in denoting this concept. Some authors are trying to encompass the complex nature of digital inequalities by introducing the "digital inequality stack" concept (Robinson et al., 2020), which mostly refers to first- and second-level DD. The first layer of this stack includes access to digital devices, software, and the Internet. Baseline inequalities overflow into a higher stack layer which includes way of using the Internet, digital literacy and skills, production, and programming. Universal access does not automatically ensure equality at a higher level.

It should be kept in mind that individual components of this stack change their original meaning in modern society. Thus, for example, Pawluczuk (2020) points to the fact that many programs aimed at digital inclusion of young people focus on improving their functional digital literacy and teaching them how to access online information while neglecting a very important aspect of critical data analysis. Without critical digital literacy, we will not be able to understand that the information we obtain online is neither objective nor neutral and that there are different techniques used to deliberately spread false information, troll, bot, etc. (Carmi & Yates, 2020). Apart from digital literacy inequalities, more and more attention is given to "big data divide," i.e., the asymmetric power position between those who collect and store huge amounts of data about individuals and some social groups and those who provide such data, without having an insight into its further use (Andrejevic, 2014).

The relationships between different layers of digital inequality stack, as well as their individual components, are very complex, and the factors which generate the observed inequalities need not be the same as well. A vast amount of research is aimed at identifying and comprehending the nature of different DD determinants.

1.1.1 Digital Divide Determinants

Most research papers on digital inequalities are limited to sociodemographic (e.g., age, gender, difference between urban and rural areas) and economic (e.g., income, employment, education level) DD determinants (Scheerder et al., 2017).

Gender-based gap was particularly pronounced at the very beginning of digital revolution when women used ICTs less frequently and had less access to the Internet than men (Robinson et al., 2020). Research conducted in 28 EU countries shows that there are currently no differences between men and women in the use of e-services and social networks (Elena-Bucea et al., 2020). A reverse trend was observed in Russia in the period between 2008 and 2018, when women started using the Internet more than men (Grishchenko, 2020). However, large gender-based DD is still evident in the least developed countries, as well as in developing countries (ITU, 2020). Empirical research indicates that younger people are more likely to use the Internet and ICTs than older ones (e.g., Elena-Bucea et al., 2020; Huxhold et al., 2020). At the end of 2014, Denmark implemented e-government strategy with the aim to address the issues related to pension, different social benefits, paying taxes, etc. online, with the possibility for citizens who prefer the classic offline way of communication to be excluded from digital communication. More than 80% of the total number of people who stated they did not want to use e-government services were over 65 years of age. Research conducted on a large sample of over 3000 participants shows that age, gender, and socioeconomic status are related to the use of ICTs. However, these determinants lose their explanatory power when the users' attitudes and motivation to use digital technologies are taken into account (Siren & Knudsen, 2017). Complex interrelations of different variables, such as belonging to a certain age cohort, socioeconomic inequalities, gender, ageism, cognitive abilities, etc., play an important role in maintaining age-related DD. Many studies have found a great difference between urban and rural areas in the use of modern digital technologies and Internet access, which is particularly pronounced in underdeveloped and developing countries (Adeleke, 2020; Grishchenko, 2020; ITU, 2020).

Economic class and education level are significant predictors of DD (Ma et al., 2019; Robinson et al., 2020; Song et al., 2019). If we only consider aggregated data, we can easily come to a misleading conclusion that the digital gap in richer countries is inevitably smaller than in poorer ones. However, it should be borne in mind that socioeconomic inequalities which determine DD in certain social strata exist even in the most developed countries. Thus, for example, the citizens of Austria and Ireland are above the European mean in general ICT adoption, eLearning, cross-border eCom, and civic participation. Nevertheless, the least educated residents of these countries lag significantly behind the European mean in all mentioned areas of digital participation (Cruz-Jesus et al., 2016). Research in the field of third-level DD shows that better educated individuals with high incomes use the Internet more efficiently for finding well-paid jobs, earning money, buying goods and services at reasonable prices, and other economic outcomes, which means that the use of modern technologies further increases the existing social inequalities (Van Deursen & Helsper, 2015).

In an extensive review of 126 research studies on different DD determinants in the area of Internet skills, uses, and outcomes, Scheerder et al. (2017) found that more than 60% of all identified determinants belonged to the stated sociodemographic and economic categories, while only 8.8% of DD determinants belonged to the category of personal factors (Table 1.1).

Table 1.1 Overview of categories and subcategories of DD determinants

Sociodemographic	Age, gender, marital status, residency, living area, living environment, urban/rural dimension, life space
Economic	Income, household income, household wealth, household poverty, family income, SES, household SES, individual SES, owning goods, financial situation, work situation, employment status, employment type, employment status parents, occupational status, social class, life stage, educational level, years of schooling, educational resources, parental education, educational level of parents, school sector, academic orientation, doing homework online, working hours, type of activity—job seeking
Social	Household composition; family size; family composition; family living arrangement; parental status; having children; parental mediation; number of children; informal networks; connected family members; connected friends; amount of Facebook friends; network size online; socializing; social activity; social support; assessing digital support networks; Facebook friends' instrumental support; formal volunteering; degree of social isolation; social orientation; loneliness; type of activity, emailing; type of activity, Facebook; type of activity, social media; type of activity, social network; type of activity, instant messaging; type of activity, social networking sites, Facebook interactions, express political content (Facebook), connections w/political actors (Facebook), political networks; type of activity, social media for political purposes, cyberpolitical participation, political orientation
Cultural	Cultural, cultural capital, cultural status, cultural possessions, religion, ethnicity, Internet use language
Personal	Type of activity, information seeking; type of activity, entertainment; type of activity, web support, groups (health related); type of activity, downloading/listening to music; type of activity, gaming; type of activity, podcast use; type of activity, online news, online news use, media use, traditional news media use, online media multiplexity, amount of media, offline news consumption, language integration, traditional literacy, literacy, language skills, English skills, previous achievements, school performance, academic performance, grade level, mastery orientation, shyness, confidence, self-efficacy, cognitive function, health status, mental health, health condition, health interests, physical activity, offline health activities, seeking offline health information, satisfaction with physician, trust in online health information; personality traits, neuroticism; personality traits, extraversion; personality traits, conscientiousness; personality traits, openness; personality traits, agreeableness, psychological distress
Material	Internet availability, Internet access, access locations, home access, home ICT access, school access, access type, access quality, number of electronic devices, PC at home, use of other technologies
Motivational	Attitude toward ICTs, attitude toward computers, Internet attitude, Internet motivation, perceived Internet relevance, Internet use, frequency of Internet use, usage frequency, (amount of) time spent online, intensity of Internet use, Internet experience, years of experience, digital skills, Internet skills, e-skills, computer skills, ICT skills, operational skills, formal skills, information skills, strategic skills, medium-related skills, creative skills, ICT competence, digital competence, media literacy, Internet literacy, digital literacy, Internet efficacy, eHealth literacy, ICT autonomy, technological efficacy, Internet use at work

Reproduced from Scheerder et al. (2017)

Personal DD determinants are diverse and, among other things, include traditional and digital literacy, school achievement, personality traits, preference in types of online activities, but also health status, cognitive functioning, and possible occurrence of disabilities. Differences in ICTs and Internet access between people with disabilities and non-disabled people became a research subject only in the first years of the new millennium, when the phrase disability digital divide (DDD) also appeared.

1.2 Disability Digital Divide

In their pioneering research on DDD, Dobransky and Hargittai (2006) compared participants with disability and non-disabled people with regard to Internet access and the way of its use. The sample included participants with five different types of physical disability. The results of this research showed that people with disability had less access to computers and the Internet in the USA. However, the influence of sociodemographic and economic factors on the frequency of Internet use was not equal in all subsamples of people with disability. It turned out that, for example, people with hearing impairment and those with difficulty in moving did not use the Internet less than non-disabled people, if the impact of their socioeconomic status was statistically controlled. After more than a decade, DDD is still very present in the USA (according to Reynolds & Leeder, 2019). Research studies conducted in countries with different degree of digitalization indicate digital disparities between disabled and non-disabled people.

Duplaga (2017) indicates a significant occurrence of DDD in using the Internet and performing specific activities in an online environment in Polish participants. Determinants of Internet use in people with disability were similar to those in non-disabled participants. Thus, for example, it was shown that the chances for highly educated individuals with disability to use the Internet were 18 times greater than for disabled people with lower level of education. In Russia, there is a trend of reducing the digital gap between certain categories of citizens estimated as a percentage of how much the advantaged group is above the disadvantaged group. However, with regard to DDD, the disparity between disabled and non-disabled people is about 30% (Grishchenko, 2020). Data for people with different types of disability were not specifically analyzed in the mentioned research studies. Since the type of disability significantly determines the frequency and manifestation of DDD, it is necessary to analyze data on people with different types of disability separately (Dobransky & Hargittai, 2006; Johansson et al., 2020; Robinson et al., 2020).

Most research papers on DDD compare participants with a specific type of disability with non-disabled participants, mainly focusing on first- and second-level DD. Research conducted in Sweden showed that adolescents with intellectual disability (ID) had less access to Internet devices and that, apart from playing video games, they were less likely to use the Internet for different purposes compared to their typically developing peers. The Internet use pattern was similar in these two groups, but with a noticeable lag in people with ID (Alfredsson Ågren et al., 2020). In Serbia, significant differences were determined in access to cell phones and their way of use between adolescents with ID and their typically developing peers (Glumbić et al., 2020a, b). Research conducted in Taiwan shows that first-level DD between students with learning disability and their typically developing peers has been closed, but that significant differences in their competencies and digital skills remain (Wu et al., 2014). The access issue is still very relevant in many countries, like in Sri Lanka where people with visual impairment do not have equal access to modern digital technologies. Employers are reluctant to hire workers with visual impairment because they do not want to increase the costs of ICT training and adaptation, and unemployment additionally complicates their social position and chances for digital inclusion (Wedasinghe, 2020). Despite the differences in sample selection, methodological design, and area in which research was conducted, all studies of this type lead to a single conclusion: disability is a significant determinant of digital inequalities in different countries; other DD determinants also affect people with disability, often increasing already existing differences.

Research studies, especially qualitative ones, targeting one specific disability group, can provide valuable insight into the nature of digital inequalities, but the possibility to generalize thus obtained data is limited. Large samples make it possible to determine how different DD determinants affect individuals with different types of disability. In Sweden, for example, DDD was examined in a sample of 771 participants with 35 different diagnoses or impairments. Of all tested groups, people who once attended special schools for students with ID had the least access to smartphones, computers, and tablets. People with autism, ADHD, and bipolar disorder used the Internet the most (Johansson et al., 2020). One of the rare research studies of this type conducted in Africa is also worth mentioning. In Namibia, only 10% of non-disabled people and only 5% of people with disability have computer access. This access is particularly low in rural areas where only 1% of people with disability use a computer (Indongo & Pempelani, 2015). The researchers used census results in which ten types of disability were identified. Computers and the Internet were least frequently used by blind people and people with hearing impairment, while people with albinism used modern ICTs the most.

Tsatsou (2019) believes that existing research studies which compare the degree of digital inclusion in people with different types of disability often rely on the medical model of disability. As an alternative, she suggests an interactionist approach within which dynamic relations of biological, psychological, and social factors could explain the observed differences in the degree of digital inclusion among people with different types of disability, as well as the variability which exists within a group of participants with the same type of disability.

1.3 ICTs and Autism

Modern ICTs have numerous advantages over traditional, non-digital approaches in teaching and treatment of people with autism spectrum disorder (ASD). A digital environment is controlled and predictable since performed actions, such as pressing a certain key, launching an application, or storing certain content, almost always have the same results. A multisensory environment with particularly prominent visual content is suitable for most people with autism whose cognition predominantly relies upon visual information processing. Computers are monotropic, i.e., full attention is given to isolated objects, out of context, which is in accordance with the tendency of many people with autism to pay attention to detail. With little effort, ICTs can be adapted to individual needs of each individual with autism, so that they are motivated to use them. Various reinforcement strategies keep their attention and motivation and reduce frustration due to possible mistakes. Using visual representations, adapting the dynamics of teaching content to individual needs of students with autism, eliminating time and space barriers between teachers and students, and structuring the environment provide practically unlimited possibilities for using ICTs in the process of education (Sanromà-Giménez et al., 2017). In a review analysis of 94 studies on the use of ICTs in educating people with autism, Valencia et al. (2019) found that most studies (36.17%) dealt with social skills development and slightly less than 30% examined the effects of using ICTs on general skills development (e.g., labeling, demonstrating, matching), while a quarter of the studies focused on conceptual skills. Almost three quarters of the studies were actually case reports.

In addition to educational purposes, ICTs can also be used to improve the existing capacities and treat difficulties inherent in ASD. Numerous applications have been developed for the purpose of enhancing theory of mind, social relations, verbal and nonverbal communication, spatial and temporal orientation, better understanding of emotions, developing independence, better use of free time, professional training, etc. Some skills which are spontaneously acquired in a complex and sometimes confusing social context can be gradually practiced in a simple and safe virtual environment, thanks to ICTs. Daily use of ICTs significantly affects way of life of not only people with autism but also their parents, other family members, and professionals who provide them with support (Guillén et al., 2016; Montes et al., 2019).

Naturally, the use of ICTs in people with autism also has a negative side: self-isolation and excessive use of computers leading to sedentary lifestyle with consequent increase of body mass index and other negative consequences (Guillén et al., 2016; Mazurek et al., 2012; Pans et al., 2019), involvement in cyberbullying and other forms of electronic aggression (Phillips & Anderson, 2020; Sallafranque-St-Louis & Normand, 2017), pathological game use (Engelhardt et al., 2017), etc. Most research studies on ICTs in people with autism refer to educational context and forms of treatment, and fewer research projects focus on problematic use of modern technologies and the Internet, while studies dealing with habits in using

ICTs in people with autism and usually only tangentially addressing complex DD issues are scarce.

Mazurek et al. (2012) examined screen-based media use in a representative sample of young people with autism in the USA. It was shown that over 40% of young people with ASD spent most of their free time playing video games. The percentage of high users with autism was much higher than in comparison groups of participants with speech and language disorders, learning disabilities, ID, and typically developing ones. Young people with ASD used social media, such as email or Internet chats, significantly less frequently than other participants with disability. As expected, participants who did not usually use social media were the ones with severe cognitive and communication disorders. By contrast, people with high-functioning autism were prone to searching the Internet, sending emails, and chatting.

Similar results were obtained by Benford (2008), who analyzed Internet-based communication in 138 participants with high-functioning autism in his PhD thesis. The obtained results point to the fact that email communication was more popular than direct face-to-face communication in these participants, even when interaction with family members and friends was concerned. Apart from sending emails, more than 70% of the participants used the Internet for browsing; more than half of the participants used the Internet for surfing, reading news, and doing research; and about one third searched for health-related information and participated in online shopping, while only 9% used the Internet to attend educational courses. An in-depth interview conducted in a subsample of participants with high-functioning autism showed that the Internet brought them a sense of liberation and that some of the social communication barriers were torn down by using computer-mediated communication (CMC).

The importance of the Internet for people with high-functioning autism is sometimes compared to the significance of sign language for the deaf community (Blume, 1997). The Internet is relatively predictable and based much more on text messages than on verbal communication. The dynamics of messaging can be adapted to users' needs. Nonverbal signals, which are highly dependent on a social context, are very significant in offline communication. By contrast, CMC is largely free of such signals, and people with autism can use emoticons and other strategies which make nonverbal aspects of communication more explicit and comprehensible. The Internet provides a certain social and emotional distance which significantly facilitates communication for all people with disability in the field of social communication (Benford, 2008).

Internet use for social purposes is most pronounced in women with high-functioning autism. They use the Internet to send emails and chat very frequently (Benford, 2008; Mazurek et al., 2012); they like to participate in online groups, leave posts on Facebook, and write blogs even more than neurotypical women (Johansson, 2019; Johansson et al., 2020). According to their own statement, 5% of women in the general population and only 2% of women with autism are not included in the digital society in Sweden.

On the contrary, people with autism are at great risk of digital exclusion in societies with a low degree of digitalization. Thus, for example, only 10% of the population in Namibia have computer access. This access is even lower in people with autism since only 4.1% of these people use a computer and only 3.2% use the Internet. Research results showed that out of ten groups of people with disability, blind participants and those with ID and ASD used cell phones the least (Indongo & Pempelani, 2015).

Physical access to ICTs is only the first step in achieving digital inclusion of people with autism. The next step would be to provide an accessible interface for people with ASD. Research conducted in Brazilian public schools showed that students with autism often refused to use laptops for educational purposes because of the abstract and complex operating system and poor user interface (Santarosa & Conforto, 2015). According to these authors, interaction with tablets is far more intuitive since the way of collecting objects by touching the screen is much more natural. All applications, regardless of whether they are designed for a wider range of potential users or specifically for people with autism, should be subject to usability testing. Eye-tracking systems, EEG, focus groups, and questionnaires applied after the intervention can be used for this purpose (Valencia et al., 2019).

Lussier-Desrochers et al. (2017) designed a conceptual model of digital participation with the following key points: access to digital devices; sensorimotor, cognitive, and technical requirements; and the comprehension of codes and conventions. The authors' original idea was to present the given dimensions as an accessibility pyramid, but such presentation indicated a higher significance of the dimensions which were closer to the base. In order to eliminate the possibility of misunderstanding and point to the dynamic relation of digital access dimensions, Lussier-Desrochers et al. (2017) presented the given dimensions in the form of cogwheels. The central cogwheel represented personal and environmental resources which activated peripheral cogwheels. In this way, interrelationship of personal competencies and environmental factors, which may be both facilitators and obstacles, affects each of the five dimensions of the digital society. Harmonized functioning of all cogwheels leads to full digital participation.

Research in the field of digital participation of people with autism mainly focuses on the development of certain skills, as well as on the detection of some environmental factors which could facilitate the process of learning. Although of great importance, research studies examining the influence of different technologies on the improvement of autism or certain abilities mostly consider the role of technology as a cognitive or behavioral prosthesis (Parsons et al., 2020). People with autism need to be active research participants and not just objects in a particular intervention. It is also necessary to make further steps toward integrating different perspectives in perceiving digital participation of people with autism.

1.4 Digital Citizenship

Although there is no generally accepted definition of digital citizenship (DC), most authors agree that a digital citizen should use the online environment in an appropriate, responsible, and efficient way; actively participate in online platforms, communities, and networks; and have a sense of belonging to the digital community (Curran & Ribble, 2017; Kim & Choi, 2018; Richardson & Milovidov, 2019). One of the most prominent researchers in this field, Ribble (2011), believes that DC has the following components: digital access, digital commerce, digital communication, digital literacy, digital etiquette, digital law, digital rights and responsibilities, digital health, and digital security. This is a very wide range of online activities and behaviors which include full participation in the digital community and competencies for overcoming digital exclusion; very complex ethical issues in the online space, the so-called netiquette (protection of intellectual property, rights, responsibilities of online community members, cyberbullying, etc.); various forms of digital and, more broadly, media literacy; digital buying and selling; active and participatory use of digital media; safe behavior; understanding health risks and improving mental and physical health; etc.

A digital citizen is not just a passive member of the online environment but also an active factor of changes in the digital community. Therefore, it is very important for the mentioned DC components to be incorporated into the educational process, in order to respond to the needs of a digital citizen in the future. Curran and Ribble (2017) organized nine DC components into three categories, respect, educate, and protect, pointing out the need for these thematic units to be repeated throughout the whole process of education, from preschool to university, in accordance with the abilities and needs of students of different ages. Research on different DC aspects is mainly limited to formal education and typically developing children. Papers dealing with the development of competencies in people with autism as digital citizens are scarce.

Good and Fang (2015) created a training program which covers all nine DC areas, aimed at children with neurodevelopmental disorders (learning disability, ADHD, and autism) and their parents. Unlike most other programs in which older individuals teach younger ones, this form of education is based on intergenerational, collaborative learning, which nurtures a sense of shared responsibility of young people with autism and their parents for safe and active participation in the digital environment. People with autism often do not have the opportunity to express their capacities and strengths and are almost always seen as a vulnerable social group. In this training program, participants with autism were given the opportunity to pass their knowledge in using modern ICTs on to their parents and to develop skills needed for active participation in the digital society in 90-min sessions over 6 weeks.

Being aware of the fact that different interventions of emotional and social learning in students with autism are still based on face-to-face communication, Probst (2017) designed a form of intervention based on the example of a "provocative selfie" which develops basic emotional and social competencies needed for critical analysis of content presented on Instagram. Through a series of carefully guided questions, a girl with autism was encouraged to understand the motives of a person who posted a provocative photograph (What does that person want to say in that way? What kind of audience is the photograph intended for?), but also her own mental states (How do I feel about that person? How do I think I look when I compare myself to her? Do my feelings affect my judgement?). This content was incorporated into the Individual Education Plan of students with autism and their peers with emotional and behavioral disorders.

Educational programs of public libraries have been developed outside the formal education environment in order to encourage digital skills in their users with ASD. These programs focus on the perception and experience of cyberbullying and the possible role of librarians in supporting people with autism to understand their position as perpetrators, victims, or observers of peer violence in the online environment (Anderson & Phillips, 2019).

We must keep in mind that people with high-functioning autism are not the only participants in the digital space. It will be very challenging for scientists and practitioners in the future to create special intervention programs designed to develop responsible and efficient behavior in the digital world and for people with more severe forms of autism.

1.5 Digital Bubbles

Unlimited digital space provides numerous possibilities to get acquainted with different opinions and attitudes. By analyzing the opposing arguments, we could choose the ones which are closest to our understanding of a certain problem. However, exactly the opposite happens in praxis. Many Internet users select information according to their beliefs, with a pronounced tendency to strongly criticize, or at least ignore, all opposing opinions. This is how a digital bubble is formed which distances its "inhabitants" from reality or at least from some perceptions of reality. Proponents of same or similar ideas further corroborate our perception of reality, and the observed echo-chamber effect additionally polarizes attitudes of people who "inhabit" different digital bubbles. For example, Schmidt et al. (2018) concluded that users of social networks directed their attention either only on the content which is in favor of vaccination or, quite the opposite, only on the content supported by members of the anti-vaccination movement. Very few people are willing to compare different views, which is why campaigns to provide accurate information about the relation between vaccination and autism through social media have practically no effect.

Digital citizens of the future should be aware of such bubbles and their position in them and should try to distance themselves from the central point of the same digital tribe. This is especially challenging for people with ASD due to their difficulties in the theory of mind. There is fear that modern technologies will distance individuals with autism from the real world, creating some kind of a social bubble which further distances them from direct communication with others. However, there are some forms of a digital social bubble which may have a positive meaning for a person with autism. This primarily refers to the neurodiversity movement and self-advocacy groups created in the digital space (Memisevic et al., 2022; Parsons et al., 2015).

A series of seven seminars with the title "Innovative technologies for autism: Critical reflections on digital bubbles" was held in the UK between 2014 and 2016. By summarizing the results of the presented papers, we concluded that digital bubbles may be observed from different aspects. In addition to already mentioned social bubbles, there are also methodological bubbles inhabited by scientists whose research topics are largely dependent on the discipline they belong to (engineering sciences, psychology, education, etc.). They do not cooperate enough with researchers from other scientific fields, and even less with end-user stakeholders, selecting topics not relevant enough from the aspect of the autistic community. The walls of methodological bubbles are further strengthened by the tendency to choose participants of a certain age, ability level, and other selection criteria. Furthermore, the significance of technology for people with autism is often considered from a neurotypical perspective, which can be overcome by including people with autism and their parents, siblings, and friends in all research phases (Parsons et al., 2015, 2017, 2020).

References

Adeleke, R. (2020). Digital divide in Nigeria: The role of regional differentials. *African Journal of Science, Technology, Innovation and Development*, 1–14. https://doi.org/10.1080/20421338.2020.1748335

Alfredsson Ågren, K., Kjellberg, A., & Hemmingsson, H. (2020). Digital participation? Internet use among adolescents with and without intellectual disabilities: A comparative study. *New Media & Society, 22*(12), 2128–2145. https://doi.org/10.1177/1461444819888398

Alliance for Affordable Internet. (2020). *Affordability report*. https://a4ai.org/affordability-report/report/2020/#what_is_the_state_of_internet_affordability_and_policy

Anderson, A., & Phillips, A. (2019). "Getting basic information isn't as helpful as the nuanced advice we can give each other": Teens with autism on digital citizenship education. *The Journal of Research on Libraries and Young Adults, 10*(3).

Andrejevic, M. (2014). The big data divide. *International Journal of Communication, 8*, 1673–1689.

Benford, P. (2008). *The use of Internet-based communication by people with autism*. Doctoral dissertation, University of Nottingham. http://eprints.nottingham.ac.uk/10661/1/thesis_post_viva_version_2.pdf

Blume, H. (1997, June 30). Autistics are communicating in cyberspace. *The New York Times* (p. 6). https://archive.nytimes.com/www.nytimes.com/library/cyber/techcol/063097techcol.html#:~:text=Yet%20anyone%20who%20explores%20the,enables%20them%20to%20do%20so

Brandtzæg, P. B., Heim, J., & Karahasanović, A. (2011). Understanding the new digital divide – A typology of Internet users in Europe. *International Journal of Human-Computer Studies, 69*(3), 123–138. https://doi.org/10.1016/j.ijhcs.2010.11.004

Carmi, E., & Yates, S. J. (2020). What do digital inclusion and data literacy mean today? *Internet Policy Review, 9*(2). https://doi.org/10.14763/2020.2.1474

Cruz-Jesus, F., Vicente, M. R., Bacao, F., & Oliveira, T. (2016). The education-related digital divide: An analysis for the EU-28. *Computers in Human Behavior, 56*, 72–82. https://doi.org/10.1016/j.chb.2015.11.027

Curran, M. B., & Ribble, M. (2017). P–20 model of digital citizenship. *New Directions for Student Leadership, 2017*(153), 35–46. https://doi.org/10.1002/yd.20228

Dewan, S., & Riggins, F. J. (2005). The digital divide: Current and future research directions. *Journal of the Association for Information Systems, 6*(12), 298–337.

Dobransky, K., & Hargittai, E. (2006). The disability divide in internet access and use. *Information, Communication & Society, 9*(3), 313–334. https://doi.org/10.1080/13691180600751298

Duplaga, M. (2017). Digital divide among people with disabilities: Analysis of data from a nationwide study for determinants of Internet use and activities performed online. *PLoS One, 12*(6), e0179825. https://doi.org/10.1371/journal.pone.0179825

Elena-Bucea, A., Cruz-Jesus, F., Oliveira, T., & Coelho, P. S. (2020). Assessing the role of age, education, gender and income on the digital divide: Evidence for the European Union. *Information Systems Frontiers*, 1–15. https://doi.org/10.1007/s10796-020-10012-9

Engelhardt, C. R., Mazurek, M. O., & Hilgard, J. (2017). Pathological game use in adults with and without Autism Spectrum disorder. *PeerJ, 5*, e3393. https://doi.org/10.7717/peerj.3393

Glumbić, N., Brojčin, B., Žunić Pavlović, V., & Đorđević, M. (2020a). Problematic mobile phone use among adolescents with mild intellectual disability. *Psihologija, 53*(4), 359–376. https://doi.org/10.2298/PSI190729014G

Glumbić, N., Brojčin, B., Đorđević, M., & Žunić-Pavlović, V. (2020b). Characteristics of mobile phone use in adolescents identified with mild intellectual disability who attend special schools in Serbia and their non-disabled peers in mainstream schools. *British Journal of Learning Disabilities, 49*(2), 217–229. https://doi.org/10.1111/bld.12358

Good, B., & Fang, L. (2015). Promoting smart and safe internet use among children with neurodevelopmental disorders and their parents. *Clinical Social Work Journal, 43*(2), 179–188. https://doi.org/10.1007/s10615-015-0519-4

Grishchenko, N. (2020). The gap not only closes: Resistance and reverse shifts in the digital divide in Russia. *Telecommunications Policy, 44*(8), 102004. https://doi.org/10.1016/j.telpol.2020.102004

Guillén, S. G., Rojas, D. G., & Fernández, S. J. (2016). Uso de las TIC en el Trastorno de Espectro Autista: Aplicaciones. *Edmetic, 5*(2), 134–157. https://doi.org/10.21071/edmetic.v5i2.5780

Gunkel, D. J. (2003). Second thoughts: Toward a critique of the digital divide. *New Media & Society, 5*(4), 499–522. https://doi.org/10.1177/146144480354003

Hargittai, E. (2002). Second level digital divide: Differences in people's online skills. *First Monday, 7*(4). https://doi.org/10.5210/fm.v7i4.942

Huxhold, O., Hees, E., & Webster, N. J. (2020). Towards bridging the grey digital divide: Changes in internet access and its predictors from 2002 to 2014 in Germany. *European Journal of Ageing, 17*(3), 271–280. https://doi.org/10.1007/s10433-020-00552-z

Indongo, N., & Pempelani, M. (2015). ICT barriers for people with disability in Namibia: Evidence from the 2011 Namibia Population and Housing Census, *11*(1), 51–67. http://hdl.handle.net/10125/58619

ITU. (2020). *Measuring digital developments: Facts and figures*. https://www.itu.int/en/ITU-D/Statistics/Documents/facts/FactsFigures2020.pdf

Johansson, S. (2019). *Design for participation and inclusion will follow: Disabled people and the digital society*. Doctoral dissertation, KTH Royal Institute of Technology. http://urn.kb.se/resolve?urn=urn:nbn:se:kth:diva-262819</div>

Johansson, S., Gulliksen, J., & Gustavsson, C. (2020). Disability digital divide: The use of the internet, smartphones, computers and tablets among people with disabilities in Sweden. *Universal Access in the Information Society*, 1–16. https://doi.org/10.1007/s10209-020-00714-x

Kim, M., & Choi, D. (2018). Development of youth digital citizenship scale and implication for educational setting. *Journal of Educational Technology & Society, 21*(1), 155–171. http://www.jstor.org/stable/26273877

Lee, H., Park, N., & Hwang, Y. (2015). A new dimension of the digital divide: Exploring the relationship between broadband connection, smartphone use and communication competence. *Telematics and Informatics, 32*(1), 45–56. https://doi.org/10.1016/j.tele.2014.02.001

Lussier-Desrochers, D., Normand, C. L., Romero-Torres, A., Lachapelle, Y., Godin-Tremblay, V., Dupont, M. È., Roux, J., Pépin-Beauchesne, L., & Bilodeau, P. (2017). Bridging the digital divide for people with intellectual disability. *Cyberpsychology: Journal of Psychosocial Research on Cyberspace, 11*(1). https://doi.org/10.5817/CP2017-1-1

Ma, J. K. H., Vachon, T. E., & Cheng, S. (2019). National income, political freedom, and investments in R&D and education: A comparative analysis of the second digital divide among 15-year-old students. *Social Indicators Research, 144*(1), 133–166. https://doi.org/10.1007/s11205-018-2030-0

Mazurek, M. O., Shattuck, P. T., Wagner, M., & Cooper, B. P. (2012). Prevalence and correlates of screen-based media use among youths with autism spectrum disorders. *Journal of Autism and Developmental Disorders, 42*(8), 1757–1767. https://doi.org/10.1007/s10803-011-1413-8

Memisevic, Djordjevic, & Glumbić. (2022). Quality of life in autism spectrum disorder. In J. L. Matson (Ed.), *Handbook of autism and pervasive developmental disorder*. Springer.

Montes, C. D. P. G., Cara, M. J. C., & Fuentes, A. R. (2019). Perspectiva actual sobre el uso de tecnologías de la información y la comunicación en personas con trastorno del espectro autista: Sistematización de experiencias. *HAMUT'AY, 6*(3), 50–61. https://doi.org/10.21503/hamu.v6i3.1846

NTIA. (1999). *Falling through the net: Defining the digital divide*. National Telecommunications and Information Administration. https://www.ntia.doc.gov/legacy/ntiahome/fttn99/contents.html

Pans, M., González, L. M., Úbeda-Colomer, J., & Devís-Devís, J. (2019). Screen time among Spanish university students with disabilities: A self-organizing maps analysis. *BMC Public Health, 19*(1), 995. https://doi.org/10.1186/s12889-019-7339-3

Parsons, S., Yuill, N., Brosnan, M., & Good, J. (2015). Innovative technologies for autism: Critical reflections on digital bubbles. *Journal of Assistive Technologies, 19*(2), 116–121. https://doi.org/10.1108/JAT-03-2015-0005

Parsons, S., Yuill, N., Brosnan, M., & Good, J. (2017). "A child with autism only has one childhood": Main themes and questions for research from the "Digital Bubbles" seminar series. *Journal of Enabling Technologies, 11*(3), 113–119. https://doi.org/10.1108/JET-07-2017-0023

Parsons, S., Yuill, N., Good, J., & Brosnan, M. (2020). 'Whose agenda? Who knows best? Whose voice?' Co-creating a technology research roadmap with autism stakeholders. *Disability & Society, 35*(2), 201–234. https://doi.org/10.1080/09687599.2019.1624152

Pawluczuk, A. (2020). Digital youth inclusion and the big data divide: Examining the Scottish perspective. *Internet Policy Review, 9*(2), 1–18. https://doi.org/10.14763/2020.2.1480

Phillips, A. L., & Anderson, A. (2020). Cyberbullying, digital citizenship, and youth with autism: LIS education as a piece in the puzzle. *The Library Quarterly, 90*(3), 264–282. https://doi.org/10.1086/708957

Plotichkina, N. V., Morozova, E. V., & Miroshnichenko, I. V. (2020). Digital technologies: Policy for improving accessibility and usage skills development in Europe and Russia. *Mirovaia ekonomika i mezhdunarodnye otnosheniia, 64*(4), 70–83. https://doi.org/10.20542/0131-2227-2020-64-4-70-83

Probst, D. (2017). Social media literacy as an IEP intervention for social and emotional learning. *Journal of Media Literacy Education, 9*(2), 45–57. https://doi.org/10.23860/JMLE-2019-09-02-04

Reynolds, R. B., & Leeder, C. (2019). Digital divide and web-use skills. *The International Encyclopedia of Media Literacy*, 1–12. https://doi.org/10.1002/9781118978238.ieml0244

Ribble, M. (2011). *Digital citizenship in schools*. International Society for Technology in Education.

Richardson, J., & Milovidov, E. (2019). *Digital citizenship education handbook: Being online, well-being online, and rights online*. Council of Europe.

Robinson, L., Schulz, J., Blank, G., Ragnedda, M., Ono, H., Hogan, B., Mesch, G., Cotton, S. R., Kretchmer, S. B., Hale, T. M., Drabowicz, T., Yan, P., Wellman, B., Harper, M.-G., Quan-Haase, A., Dunn, H. S., Casilli, A. A., Tubaro, P., Carveth, R., et al. (2020). Digital inequalities 2.0: Legacy inequalities in the information age. *First Monday, 25*(7). https://doi.org/10.5210/fm.v25i7.10842ff

Sallafranque-St-Louis, F., & Normand, C. L. (2017). From solitude to solicitation: How people with intellectual disability or autism spectrum disorder use the internet. *Cyberpsychology: Journal of Psychosocial Research on Cyberspace, 11*(1). https://doi.org/10.5817/CP2017-1-7

Sanromà-Giménez, M., Lázaro-Cantabrana, J. L., & Gisbert-Cervera, M. (2017). La tecnología móvil: Una herramienta para la mejora de la inclusión digital de las personas con TEA. *Psicología, Conocimiento y Sociedad, 7*(2), 173–192. https://doi.org/10.26864/pcs.v7.n2.10

Santarosa, L. M. C., & Conforto, D. (2015). Tecnologias móveis na inclusão escolar e digital de estudantes com transtornos de espectro autista. *Revista Brasileira de Educação Especial, 21*(4), 349–366. https://doi.org/10.1590/S1413-65382115000400003

Scheerder, A., van Deursen, A., & van Dijk, J. (2017). Determinants of Internet skills, uses and outcomes. A systematic review of the second-and third-level digital divide. *Telematics and Informatics, 34*(8), 1607–1624. https://doi.org/10.1016/j.tele.2017.07.007

Schmidt, A. L., Zollo, F., Scala, A., Betsch, C., & Quattrociocchi, W. (2018). Polarization of the vaccination debate on Facebook. *Vaccine, 36*(25), 3606–3612. https://doi.org/10.1016/j.vaccine.2018.05.040

Siren, A., & Knudsen, S. G. (2017). Older adults and emerging digital service delivery: A mixed methods study on information and communications technology use, skills, and attitudes. *Journal of Aging & Social Policy, 29*(1), 35–50. https://doi.org/10.1080/08959420.2016.1187036

Song, Z., Song, T., Yang, Y., & Wang, Z. (2019). Spatial-temporal characteristics and determinants of digital divide in China: A multivariate spatial analysis. *Sustainability, 11*(17), 4529. https://doi.org/10.3390/su11174529

Tsatsou, P. (2019). Digital inclusion of people with disabilities: A qualitative study of intra-disability diversity in the digital realm. *Behaviour & Information Technology, 39*(9), 995–1010. https://doi.org/10.1080/0144929X.2019.1636136

United Nations E-Government Survey. (2018). *Gearing E-government to support transformation towards sustainable and resilient societies*. United Nations. https://www.unescap.org/resources/e-government-survey-2018-gearing-e-government-support-transformation-towards-sustainable

Valencia, K., Rusu, C., Quiñones, D., & Jamet, E. (2019). The impact of technology on people with autism spectrum disorder: A systematic literature review. *Sensors, 19*(20), 4485. https://doi.org/10.3390/s19204485

Van Deursen, A. J., & Helsper, E. J. (2015). The third-level digital divide: Who benefits most from being online? In *Communication and information technologies annual* (pp. 29–52). Emerald Group Publishing Limited. https://doi.org/10.1108/S2050-206020150000010002

Van Dijk, J. A. (2017). Digital divide: Impact of access. *The International Encyclopedia of Media Effects*, 1–11. https://doi.org/10.1002/9781118783764.wbieme0043

Warren, M. (2007). The digital vicious cycle: Links between social disadvantage and digital exclusion in rural areas. *Telecommunications Policy, 31*(6–7), 374–388. https://doi.org/10.1016/j.telpol.2007.04.001

Wedasinghe, N. (2020). *Bridging the disability digital divide of visually impaired community in Sri Lanka: A framework to overcome the issues*. Doctoral dissertation, General Sir John Kotelawala Defence University.

Wei, K. K., Teo, H. H., Chan, H. C., & Tan, B. C. (2011). Conceptualizing and testing a social cognitive model of the digital divide. *Information Systems Research, 22*(1), 170–187. https://doi.org/10.1287/isre.1090.0273

Wu, T. F., Chen, M. C., Yeh, Y. M., Wang, H. P., & Chang, S. C. H. (2014). Is digital divide an issue for students with learning disabilities? *Computers in Human Behavior, 39*, 112–117. https://doi.org/10.1016/j.chb.2014.06.024

Chapter 2
Participatory Design

2.1 What Is Participatory Design?

Participatory design (PD) is an approach and a vision advocating that people who will be affected by technologies should participate in their design (Frauenberger et al., 2017). It is usually defined as a set of theories, practices, and methods that encourage the participation of end users or other stakeholders in designing technological artifacts or services (Frauenberger et al., 2012a). PD involves many non-designers in various activities during the design process. The term non-designers refers to potential users, other external stakeholders, and/or people who are team members but are not designers (e.g., marketing experts, engineers, salespeople, etc.). The PD process usually involves people of different backgrounds, experiences, interests, and roles they have in the project. Thus, it is essential to find an appropriate way to engage and involve them in PD activities (Sanders et al., 2010).

In traditional design methods, trained researchers observe or interview passive users whose contribution is to perform a task or give opinions on a product designed by others. On the other hand, PD designers see users as project co-designers who are experts in daily life experiences. All team members cooperate in finding solutions, and a researcher's role is to facilitate user involvement in the co-creation process (Sanders & Stappers, 2008). The premise behind PD is that users are best qualified to determine how to improve their own work and that their perception of technology is equally important as the technical characteristics of a product (Carmel et al., 1993). The PD methodology is based on the decision-making power of co-designers and incorporating their values in the design process and its outcomes, which can be a prototype of products or services, a new way of organizing work or designing space. In this approach, the designing process is equally important as the final result. PD is seen as a collective "reflection-in-action" process involving several participants in research, reflection, and learning. The participants usually take on the roles of both users and designers, where designers are trying to learn about

N. Glumbić et al., *Digital Inclusion of Individuals with Autism Spectrum Disorder*, Autism and Child Psychopathology Series,
https://doi.org/10.1007/978-3-031-12037-4_2

the reality of users and users are trying to articulate the desired goals and learn about appropriate technological tools to achieve them (Robertson & Simonsen, 2012; van der Velden & Mörtberg, 2015).

PD examines unspoken, invisible aspects of human activity. It assumes that these aspects can be productively and ethically examined through a design partnership with participants, in which a researcher-designer and other participants jointly design artifacts, workflow, and working environment. This partnership must be implemented iteratively so that researchers-designers and other participants can improve their own understanding of the activity (Spinuzzi, 2005).

The principles of social justice, which are the basis of PD, oppose the hierarchical structure of the traditional design process, in which experts create technology that should support users. Instead, users, designers, and theorists collaborate in designing and evaluating technologies. In authentic participatory collaboration, the boundaries between these roles are blurred, and all participants are encouraged to collaborate as co-designers in all aspects of the design process. However, the degree to which users are truly empowered to make a change often lags behind the ideal since it can be difficult to establish successful collaboration and reconcile different and sometimes opposing perspectives (Sturm et al., 2019).

Motivation to use PD ranges from the pragmatic need to increase the compatibility between technology features and user demands to an ideological agenda for empowering people, democratizing innovations, and designing an alternative future (Frauenberger et al., 2017). Regardless of these differences, PD essentially deals with facilitating creative processes to create alternative visions of the future (Makhaeva et al., 2016).

2.1.1 The Principles

The main principles of PD were established mainly in Scandinavia in the 1970s:

- *Equalizing power relations*—finding ways for those who are invisible or weaker in the power structure of an organization or society to express their views.
- *Situation-based actions*—direct work with individuals or their representatives at work, at home, or in public space to understand activities and technologies in the natural environment.
- *Mutual learning*—encouraging and empowering the understanding of different participants by finding common ground and ways of working.
- *Tools and techniques*—which in practical, specific situations help various users to express their needs and visions. PD implies doing something concrete and tangible. The "design by doing" method, such as modeling and prototyping, is one of the major determinants of PD since it enables an "ordinary worker" to use practical skills when participating in the design process. PD has developed various tools and techniques to support "reflection-in-action" that allows users to participate in the design.

- *Alternative visions about technology*—ideas that generate equality at the workplace, at home, in public space, or other places.
- *Democratic practices*—using practices and models of behavior that promote equality among "stakeholders" (Greenbaum & Loi, 2012; Kensing & Greenbaum, 2013; Luck, 2018).

The principles of PD prevent the design process from being merely an instrumental phase for obtaining user input on the final product. Since they encourage authentic participation and engage the experience, skills, needs, and values of co-designers, the design process becomes a space in which alternative visions about technology are developed. Through the creative use of participatory methods, PD enables the use-before-use scenario, in which co-designers can test the outcomes before the final product is made or used. This process results in products or services that incorporate the values and needs of co-designers, which become materialized in the design (van der Velden & Mörtberg, 2015).

2.1.2 The Methods

The concept of methods in PD refers to a coherent set of principles and general guidelines on how to implement the design process from start to finish from the PD perspective (Bratteteig et al., 2013).

There is no single PD method that can be applied to all situations. Each PD project is related to local characteristics, and therefore there is no universal PD process that can be transferred from one situation to another. According to Luck (2018), PD is not defined by formulas, rules, and strict definitions but rather adherence to the basic principles of design participation. Thus, PD is not one approach but a set of design practices that vary in rigidity and validity and rely on different methods, tools, and techniques (Brandt et al., 2013). Consequently, PD is often referred to as a research orientation or a field within human-computer interaction rather than strictly research methodology (Van Mechelen, 2016).

The PD methodology results from participatory action research. Designers see themselves as facilitators trying to encourage users to make their own decisions. To achieve this goal, PD emphasizes joint research and co-design: researchers-designers make conclusions collaborating with users. This is an iterative process that allows users and researchers to critically examine the influence of these gradual improvements. Most research studies identify three main stages: initial exploration in which designers meet the users; discovery processes when various techniques are used to understand and determine priorities and form a vision of a future process or product; and prototyping in which designers and users iteratively shape technological artifacts to match them with the vision developed in the second phase (Spinuzzi, 2005).

Sanders et al. (2010) propose a methodological framework that consists of three dimensions: form, purpose, and context. The *form* describes the type of action between participants in an activity: making, telling, and/or enacting. Making tangible things refers to using two-dimensional collages and maps and making three-dimensional models from foam, clay, Lego bricks, or Velcro modeling. Talking, telling, and explaining include stories and storyboarding through writing, drawing, blogs, photographs, videos, etc. Diaries, daily logs, and maps for organizing, categorizing, and prioritizing also belong to this category. Finally, acting, enacting, and playing involve playing different games (e.g., game boards), props and black boxes, participatory envisioning and dramatizing by asking the users to envisage themselves in future situations, and improvisation. The *purpose* explains, from four aspects, what the tools and techniques will be used for: (1) probing participants, (2) priming participants to engage in their field of interest, (3) better understanding participants' existing experience, or (4) generating ideas or design concepts for the future (e.g., by creating and researching future scenarios). Each form can be used for any purpose. The *context* defines where and how the tools and techniques are used. It is described by group size and composition, face-to-face vs. online implementation, the venue, and stakeholder relationships.

The PD process usually includes people of different backgrounds, experiences, interests, and roles in the project. Therefore, it is important to find an appropriate way for them to be engaged and included in PD activities (Sanders et al., 2010). Walsh et al. (2013) set a framework that describes PD techniques in working with children through eight dimensions (Octoract). Two dimensions refer to intergenerational participants (previous design experience and ability), and two refer to the design goal (design space and maturity of the design goal), while four dimensions refer to the technique (cost, portability, technology level, and physical interaction).

2.2 Participation of People with ASD in PD

PD is especially significant in creating technologies for groups usually marginalized in design and whose way of life is far from designers' or researchers' (Frauenberger et al., 2017). There are three reasons why PD is important for children with disabilities. First, the world and life experience of children with disabilities differ from the experience of designers or researchers who do not have disabilities, which makes it difficult to show empathy or a deeper understanding of the needs and requirements of children with disabilities when creating technologies. Then, the participation of children with disabilities in developing technologies allows having realistic expectations, which increases the chances that the technology will be accepted and used. Finally, the participation of children with disabilities in designing technologies gives them a sense of involvement and empowers them (Frauenberger et al., 2012a). Participating in some design activities can encourage positive behaviors such as greater responsibility or engagement. Also, participation can have a lasting influence on children providing them with opportunities to develop skills such as creativity, social skills, teamwork, narrative, and technical skills that can be useful in other spheres of life (Benton & Johnson, 2015).

Although engaging people with ASD in all aspects of technology design and evaluation can significantly improve adapting technology to their needs and views, most technologies for people with ASD have been developed without their contribution or with a very limited one (Sturm et al., 2019).

The explanation is, in part, probably related to the difficulties researchers face when including people with ASD in the design process. These difficulties include narrowed interests, perfectionism, social anxiety (Makhaeva et al., 2016), variations in skills in different people with ASD (Sturm et al., 2019), difficulties in social communication and interaction, and lack of trust that people who do not have autism can design technology for them (Jarosinski, 2019).

Frauenberger et al. (2012a) distinguish between three ways in which children with disabilities participate in the design process. The first involves *non-participatory approaches* where system design relies on theories, best practices, or previous experience related to disability characteristics, but children with disabilities are not directly involved in the process. *Participation via proxy* is an approach in which information about the needs of children with disabilities is obtained from people who know the children well, such as parents, teachers, or education professionals. Finally, *full participation* includes any form of engagement that allows children with disabilities to influence the outcomes directly.

The following review includes only the papers in which children and adults with ASD were directly involved in the design process.

The Frauenberger et al. (2016, 2017, 2019) project OutsideTheBox aimed to enable children with ASD to manage the design process by expressing wishes and ideas arising from their understanding of the world.

Frauenberger et al. (2017) recommend combining, merging, reinterpreting, and adapting elements of different methods. In that sense, they offer a visual tool that enables the merging of methodological building blocks and their alignment from five perspectives: a child, designers, the context, previous outcomes, and the available methodological repertoire. The tool shape is inspired by a board game with hexagonal cards of different colors that can be arranged and rearranged to get a complete picture of various perspectives that affect planning.

Cards belonging to each of the five perspectives can be combined in the central field. There are two methodological repertoires from which a designer can choose tools and techniques to start planning. One is the general repertoire that includes techniques and tools familiar to the designer or that exist in the literature. The other repertoire is developed while collaborating with a specific child. Cards related to previous outcomes include ideas, issues, prototypes, or scenarios that can be referred to or based on which the process can be created. Context cards describe the physical settings in which the process takes place, available raw materials, and a broader relevant context (the structure of the project, school, etc.). The last group of cards describes designers' perspectives, especially their goals, expertise, skills, and different roles they take on in collaboration.

The design process relies on two interrelated concepts: creativity in autism and Handlungsspielraum (Action-Play-Space). The authors recommend maintaining a delicate balance between structure and freedom that allows children to think creatively about technology. Structure is provided through familiar materials, routines, and roles. Freedom is offered through the opportunity for children to step out of their comfort zones and create something new, occasionally in the form of new materials or activities. The authors use the German compound Handlungsspielraum to refer to this space that consists of structure and freedom (Makhaeva et al., 2016). With this term, they want to describe children's engagement in a creative process in which they will not be overburdened. The process begins with children's specific interests that are carefully redirected and used to include them in the creative process. They consider creativity in autism to be situational, continuous, cumulative, experience-based, and embodied.

The children who participated in the project, 6–8 years of age, had well-developed language skills and no significant intellectual disabilities. The children were engaged in three cycles during the project, each lasting throughout one school year. Smart objects were developed through various PD processes and individual work with nine children. Different methods were used to map the ones allowing meaningful inclusion of these children in PD.

The following procedure was followed for each child, Contextual Inquiry, which included interviews with guardians, teachers, and children, observations, and probes; design a child worked on by using one out of six different methods; and evaluation phase after the product was created (with viewpoints of people with disabilities being especially important). Although individual procedures differed significantly, the overall framework and design brief were common to everyone.

Two researchers attended each 2-week session. The Active Observer facilitated the sessions, determined the schedules, kept track of time, provided materials and feedback, and structured the sessions. The second, Play Partner, followed Active Observer's instructions, worked together with the child, and provided support in exhibiting skills (Frauenberger et al., 2019).

An earlier Frauenberger et al. (2010, 2011, 2012b, 2013) project called ECHOES included typically developing (TD) children and children with ASD who attended regular schools. Students with ASD had developed speech and preserved cognitive potentials. This project aimed to design technology that would support the development of social skills in both TD children and children with high-functioning autism.

The learning environment within the project was modeled on a large multi-touch surface with computer power adequate to create a virtual world in real time and provide high-quality sound, visual emotion recognition, and webcam eye-tracking (Fig. 2.1).

Describing the challenges of working with children with ASD, Frauenberger et al. (2010) state that these children's ideas cannot be literally converted into design since they are influenced by direct experience, memories, television, games, and knowledge of the environment. Instead, they seek to identify basic phenomenological qualities that can be converted into numerous design concepts and incorporated into a virtual environment. They state the following key points of the PD process when children with ASD are concerned: establishing strong and long-lasting student relationships, facilitating communication, providing a creativity encouraging environment, reinterpreting and translating the ideas of children with ASD, and

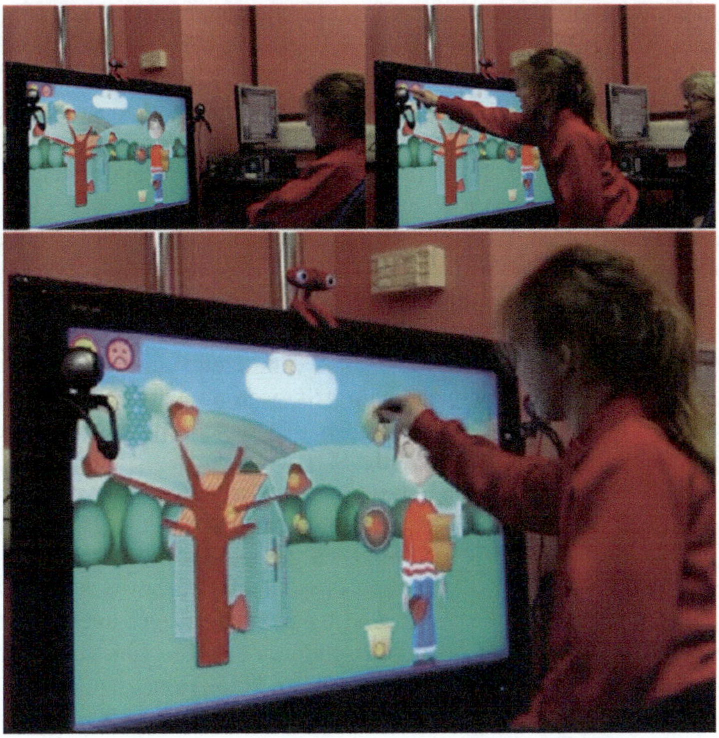

Fig. 2.1 Multi-touch surface monitor. (Reproduced from Frauenberger et al., 2013)

using a structured approach and action research in research design (Frauenberger et al., 2012a).

According to these authors, tools in the PD process involving children with ASD should be fun and easy to use, visual support should scaffold interaction, aims and activities should be structured, children should be allowed to express themselves less directly and potentially nonverbally, and the complexity of activities should be reduced. Based on these characteristics, a tool was developed that allowed a child to mark scenes in a virtual environment to give feedback within a design critique activity. A simple "stamping" mechanism was used, allowing the child to choose one out of three facial expressions (smiley, frowny, confused) to mark the object in a scene. This provided children with different choices in giving feedback on the environment, visual reminders, and a way to express feelings without open-ended questions (Frauenberger et al., 2013).

In 1 of the studies (Frauenberger et al., 2011), the development of ECHOES learning environment involved 36 typically developing children 5–7 years of age, 2 boys with ASD, and 1 girl with undiagnosed social and language difficulties. Four sessions were organized with each group, and each session lasted for about an hour.

The first session, called Desert Island, examined how children interacted with objects. Starting from the Fictional Inquiry technique, the authors developed a plot where the children were on a desert island. They had enough food, but they began to get bored. The children found a treasure chest and were asked to think of what they could do with the magic items from the chest to have fun until the rescuers arrived. The children were divided into five groups. Each group sat around a table on which there was a large piece of paper with a palm tree as a desert island symbol. Each group got a "treasure chest" (a black plastic box) containing ten items. The children were encouraged to draw and write while developing ideas. One member of each group was chosen to be a reporter going on an expedition to interview other groups about their items and games. Each "reporter" got an audio recording device. The following day, each child drew a favorite item on a piece of paper. Particularly motivating affordances were identified and included in subsequent PD activities. The children were more engaged in the items with interesting functions or specific perceptive qualities. The participants with ASD were more repetitive in the game. However, not many indications of imaginative play or starting a narrative were identified in any of the groups (both TD and ASD).

The second session implemented the Odd-One-Out activities developed to examine how children interacted with objects when given a task frame. The children were divided into groups of six or seven, and each group got a set of three items and a worksheet. The task was to circle the odd-one-out and draw or write why they had circled that particular item. The children with ASD focused on perceptual characteristics and details (e.g., color), while TD children selected functional features to indicate the differences between the items (e.g., it bounces).

The third activity, called The Comic, aimed to provide a deeper insight into the role of imaginative play and emergent narrative. It was based on Gray's (1998) social stories and comics for children with ASD, in which children developed their own stories. The children completed the empty frames between the given beginning and end of the comic (picture and text). The plot of this story was as follows: "The princess has been locked up by the nasty dragon, can you help to free her? The key to her freedom lies in this thing you were given by the great magician. It has special powers that you will need to use to free the princess and lock up the dragon." The template also provided space where the children could write why they found the chosen item special. This activity was performed only with TD children. The children were divided into groups of six, and each group was given one item familiar from previous activities. Most children described the used items but did not incorporate them in the story. A clear, functional role of the items in the story was determined in only six children. The authors concluded that the plot should be more structured and easier to understand.

The last activity, called Into the digital, took place in a virtual environment. The session involved giving each group of children a series of prototypes. The aim was to examine the possibilities of a virtual environment that could not be examined in physical reality.

Finally, a 5-min video was recorded to emphasize the children's crucial role in the project. The video summarized all activities the children participated in, and each child was given a personalized certificate. The video was presented at the end of the school year celebration that the parents also attended.

Sturm et al. (2019) write about PD of a hybrid two-player Kinect game that encourages the recognition of complex emotions and collaboration between people with ASD and their TD peers. The main goal of Connecting through Kinect is to obtain insights from people with ASD who can speak to develop a game for children with ASD who cannot successfully express their preferences.

In the game, the players stand next to each other and move the pieces of a jigsaw puzzle using hand movements. Each jigsaw shows outlines of a figure in an emotionally saturated context. After putting together the body, the players need to agree on the appropriate emotion for the figure's face and select it from the given options. The emotions become more and more complex throughout the game. After each level, the players can jointly choose an audio-video clip or a collaborative mini-game as a reward.

Ten college students with ASD, three of their mentors, and one deaf student were selected to give feedback on the game design. The participants with ASD did not take part in developing the general goals of the game, but they were asked to guess the purpose of the game and state whether it was important to teach emotion recognition skills to young people with ASD. The students chose the level for them to get involved—some of them only wanted to play the game in a specific phase of development and then provide feedback, while others also participated in exchanging opinions with the whole team of designers and developers. Only one student with ASD chose to take on the role of a paid part-time research assistant, while others believed that they did not have the necessary design and/or programming skills or enough time due to other obligations. The students played the game with their mentors or a lab assistant, and the sessions were recorded on camera.

A structured interview was conducted after each level. It included questions about the game appearance, feelings experienced while playing, and specific questions about the protagonists' feelings. The students were asked what they liked and disliked, what they would change, and why. Their experience as players was taken into account, and they were asked to give ideas from previously played commercial games. The students were given positive feedback, and they were informed when their ideas would be used. Based on the recordings, five 30- to 60-min videos were coded, in which a student with ASD and a student without ASD played the game. Seven behavior categories of students with ASD were coded: (1) looking at the screen, (2) looking at the partner, (3) showing positive emotions (e.g., a smile), (4) expressing frustrations, (5) asking for help, (6) turn taking behavior, and (7) conversation/commenting.

Iterative design/evaluation was developed through the following stages: initial prototyping, design feedback, coded evaluations, extensive design changes (in which only developers participated), design feedback, and coded evaluations. At the end of the process, information was obtained from ten teenagers with ASD who were only informants (they were not design partners). Instead of mentors, the adolescents with ASD played the game with other students with ASD or the research assistant, who followed their moves.

Most students with ASD felt that their contribution to the project was highly appreciated and would recommend a friend with ASD to participate in the Kinect project. They were very pleased that their ideas were included in the game design and improved the game in different ways. However, a significant limitation was that most students chose to be only informants rather than taking on the role of design partners.

The authors suggest that future research on involving students with ASD in technology design should include a clearer structure, more frequent and regular meetings, training for all team members in how to communicate and plan team functioning, more low-tech engagement opportunities, computing opportunities that are available to new programmers, finding more mentors, and formal training in animation and programming for those who are interested.

Malinverni et al. (2016) suggest using a multimodal analysis in PD involving children with ASD. This means collecting and interpreting information from various resources a person uses (e.g., gestures, looks, movement, etc.) to construct meaning. Thus, the analysis expands beyond intentional communicational prompts, which enables overcoming the barriers in communication and expression. They illustrate this approach by developing the "Land of Fog" game to improve social initiation and collaboration. The game is based on cognitive theories that emphasize the relationship between physical activities and cognitive processes, known as Embodied Cognition. This theory points out the role of the body and sensorimotor activities in developing cognitive processes. The authors believe that body movements in multiplayer settings increase the social nature of the playing experience. Also, the game is based on the assumption that children's exploration and discovery lead to a surprise and the need to talk about that feeling.

The "Land of Fog" combines virtual and real space (a circular 6-meter-wide projection on the floor filled with fog). Four boys with high-functioning ASD (10–12 years of age) filled that space.

Children participated in three sessions, each lasting for an hour and a half. The first session, the only one described in the paper, focused on children's embodied interaction and interpretation of the environment. The remaining two sessions dealt with the visual aspects of the game and its characters' behavior.

The first "Land of Fog" prototype consisted of a fog-covered surface with no visual elements, contents, or game mechanisms and was therefore completely open to children's suggestions. The floor under the fog contained surfaces of different colors to evoke a sense of movement through various types of scenery. The children were divided into pairs—the "explorers" and the "detectives." One child in the pair of "explorers" had a butterfly net, while the second had a camera. The "explorers" were asked to walk over the projection on the floor and explore the space together. The butterfly net served as a magic wand that created circular holes in the fog. The child with the camera was instructed to take photographs of everything he found interesting (Fig. 2.2). The "detectives" were placed on the balcony overlooking the whole room. They were asked to try and imagine what the environment looked like, what creatures might inhabit it, and what their peers should do while exploring. After 15 min, the pairs switched their roles—the "explorers" became "detectives" and vice versa.

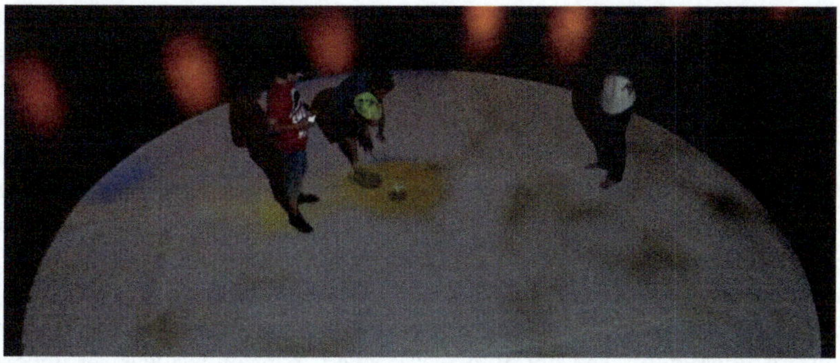

Fig. 2.2 Children exploring the "Land of Fog". (Reproduced from Malinverni et al., 2016)

After exploring the environment, the children were asked to use art materials and make what they would like to see in the fog. The authors made video recordings and coded the children's movements through the space and their gaze direction. The children's attention was quantified by following the routes and photographs they made while moving through the space.

In a related paper, Mora-Guiard et al. (2017) described how participants with ASD defined esthetics and chose the Land of Fog inhabitants. Each child first designed their own environment. All ideas were later discussed and integrated into the final design of the environment. Then, the children suggested elements and creatures that would inhabit the world they designed and how they would behave and interact with each other. Finally, the children had the opportunity to try out the gameplay of the full-body interaction system in the Wizard-of-Oz activity (a technique in which children think they directly interact with the computer, but actually a researcher interprets their actions and interacts with the computer, Höysniemi et al., 2004). In the next stage, other students with ASD piloted the game and, through interviews, gave feedback on the design. New changes were made after piloting, followed by an evaluation in which TD children partnered the children with ASD. Improvements were found in the children's engagement, socialization, and collaboration while playing.

Malinverni et al. (2014, 2017) describe an inclusive design model that aims to develop games children enjoy but are at the same time therapeutically effective. They suggest designing co-located multi-user games to encourage social interaction. Within this approach, children are directly confronted with situations that require social interactions with peers, unlike simulation-based environments where children interact only with a virtual environment. The proposed model includes four steps: (1) professionals determine therapeutic goals and strategies, (2) children are encouraged to state their interests and motives, (3) integrating professionals and children's contributions to define game mechanics and experiences, and (4) conducting an exploratory evaluation of a game.

The authors described the development and design of a Kinect-based game called "Pico's Adventures" that aimed to facilitate the development of social initiation skills in children with ASD. Five participatory sessions were conducted to identify the preferences, interests, and motivation of boys with ASD. The sessions took place weekly and lasted for 1 h. Four boys with ASD, 9–10 years of age, participated. All four had typical cognitive abilities and functional language. Although they were older than the children the game was intended for, their age was assessed to be more suitable for PD activities. As additional motivation, the boys were told that they were helping create a game for younger children. Each session was designed to respond to specific aspects of the game design. All workshops included stories about the main character's journey. At the sessions, the boys were given "scene cards" that described simple scenarios based on specific locations, goals, and conflicts of characters. The children were asked to provide ideas on unspecified aspects of the scene using modalities of their choice (speech, drawing, enactment, etc.). With this approach, the researchers improved narrative elements and game mechanics and identified potential rewards and resources in the game.

Initial evaluation was conducted with the children that participated in the design development through two additional sessions after the workshops. It was examined whether the game met the children's expectations, and problems with using the application were identified. An additional exploratory study was conducted with ten younger boys with ASD (4–6 years of age). These children also accepted the game well and showed some behaviors related to social initiation.

When PD is concerned, the authors recommend using narrative resources (i.e., narrative structure, game back-story, scene cards) as a framework to which both children and professionals can contribute. Furthermore, they believe that experts' requirements should be used to define goals and structure, while children contribute to specific sequences of the game.

Bossavit and Parsons (2016, 2018) describe the participatory design of a two-player game for teaching geography. The game is based on the natural user interface and uses Kinect technology to compare cooperative and competitive modes. They used The Body Menu, a technique that associates virtual menu items with different body parts and selects them when the user reaches these zones with hands.

Four high-functioning teenagers with ASD were invited to participate in the design team, but only two attended the sessions regularly. The students' teachers contributed by giving feedback before and during the design process.

Six sessions were held. In the first session (foundation session), the researchers introduced The Body Menu to the teachers, and they jointly discussed how this technique could be used in school settings. The students participated in the second session (context setting session) as informants and users. They got acquainted with the project and played on the Kinect using The Body Menu. Later, they expressed their preferences regarding the game through a visual questionnaire, which was used to narrow down the ideas for prototyping. Although the researchers provided visual schedules for planning future meetings and blank papers for writing down ideas and sketching prototype screenshots, none of the boys used them.

In the third and fifth sessions (idea generation sessions), the students, as co-designers, generated ideas for competitive and cooperative modes through discussion. Since the students found it difficult to design the game from the beginning, the researchers gave them a video example of a geography-related game. A researcher verbally integrated each new idea into the scenario, taking into account possible causes and consequences. If the idea did not fit into the scenario, the researcher rejected it with the consent of all stakeholders or modified it if the team members considered it important. When there were no more new ideas, the researcher asked questions about the game characteristics to encourage discussion. All ideas were shown with gestures or verbally described. The students had the roles of testers and co-designers in the fourth and sixth sessions (iteration sessions) when they played with the prototype and provided feedback on its characteristics.

The authors emphasized that true equality between the students and other team members was not achieved. The researchers made decisions regarding content and values, while the students mainly decided on implementation. The authors pointed out the significance of enabling students to determine on their own what their contribution would be, even when some of them wanted to participate for only a short time. According to them, equality in design partnership implies respecting different types of expertise that each partner brings into the design team. The authors also noticed that students with ASD were easily discouraged because they were often marginalized in the past.

Van Rijn and Stappers (2008) consider the ways to motivate users to participate in the PD process. They believe that "psychological ownership" of users will be improved if appropriate tools and techniques are used to encourage expression, if their expressions (e.g., notes, handwriting, pictures) are present in the results, and if their messages are taken into account, which would show that their contribution was recognized and appreciated.

The authors included three boys with ASD, their parents, teachers, and other professionals in designing a language-learning toy. The project had three phases: exploration, concept development, and prototype testing. The users were involved in the first and the third phases. After each phase, the designer visited the users to discuss the results, such as reports, prototypes, and presentations.

The designer observed the boys at home, at school, and in speech therapy during the exploration phase. The parents reported their personal experiences with autism through interviews. Professionals were also involved in this phase. Several expression tools were used, such as workbooks and collage-making kits and a script-providing tool. The users' original expressions, such as stories, artifacts, and videos, were included in the report to give the users a sense of ownership. Conclusions were written using the users' notes and handwriting so that they could recognize their contributions. At the end of this phase, the parents and teachers were shown preliminary reports they discussed with the designer.

In the testing phase, the boys and their parents evaluated the prototype during home visits when they played with it for about an hour. The parents were asked to take on the role of a co-researcher due to their expertise in knowing the child. The designer used the prototype and the workbook to confirm to parents they had expert roles. The prototype reflected the users' opinions. Finally, the users received the report and an invitation to a presentation where they could answer the questions from the audience. The authors concluded that the signs of users having a sense of belonging and motivation included the following: willingness to participate in the design process, taking the initiative, feeling proud of the results, and having a sense of responsibility for them.

Benton et al. (2011, 2012, 2014) developed the Interface Design Experience for the Autistic Spectrum (IDEAS) to include children with ASD in PD of a math game. IDEAS combines PD strategies developed for children without autism with the TEACCH (Treatment and Education of Autistic and related Communication handicapped Children) program used in the education of these children (Mesibov et al., 2004), with a focus on alleviating sensory difficulties, using students' interests, and improving abstraction and generalization.

The original IDEAS method (Benton et al., 2011) was designed for individual work with children during one session consisting of (1) an introduction to a design topic, (2) a discussion on previous experience/demonstration of similar software, (3) communicating one's own ideas on the design and writing them down in the prepared template, and (4) summarizing the best ideas regarding the interface design. Visual schedules were also used to show sequences of these activities and served as a checklist for documenting children's progress. In this version, IDEAS was tested with ten high-functioning children with ASD (10–14 years of age) who gave their ideas on designing a math game interface. The level of support in each session (including sample ideas and template interface designs) was in accordance with the needs of each child. It was found that children with ASD could participate in creative activities but needed additional support in some of them to achieve full participation, especially the children who had idea generation difficulties.

The same authors (Benton et al., 2012) later extended the application of IDEAS to support children with ASD in collaborating with the design team. The extended method included similar activities but over six sessions in which an idea led to a working prototype. Whiteboards were used to write down visual schedules in which students marked the completed tasks and other information about the session. The design team included children with ASD, teachers, and two researchers (one with the technical knowledge needed to make a computer prototype and the other with knowledge about autism). When needed, adults provided assistance to the children, directed social interaction, and insisted on respecting social rules such as turn-taking and listening to others.

Two teams were formed, each including three high-functioning young people with ASD. They met once a week, over 6 weeks, to develop a math game. Each session began with an introduction and explanation of the task, a reminder of the rules they had made at the first meeting, and a visual reminder of previous sessions. The sessions focused on (1) building a team; (2) talking about previous experiences regarding feedback and rewarding at school, as well as playing and talking about the existing math games; (3) generating ideas using templates and making paper prototypes to improve the feedback and rewarding system in the game; (4) discussing how to animate the adapted computerized versions of the game developed by a researcher based on the team's ideas; (5) fine-tuning of the first animated computer version with printed storyboards; and (6) evaluating the final prototype and completing a questionnaire on the PD process they participated in. The authors pointed out the need to connect design activities with the existing knowledge of students and the selection of content consistent with student abilities, regular meetings, and providing opportunities for different ways of expression.

The next thing that interested researchers was whether IDEAS could also be applied to TD children. Benton and Johnson (2014) used the same methodology as Benton et al. (2012). The team structure, task, number, and content of sessions remained the same. However, this time, two design teams included children with ASD, while the other two included TD children. The authors report that both TD children and children with ASD may benefit from a structured and supportive approach to PD. However, these benefits can vary between different groups and also within different groups. Some children may need additional structure and support more than others. TD children can also need additional support due to literal interpretations, difficulties in reaching a compromise, aspiration to be dominant in the group, and problems with creativity and concentration.

In a more general approach also based on TEACCH, Benton et al. (2014) deal with a full range of neurodiverse children. This approach, called Diversity for Design (D4D), is also based on a child's strengths and relies on four principles:

1. *Understanding culture*—which, for example, refers to characteristics and predictable patterns of thinking and behaving.
2. *Tailoring to the individual*—the approach application should be flexible and individualized, which enables the use of various concepts and methods relevant to a wide range of developmental levels and behavioral profiles.
3. *Structuring the environment*—to reduce the impact of the environment on a person's abilities, understanding, and learning.
4. *Providing supports*—so that a person could understand certain activities better (e.g., attaching visual representations and physical demonstrations to verbal presentations).

Grawemeyer et al. (2012) developed an intelligent math tutoring system, which included an educational pedagogical agent (EPA). EPA are virtual characters that have a body and can, for educational purposes, interact and communicate through voice, gestures, and facial expressions (Grivokostopoulou et al., 2020). The EPA development kit (EPA DK) that directly transforms, on-the-fly, EPA sketches into functional prototypes was used to develop this system. EPA DK allows the presentation of various layouts and provides opportunities for feedback, interaction, and changes in the EPA appearance using different media, such as screen printouts and drawing software.

PD involved a three-step process: individual generation of ideas, mixing ideas, and integration into a "big idea." This process was complemented by the on-the-fly fast prototype change that was facilitated by EPA DK during the design sessions. The sessions were conducted at school and included six young people with ASD, 11–15 years of age, divided into two groups.

The students were asked to individually design the EPA for a math tutor using crayons, pencils, and blank papers. At the end of the first session, the participants were asked to explain their idea to other group members. This was followed by

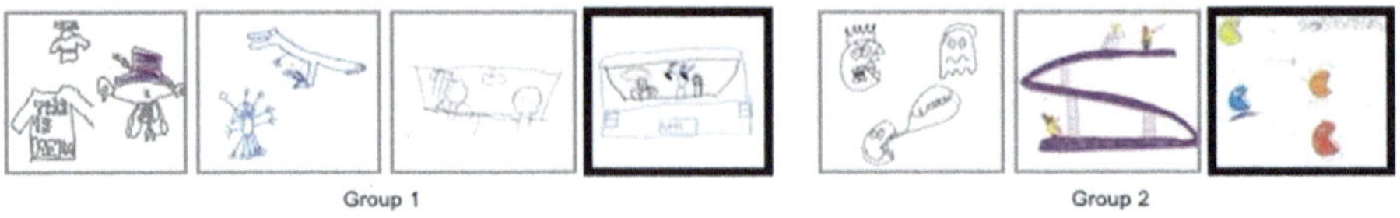

Fig. 2.3 Examples of individual and combined group (bold frame) EPA ideas. (Reproduced from Grawemeyer et al., 2012)

combining individual ideas into a common group idea they then drew on a paper (Fig. 2.3). Two group ideas were combined into one "big EPA idea" in the next step. Representatives of one group explained their group's idea to members of the other group, while the researcher noted down the main characteristics of the EPA design on the whiteboard. The features liked by members of the opposite group were especially emphasized. Then, the participants decided on the "big EPA idea" that included all characteristics the students liked the most. Finally, EPA was made of art materials.

All six participants were involved in an all-day prototyping session, in which EPA DK was used for the visualization and development of the EPA idea. The "big EPA idea" was used as a basis. The EPA prototype was presented, as well as various feedback options and interaction styles. The students stated what they liked and disliked. The options they did not like were removed right away during the design session. Then, the students were asked to refine the EPA design according to their wishes. They were given an electronic version of the external representation of EPA shown in the prototype. The improved design was included in the EPA prototype and presented to the participants. Finally, the students were asked to provide ideas for verbal character interaction using screen printouts that show the EPA design.

In a one-semester study, Foss et al. (2013) examined the use of Cooperative Inquiry in school. The research included ten boys with special educational needs, 10–12 years of age, two of whom had ASD. They participated in designing a browser-based computer game over six sessions. The boys generally had positive experiences and managed to develop a partnership with adults while designing the game. Based on the results, the authors gave recommendations for the use of Cooperative Inquiry in special classes: extra time for informal activities during design sessions, maintaining a high adult-to-child ratio, providing simple instructions in oral or written form, and ensuring high engagement of students.

Millen et al. (2010) developed a "design a game" procedure they first tested in TD students and then, with adaptations, in students with ASD. The procedure was used in designing a serious game, Block Party, based on joint problem-solving. The children paired up, and each child accessed the virtual environment from different laptops. A pair could communicate through an avatar. The task was to build a tower of blocks jointly. However, each block had two colors, and each child had their own color pattern to make. To complete the task, the children had to communicate with each other to jointly choose a block with the combination of colors that suited both players.

The prototype review session included five students with ASD, 16 and 17 years old. The session was implemented in an information and communications technology class with the teacher's help. The Block Party training scenario was projected on an interactive whiteboard. The keyboard and mouse were connected to the laptop with a long cable so that all students could interact with the virtual environment from their places. Each student was given a feedback sheet with screenshots of different Block Party stages and the accompanying columns for "Like," "Dislike," and "Not sure." Feedback posters, which were enlarged copies of individual feedback sheets, were placed on the walls next to whiteboards. These posters were used to collect feedback from the whole group, and the students, one by one, commented on them. Members of the group took control in turn or told the teacher what to do next. The teacher paused the program at different levels and asked the students what they thought of it. These pauses corresponded to screenshots on feedback sheets in which the students wrote the answers (Fig. 2.4). The students were encouraged to write both positive and negative comments and were repeatedly told there were no right or wrong answers. One student was asked to write group comments on the posters. The authors pointed out that it was methodologically important for worksheets and learning materials to be consistent and precise since the students with ASD tended to find minor inconsistencies that hindered their work.

The scenario design method was tested in three 13- and 14-year-old students with ASD who attended a regular school. The activity, which was prolonged from

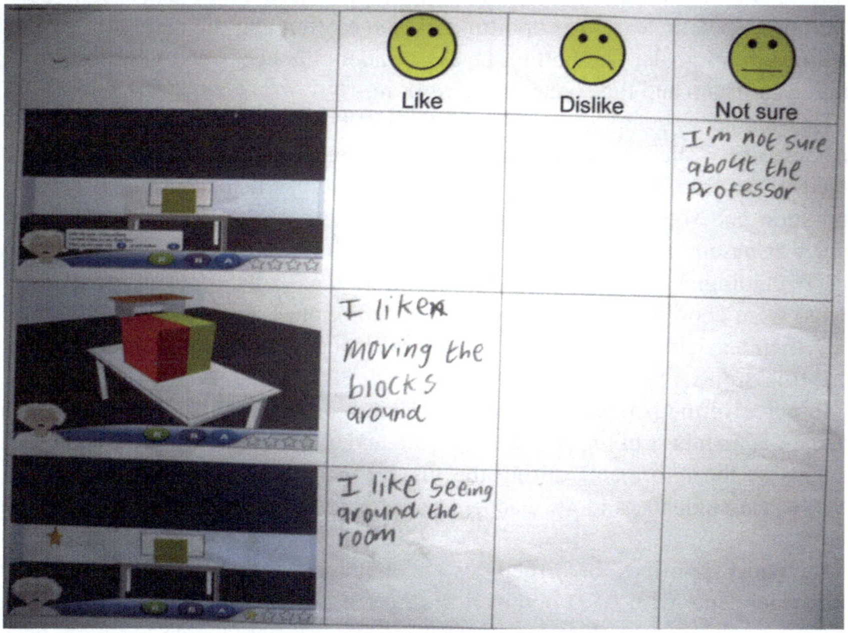

Fig. 2.4 Individual feedback worksheets used in the review session of the serious game Block Party prototype. (Reproduced from Millen et al., 2010)

the planned one to about 2 h at students' initiative, was divided into six parts. The students were first encouraged to think about different types of computer games they played. Then, they were directed to consider what they liked or disliked in those games and then generate ideas for computer game design. After that, the students and the researcher talked about friendship, what it meant to be a good friend, and why we liked to play computer games with friends. The last two parts focused on the game design. The students were asked to provide ideas for different aspects of playing the game and were then encouraged to draw some of them.

According to the authors, this method proved to be successful for several reasons—the depth of understanding the task, the quality of students' ideas, and the time spent working on the task. They emphasize that the tasks should be structured, clear, and focused and that we should be flexible when unplanned circumstances arise.

Parsons and Cobb (2014) wanted to examine how inclusive research functioned in education and recognize the limits of inclusivity of this process. They investigated how collaboration in a multidisciplinary team affected the learner-centered design process. They illustrated this process through cooperation between children with ASD and their teachers on the development of technologies that support social conversation and collaboration.

They conceptualized the complexity of the process as a "triple-decker sandwich" consisting of theory, technologies, and thoughts. The upper layer represents a top-down theoretical approach in developing educational tasks. The middle layer, technologies and their affordances, refers to the type of technology that will be used or developed, specific learning opportunities it can offer, and the nature of the developed tasks and goals. The bottom layer considers the needs and viewpoints of the target user group and the context they work in.

This model was applied within the COSPATIAL (Communication and Social Participation: Collaborative Technologies for Interaction and Learning) project that aimed to develop collaborative technology prototypes that would help teach collaboration and social conversation to children with ASD. The upper, theoretical, layer was based on constructivism and the principles of cognitive behavioral therapy. Technologies that encourage collaboration (e.g., collaborative virtual environments) were chosen for the middle layer. The bottom layer included children with ASD, their teachers, social and organizational school factors, and the existing school infrastructure.

To perceive the perspective of target group members, the authors included five teachers as members of the core design team and five students with ASD and six TD students as the informants during the first year of the project. Six students with ASD, 8 TD students, and 40 teachers participated in usability testing in the second year.

The paper describes the difficulties encountered in incorporating some suggestions of students with ASD obtained during the evaluation of an early prototype. Children's wishes to explore a virtual environment differed from teachers' desires for a more limited environment that would be less distracting when learning. The designers decided to follow the teachers' ideas, which resulted in the most capable students feeling deprived or bored in limited activities. The authors considered to what extent the focus on outcomes (the impact of technology on children) was compatible with the cooperative, empowering PD approach.

Within the COSPATIAL project, Millen et al. (2012) developed a collaborative virtual environment, Island of Ideas. This place is designed as a virtual island where a researcher participates in PD activities with children to discover their opinions about the game design. The children and the researcher can access a virtual room from different laptops and communicate with each other using headphones and microphones. Users can be presented as avatars or "video pods." Before entering the virtual environment, a student may choose a male or female avatar with various hair colors and t-shirts. Video communication is in real time. Within the virtual environment, five stops are placed around the island, where various activities or discussions related to the game design take place. The stops enable the researcher to structure the sessions clearly and logically, making it easier for the student to understand the activities. The student can move freely through the virtual environment but is required to move from stop to stop with the researcher. Each stop usually consists of three surfaces. The first surface explains the activity that will be performed at the station. The activity takes place at the middle one. At the last surface, the activity is summarized, and the student is directed to the next stop. The initial and final surfaces correspond to the virtual schedule shown at the first stop that structures the activity and helps the students to understand what is expected of them in each part of the session.

A study conducted to evaluate the usability of "Island of Ideas" as a PD resource included 12 students with ASD, 11–14 years of age. All students had developed speech and attended regular schools.

Each student participated in four 60-min sessions. The first session was introductory, where the researcher got to know the student. Over the next two sessions, the following activities were performed using "Island of Ideas": (1) showing the visual schedule to the student and explaining the goal of the session, (2) playing a commercial game for 10 min, (3) having an interview with the researcher (discussing design characteristics of the played game), (4) drawing ideas for a new game level (in paint), and (5) considering the student's ideas in a virtual gallery of texts and images. A different game was played in each of these two sessions, and the interview was conducted using avatars or video pods. The final, fourth session was evaluative, and the students were asked to critically review "Island of Ideas" with the researcher.

The authors reported that the students were excited to use tablets and digital pens for drawing. Some of them initially doubted their drawing skills, but the researchers explained they were not important and showed them how to erase parts of drawings easily. The students were able to generate different ideas regarding new levels, obstacles, rewards, and ideas for representing life in the game. The gallery of ideas was motivating for students, which enabled the researcher to ask questions about their ideas and get additional explanations. The initial results slightly favored using video pods in PD during the virtual island sessions.

Roper et al. (2019) started from the assumption that difficulties of children with ASD related to PD could be alleviated if face-to-face communication was replaced by collaborative virtual environments where avatars represented participants. In such an environment, three groups of children (TD children, high-functioning children with ASD, and low-functioning children with ASD) evaluated the existing computer games and gave suggestions for their further development. TD participants were 8–9 years old, while participants with ASD were 12–14. Within collaborative virtual environments, the players were represented as computer-generated avatars or video pods (what the authors call a mixed reality condition). These two conditions were compared to face-to-face communication.

Each student participated in three 60-min sessions over 3 weeks. All sessions included the same facilitator, who was a pair to each child individually. The sessions had the same structure and consisted of four main components. In the introductory part, the facilitator explained the session structure to a student and what was expected of him. The facilitator and the student discussed the main goals of the session. A printed schedule with visual prompts was used to make it easier for the student to understand the purpose of activities and relieve anxiety related to the upcoming activities. The next phase involved playing commercially available computer games for 10 min. Simple games with some common design characteristics (e.g., characters, rewards, lives, and obstacles) were selected. This enabled the student to go through the selected game several times in a short while. Finally, in the third part of the session, the student was asked questions about the design characteristics of the game and ideas for developing a new game. Members of all three groups reviewed all three games, and the interviews were conducted in one of the three previously mentioned conditions (avatar, video pods, face-to-face).

A questionnaire completed by the students (enjoyment during the session, choosing an interview method they liked) was used for evaluation. The students also assessed how much they liked the conditions in a particular session using a five-point Likert "smiley" scale. The facilitators evaluated three categories (student engagement, ability to critique, ability to generate ideas) based on the analysis of video recordings.

The results showed that TD students performed best in the face-to-face condition. Although students with ASD generally had better achievements in computer-mediated conditions, there were also differences between them. High-functioning students with ASD performed best in the avatar condition, while low-functioning students with ASD were the most successful in the mixed reality condition. Also, the task involving critiquing and generating new ideas proved to be too difficult for low-functioning students with ASD. Regardless of the facilitator's assessment, all three groups of students showed a preference for computer-mediated conditions.

Zarin and Fallman (2011) described an interactive design process of small software applications aiming to improve social communication skills. This process involved six children, 5–8 years of age, with ASD or Down's syndrome. The system was designed with the users, their teachers, and other professionals.

The design process was divided into three phases. The design team first conducted a contextual study in which teachers and professional caregivers were interviewed. Observational data from video clips, images, and notes were collected. The second phase of the project included scenario development and iterative prototyping. Over 20 micro applications based on the Flash program were constructed. The authors chose micro applications over sketching the interface on paper, believing that would reduce the metaphorical gap between a representation and what it stood for. After several iterations, a general framework ("The Troll Forest") was chosen, which helped to create a cohesive structure of the broader system that included micro applications. During the third phase, the entire system was tested and evaluated within the class. First, the whole group explored the system together. Then, with teacher support, they were one by one encouraged to interact with each of the four micro applications. After each session, the children and teachers were asked to discuss what was happening during the session.

Madsen et al. (2009) included seven verbal adolescents with ASD, 10–17 years of age, in the initial testing of a software prototype designed to develop understanding and expressing emotions. They conducted four sessions recorded on camera and then interviewed students and their teachers.

Fabri et al. (2016) included young people with ASD in designing an online toolkit that would provide these students information and strategies for overcoming the obstacles they may encounter in higher education. They used the Design Thinking approach and its five-step model (Empathize-Define-Ideate-Prototype-Test).

The *empathize* step should enable understanding what people do and what needs affect their lives. Thus, representatives of different groups completed the online questionnaires (students with ASD, parents of students with ASD, academics, secondary school teachers, and support staff members). In addition, some of the students were interviewed to get a deeper insight into their personal experiences.

The *define* step during collaborative sessions, which brought together researchers, academics, and adults with ASD, involved segmenting data, identifying needs, and summarizing findings. Both good and bad sides of the existing practice were discussed.

During the *ideate* step, all participants were asked to suggest topics related to the problems identified in the define step. The suggestions were noted and discussed, and certain problems and questions were clarified. After the meeting, the partners voted for the topics that, in their opinion, had the greatest impact on the target group and should be included in the toolkit prototype.

The *prototype* version of the online toolkit covered numerous topics. There were variations in how a topic should be presented (e.g., long scrolling sections or short texts with previous/next navigation). The visual design of the toolkit prototype was simple, with few colors and easy navigation. Some of the content was not created online but as a paper prototype. Short video clips on three toolkit topics were made and presented in the video introduction.

In the final *test* step, three workshops were organized to evaluate the online toolkit prototype and consider the ideas regarding design characteristics. UK students participated in the first workshop, and their ideas were used to improve the prototype that was the basis of the next workshop. In the third workshop, participants from Finland evaluated the design and functionality of the English user interface version, as parts of the content translated into Finnish. The authors stated that, despite initial anxiety, students with ASD enjoyed the activities and appreciated the willingness to hear their opinions.

Discussing the design that involves adults with ASD who had limited speech and learning disabilities, Gaudion et al. (2015) suggested empathic understanding, in which each stage of the design process influences the next, rather than using predetermined methods. Instead of focusing on limitations, the authors emphasized the triad of strengths (sensory preferences, interests, and action capabilities) that affected their relationships with the environment. In order to examine a person's daily experience, it is necessary to combine data from several sources—people with ASD, designers, and parents/people who provide support. The authors observed this process of gathering information through three stages. In the first stage that involves sensory activities and mirroring interests, a designer can register facts that he may not get from other sources that focus on care, health, or safety. In the next step, the designer applies various visual mapping tools a person will use to express thoughts and preferences. The third stage includes a series of co-creation workshops, in which parents and support staff are encouraged to present their own design ideas.

Weisblatt et al. (2019) used a user-centered design with co-design elements (PD) in developing the Point OutWords software. Point OutWords, a tablet-based software, is designed to develop manual and oral motor skills that are prerequisites for communication by pointing or speaking in people with ASD with underdeveloped communicative speech. Users were included in the development of this software as co-creators, either directly through nonverbal choices or indirectly through the reports of their communication therapists.

The design, development, and evaluation of Point OutWords have so far gone through three phases involving parents, caregivers, therapists, and children with autism with very limited communication skills.

The first phase included prototyping and testing at a clinic with patients with ASD. Designers observed this phase, and therapists provided data and feedback. This phase included 31 children with ASD, 3–7 years of age, and their communication therapists. All users contributed as testers, and six child-therapist dyads participated as co-creators. The role of co-creators involved closer collaboration between children, therapists, and programmers, including an explicit choice of user interface elements, such as avatars and graphic styles, and implicitly showing preferences through their own behavior when interacting with mock-ups and prototypes. Designers came to the clinic and observed the interaction between users and their therapists while working with Point OutWords prototypes. Therapists provided feedback on their own experience and the experience of their clients. Co-creators provided feedback through unstructured interviews with therapists and direct observations of work sessions with designers' prototypes and mock-ups of the software. The prototypes were modified through several iterations, evaluated by co-creators and testers, and then improved. Other educational applications were also used to test the users in order to identify potential problems in their interaction with standard application design. Visuomotor interactions in Point Mode were tested using a mock-up. A user and a therapist sat in front of a large thick white sheet of paper on which magnets fastened pieces of a jigsaw puzzle. The designers, who could not be seen on the other side of the paper, used the magnets and moved the jigsaw pieces according to the user's instructions. The observed interaction of users with this mock-up was used to obtain qualitative data on the routes by which the children moved their fingers in contact with the surface. Interactions with the virtual keyboard in Type Mode were tested using a prototype in which feedback was emphasized through animation and the sound of a balloon bursting when the correct key was pressed.

In the second phase, focus groups were formed to consider two thematic areas—usability/acceptability and issues related to the design of a pilot study. Usability and acceptability were tested through interviews with parents. The pilot study was developed in consultation with the focus group that included four parents of nonverbal children with ASD and was facilitated by a co-investigator parent. These meetings and software presentations generated feedback on the project design, goals, and implementation.

Finally, the third phase included the pilot study and initial feasibility study to determine (1) fidelity to the recommended treatment method, (2) acceptability of the intervention for users with ASD and their caregivers, and (3) acceptability of candidate outcome measures to assess the efficacy of the Point OutWords intervention. Feedback was formally collected from parents after participating in the pilot study.

Wilson et al. (2019) developed the Co-Design Beyond Words (CDBW) approach for minimally verbal children with ASD at preschool age. This approach combines the existing co-design methods with practice-based speech-language treatment methods, in which children have the leading role and which are based on their interests so that children's activities and interactions can be understood better. Key points of the process and units of analysis are *moments of interaction*—micro instances of mutual attention, turn-taking, and imitation in which minimally verbal children with ASD convey meaning without words—through action, interaction, and focus of attention.

CDBW was used in prototyping an interactive ball (The TangiBall) that was supposed to enable children to record their own voices and sounds. The prototyping had three iterative phases: the Foundation Phase (preparation for interaction), the Interaction Phase (designing and reflecting in the moment), and the Reflection Phase (reflection-on-action).

The process included ten children with ASD, 5–8 years of age. Data were collected from videos and photographs taken during joint design sessions, field notes, and interviews with teachers and therapists who participated in these activities.

The authors believed that, in this way, children could express their insights regarding design, direct the design process, and at the same time discover their strengths, interests, and abilities.

It can be concluded that people with ASD are able to develop a partnership and significantly contribute to the design process. After initial restraint, these people enjoy the design activities and are happy their contribution is appreciated. However, during the PD process, it is necessary to find a balance between the structure, so that people with ASD do not get overburdened, and freedom that gives them space to express creativity. Also, sometimes people with ASD refuse to take on more complex roles in the design team because they doubt their own skills. Although different authors have found original methodological solutions and ingenious techniques, it is noticeable that people with preserved speech and cognitive potentials dominate the design teams. Still, few studies show that even minimally verbal people with ASD and those with learning disabilities can be included in the PD process. Furthermore, additional data on the participation of preschool children and adults with ASD in the PD process would be very significant.

References

Benton, L., & Johnson, H. (2014). Structured approaches to participatory design for children: Can targeting the needs of children with autism provide benefits for a broader child population? *Instructional Science, 42*(1), 47–65. https://doi.org/10.1007/s11251-013-9297-y

Benton, L., & Johnson, H. (2015). Widening participation in technology design: A review of the involvement of children with special educational needs and disabilities. *International Journal of Child-Computer Interaction, 3-4*, 23-40 S2212868915000033. https://doi.org/10.1016/j.ijcci.2015.07.001

Benton, L., Johnson, H., Brosnan, M., Ashwin, E., & Grawemeyer, B. (2011). IDEAS: An interface design experience for the autistic spectrum. In *CHI'11 extended abstracts on human factors in computing systems* (pp. 1759–1764). https://doi.org/10.1145/1979742.1979841

Benton, L., Johnson, H., Ashwin, E., Brosnan, M., & Grawemeyer, B. (2012, May). Developing IDEAS: Supporting children with autism within a participatory design team. In *Proceedings of the SIGCHI conference on Human factors in computing systems* (pp. 2599–2608). https://doi.org/10.1145/2207676.2208650

Benton, L., Vasalou, A., Khaled, R., Johnson, H., & Gooch, D. (2014, April). Diversity for design: A framework for involving neurodiverse children in the technology design process. In *Proceedings of the SIGCHI conference on human factors in computing systems* (pp. 3747–3756). https://doi.org/10.1145/2556288.2557244

Bossavit, B., & Parsons, S. (2016, May). "This is how I want to learn" high functioning autistic teens co-designing a serious game. In *Proceedings of the 2016 CHI conference on human factors in computing systems* (pp. 1294–1299). https://doi.org/10.1145/2858036.2858322

Bossavit, B., & Parsons, S. (2018). Outcomes for design and learning when teenagers with autism codesign a serious game: A pilot study. *Journal of Computer Assisted Learning, 34*(3), 293–305. https://doi.org/10.1111/jcal.12242

Brandt, E., Binder, T., & Sanders, E. B. N. (2013). Tools and techniques: Ways to engage telling, making and enacting. In J. Simonsen & T. Robertson (Eds.), *Routledge international handbook of participatory design* (pp. 145–181). Routledge.

Bratteteig, T., Bødker, K., Dittrich, Y., Mogensen, P. H., & Simonsen, J. (2013). Methods: Organising principles and general guidelines for participatory design projects. In J. Simonsen & T. Robertson (Eds.), *Routledge international handbook of participatory design* (pp. 117–144). Routledge.

Carmel, E., Whitaker, R. D., & George, J. F. (1993). PD and joint application design: A transatlantic comparison. *Communications of the ACM, 36*(6), 40–48. https://doi.org/10.1145/153571.163265

Fabri, M., Andrews, P. C., & Pukki, H. K. (2016). Using design thinking to engage autistic students in participatory design of an online toolkit to help with transition into higher education. *Journal of Assistive Technologies, 10*(2), 102–114.

Foss, E., Guha, M. L., Papadatos, P., Clegg, T., Yip, J., & Walsh, G. (2013). Cooperative inquiry extended: Creating technology with middle school students with learning differences. *Journal of Special Education Technology, 28*(3), 33–46. https://doi.org/10.1177/016264341302800303

Frauenberger, C., Good, J., & Keay-Bright, W. (2010, November). Phenomenology, a framework for participatory design. In *Proceedings of the 11th Biennial participatory design conference* (pp. 187–190). https://doi.org/10.1145/1900441.1900474

Frauenberger, C., Good, J., & Keay-Bright, W. (2011). Designing technology for children with special needs: Bridging perspectives through participatory design. *CoDesign, 7*(1), 1–28. https://doi.org/10.1080/15710882.2011.587013

Frauenberger, C., Good, J., & Alcorn, A. (2012a, June). Challenges, opportunities and future perspectives in including children with disabilities in the design of interactive technology. In *Proceedings of the 11th international conference on interaction design and children* (pp. 367–370). https://doi.org/10.1145/2307096.2307171

Frauenberger, C., Good, J., Alcorn, A., & Pain, H. (2012b, June). Supporting the design contributions of children with autism spectrum conditions. In *Proceedings of the 11th international conference on interaction design and children* (pp. 134–143). https://doi.org/10.1145/2307096.2307112

Frauenberger, C., Good, J., Alcorn, A., & Pain, H. (2013). Conversing through and about technologies: Design critique as an opportunity to engage children with autism and broaden research(er) perspectives. *International Journal of Child-Computer Interaction, 1*(2), 38–49. https://doi.org/10.1016/j.ijcci.2013.02.001

Frauenberger, C., Makhaeva, J., & Spiel, K. (2016, May). Designing smart objects with autistic children: Four design exposès. In *Proceedings of the 2016 CHI conference on human factors in computing systems* (pp. 130–139). https://doi.org/10.1145/2858036.2858050

Frauenberger, C., Makhaeva, J., & Spiel, K. (2017, June). Blending methods: Developing participatory design sessions for autistic children. In *Proceedings of the 2017 conference on interaction design and children* (pp. 39–49). https://doi.org/10.1145/3078072.3079727

Frauenberger, C., Spiel, K., & Makhaeva, J. (2019). Thinking outside The box-designing smart things with autistic children. *International Journal of Human Computer Interaction, 35*(8), 666–678. https://doi.org/10.1080/10447318.2018.1550177

Gaudion, K., Hall, A., Myerson, J., & Pellicano, L. (2015). A designer's approach: How can autistic adults with learning disabilities be involved in the design process? *CoDesign, 11*(1), 49–69. https://doi.org/10.1080/15710882.2014.997829

Grawemeyer, B., Johnson, H., Brosnan, M., Ashwin, E., & Benton, L. (2012, June). Developing an embodied pedagogical agent with and for young people with autism spectrum disorder. In *International conference on intelligent tutoring systems* (pp. 262–267). https://doi.org/10.1007/978-3-642-30950-2_33

Gray, C. (1998). Social stories and comic strip conversations with students with Asperger syndrome and high- functioning autism. In E. Schopler, G. Mesibov & L. Kunce (Eds.), *Asperger syndrome or high functioning autism? Current Issues in Autism* (pp. 167–198). Plenum Press.

Greenbaum, J., & Loi, D. (2012). Participation, the camel and the elephant of design: An introduction. *CoDesign, 8*(2–3), 81–85. https://doi.org/10.1080/15710882.2012.690232

Grivokostopoulou, F., Kovas, K., & Perikos, I. (2020). The effectiveness of embodied pedagogical agents and their impact on students learning in virtual worlds. *Applied Sciences, 10*(5), 1739. https://doi.org/10.3390/app10051739

Höysniemi, J., Hämäläinen, P., & Turkki, L. (2004, June). Wizard of Oz prototyping of computer vision based action games for children. In *Proceedings of the 2004 conference on Interaction design and children: Building a community* (pp. 27–34). https://doi.org/10.1145/1017833.1017837

Jarosinski, W. W. (2019). *Using co-design to develop 'Autshare', an online solution-sharing platform for Autistic individuals.* Bachelor's thesis, University of Twente. http://essay.utwente.nl/78732/1/Jarosinski_BA_EEMCS.pdf

Kensing, F., & Greenbaum, J. (2013). Heritage: Having a say. In J. Simonsen & T. Robertson (Eds.), *Routledge International Handbook of Participatory Design* (pp. 21–36). Routledge.

Luck, R. (2018). What is it that makes participation in design participatory design? *Design Studies, 59*, 1–8. https://doi.org/10.1016/j.destud.2018.10.002

Madsen, M., El Kaliouby, R., Eckhardt, M., Hoque, M. E., Goodwin, M. S., & Picard, R. (2009). Lessons from participatory design with adolescents on the autism spectrum. In *CHI'09 extended abstracts on human factors in computing systems* (pp. 3835–3840). https://doi.org/10.1145/1520340.1520580

Makhaeva, J., Frauenberger, C., & Spiel, K. (2016, August). Creating creative spaces for co-designing with autistic children: The concept of a "Handlungsspielraum". In *Proceedings of the 14th Participatory design conference: Full papers-Volume 1* (pp. 51–60). https://doi.org/10.1145/2940299.2940306

Malinverni, L., Mora-Guiard, J., Padillo, V., Mairena, M., Hervás, A., & Pares, N. (2014, June). Participatory design strategies to enhance the creative contribution of children with special needs. In *Proceedings of the 2014 conference on Interaction design and children* (pp. 85–94). https://doi.org/10.1145/2593968.2593981

Malinverni, L., Mora-Guiard, J., & Pares, N. (2016). Towards methods for evaluating and communicating participatory design: A multimodal approach. *International Journal of Human-Computer Studies, 94*, 53–63. https://doi.org/10.1016/j.ijhcs.2016.03.004

Malinverni, L., Mora-Guiard, J., Padillo, V., Valero, L., Hervás, A., & Pares, N. (2017). An inclusive design approach for developing video games for children with autism spectrum disorder. *Computers in Human Behavior, 71*, 535–549. https://doi.org/10.1016/j.chb.2016.01.018

Mesibov, G. B., Shea, V., & Schopler, E. (2004). *The TEACCH approach to autism spectrum disorders*. Springer. https://doi.org/10.1007/978-0-306-48647-0

Millen, L., Cobb, S., & Patel, H. (2010, September). Participatory design with children with autism. In *Proceedings of the 8th international conference on disability, virtual reality and associated technologies* (pp. 93–101).

Millen, L., Cobb, S. V. G., Patel, H., & Glover, T. (2012, September). Collaborative virtual environment for conducting design sessions with students with autism spectrum conditions. In *Proceedings of the 9th international conference on disability, virtual reality and associated technologies* (pp. 269–278).

Mora-Guiard, J., Crowell, C., Pares, N., & Heaton, P. (2017). Sparking social initiation behaviors in children with autism through full-body interaction. *International Journal of Child-Computer Interaction, 11*, 62–71. https://doi.org/10.1016/j.ijcci.2016.10.006

Parsons, S., & Cobb, S. (2014). Reflections on the role of the 'users': Challenges in a multi-disciplinary context of learner-centred design for children on the autism spectrum. *International Journal of Research & Method in Education, 37*(4), 421–441. https://doi.org/10.1080/1743727X.2014.890584

Robertson, T., & Simonsen, J. (2012). Challenges and opportunities in contemporary participatory design. *Design Issues, 28*(3), 3–9. https://doi.org/10.1162/DESI_a_00157

Roper, T., Millen Dutka, L., Cobb, S., & Patel, H. (2019). Collaborative virtual environment to facilitate game design evaluation with children with ASC. *International Journal of Human Computer Interaction, 35*(8), 692–705. https://doi.org/10.1080/10447318.2018.1550179

Sanders, E. B. N., & Stappers, P. J. (2008). Co-creation and the new landscapes of design. *CoDesign, 4*(1), 5–18. https://doi.org/10.1080/15710880701875068

Sanders, E. B. N., Brandt, E., & Binder, T. (2010, November). A framework for organizing the tools and techniques of participatory design. In *Proceedings of the 11th biennial participatory design conference* (pp. 195–198). https://doi.org/10.1145/1900441.1900476

Spinuzzi, C. (2005). The methodology of participatory design. *Technical Communication, 52*(2), 163–174.

Sturm, D., Kholodovsky, M., Arab, R., Smith, D. S., Asanov, P., & Gillespie-Lynch, K. (2019). Participatory design of a Hybrid Kinect game to promote collaboration between Autistic players and their peers. *International Journal of Human Computer Interaction, 35*(8), 706–723. https://doi.org/10.1080/10447318.2018.1550180

Van der Velden, M., & Mörtberg, C. (2015). Participatory design and design for values. In J. van den Hoven, P. E. Vermaas, & I. van de Poel (Eds.), *Handbook of ethics, values, and technological design: Sources, theory, values and application domains* (pp. 41–66). Springer. https://doi.org/10.1007/978-94-007-6994-6_33-1

Van Mechelen, M. (2016). *Designing technologies for and with children: Theoretical reflections and a practical inquiry towards a co-design toolkit.* Doctoral thesis, UHasselt—KU Leuven. https://lirias.kuleuven.be/1674366?limo=0

van Rijn, H., & Stappers, P. J. (2008, October). Expressions of ownership: Motivating users in a co-design process. In *Proceedings of the tenth anniversary conference on participatory design* (pp. 178–81).

Walsh, G., Foss, E., Yip, J., & Druin, A. (2013, April). Octoract: An eight-dimensional framework for intergenerational participatory design techniques. In *Proceedings of the SIGCHI conference on human factors in computing systems* (pp. 2893–2902).

Weisblatt, E. J., Langensiepen, C. S., Cook, B., Dias, C., Plaisted Grant, K., Dhariwal, M., Fairclough, M. S., Friend, S. E., Malone, A. E., Varga-Elmiyeh, B., Rybicki, A., Karanth, P., & Belmonte, M. K. (2019). A tablet computer-assisted motor and language skills training program to promote communication development in children with autism: Development and pilot study. *International Journal of Human Computer Interaction, 35*(8), 643–665. https://doi.org/10.1080/10447318.2018.1550176

Wilson, C., Brereton, M., Ploderer, B., & Sitbon, L. (2019, May). Co-design beyond words: 'Moments of interaction' with minimally-verbal children on the Autism spectrum. In *Proceedings of the 2019 CHI conference on human factors in computing systems* (pp. 1–15). https://doi.org/10.1145/3290605.3300251

Zarin, R., & Fallman, D. (2011, May). Through the troll forest: Exploring tabletop interaction design for children with special cognitive needs. In *Proceedings of the SIGCHI conference on human factors in computing systems* (pp. 3319–3322). https://doi.org/10.1145/1978942.1979434

Chapter 3
Autism and Digital Learning Environment

3.1 Introduction

Technological advances have expanded the possibilities to use computer-based devices in education. Interactive and portable devices, such as tablets and smartphones, have increased the accessibility and ease of using computer-based technology in teaching academic skills to students with different disabilities (Spooner et al., 2014).

Although instruction for students with ASD in the past focused on functional rather than academic skills, the development of inclusive education shifted the focus to teaching standards-based academic skills (Ain, 2018; Bročin, 2013; Courtade et al., 2012). Children with ASD show great interest in technology and computers, which can be used to increase their engagement and concentration in academic activities (Serret et al., 2017). Technologies such as computer-based tools, virtual/augmented reality, applications for cellphones and tablets, and robotics create a pleasant environment that fosters the learning of students with ASD (Mazon et al., 2019; Valencia et al., 2019). Unlike specialized devices, this technology is usually familiar to teachers and can thus be more easily incorporated into teaching (Knight et al., 2013; Spooner et al., 2014).

The use of information and communications technologies (ICT) can become a reliable tool in an inclusive environment since it facilitates access to knowledge, information, and learning and the interaction between students and teachers. ICT helps all students to understand, assimilate, and consolidate cognitive materials, such as math and language, better (Anagnostopoulou et al., 2021).

N. Glumbić et al., *Digital Inclusion of Individuals with Autism Spectrum Disorder*, Autism and Child Psychopathology Series,
https://doi.org/10.1007/978-3-031-12037-4_3

Computer-based technology can improve skills in various academic domains (literacy, science, math, collateral skills[1]). Furthermore, it can foster the implementation of universal design in learning principles by providing alternative pathways of representation, engagement, and expression (Yakubova et al., 2021). The *A-Class* software recognizes the computers of students with ASD based on usernames and passwords and extracts information about their interests previously stored in a database. As a result, most students in class see one interface, while it differs for each child with ASD depending on individual interests (Rahman et al., 2011).

The advantages of ICT in teaching students with ASD are numerous. Computer-based devices are available, relatively inexpensive, and intuitively used, and many are also easily portable (Hassan et al., 2011; Kagohara et al., 2013; Wright et al., 2020). Devices such as tablets and smartphones are less stigmatizing and more socially inclusive than, for example, traditional augmentative and alternative communication (AAC) devices (Hong et al., 2017; Spooner et al., 2014).

Students with ASD love to work on computers, which makes practicing academic skills more pleasant and the intervention more game-like (Caria et al., 2018; Grynszpan et al., 2014; Kagohara et al., 2013; Knight et al., 2013; Ploog et al., 2013; Ramdoss et al., 2011).

The environment is safe, controlled, and predictable, which also suits these students (Anagnostopoulou et al., 2021; Valencia et al., 2019).

Computer-based interventions can increase autonomy (Knight et al., 2013; Tsiopela & Jimoyiannis, 2014), instruction can be individualized, and content complexity can be adapted to students' abilities (Bradley & Newbutt, 2018). These are predictable rule-based systems with repetitive patterns according to which children with ASD have natural tendencies (Caria et al., 2018). Tasks can be repeated from exercise to exercise with very few changes, and the software can consistently provide encouragement and reinforcement (Hassan et al., 2011). Due to a small number of stimuli, clearly defined tasks and focused attention reduce distractions (Grynszpan et al., 2014) and enable precise, independent, and efficient learning of new skills (Ploog et al., 2013).

Compared to the usual teaching environment, the amount and complexity of student-teacher interaction are reduced, while most pieces of software are based on visual information presentation, which is the communication modality preferred by most students with ASD (Caria et al., 2018; Hassan et al., 2011; Odom et al., 2015; Ramdoss et al., 2011; Tsiopela & Jimoyiannis, 2014).

Apart from numerous advantages, there are also some potential drawbacks of computer-based interventions. It is feared that they may encourage isolation by reducing meaningful face-to-face interaction. There is also the risk of video game addiction and fostering limited patterns of behavior and ways of responding to stimuli (Bradley & Newbutt, 2018; Grynszpan et al., 2014; Ploog et al., 2013). Some authors are concerned about the development of a sedentary lifestyle and the lack of

[1] Collateral skills are defined as essential for academic skills and further general knowledge (e.g., behavior while performing tasks, engagement, asking questions in an academic context, Yakubova et al., 2021).

opportunities to practice verbal communication, social skills, joint attention, and eye contact (Jiménez-Muñoz et al., 2022; Ramdoss et al., 2011).

The following pages will discuss the use of digital technologies in a school context, primarily in some conceptual skills.

3.2 Literacy

Although there are great individual differences among children with ASD, learning to read is often difficult for them. While decoding skills are frequently described as correct, reading comprehension, although heterogeneous, is usually poor (Jones et al., 2009; Nation et al., 2006). The contributing factors include language delays, social difficulties, and behaviors that hinder a typical learning experience (Travers et al., 2011). Internal factors that can contribute to literacy difficulties include attention span and problems with concepts requiring auditory information processing, such as decoding and phonemic awareness. Learning to read and write in children with ASD can also be hindered by external factors such as the lack of appropriate instruction and low expectations (Mandak et al., 2019). Unlike the usual literacy instruction that includes informal teaching and engagement in an environment rich in reading content, children with ASD need early systematic instruction in this area.

Most software applications, especially serious games, are aimed at the global reading of words (Basil & Reyes, 2003; Mandak et al., 2019; Rasche et al., 2013; Serret et al., 2017), but some also focus on the phonics approach (Mahayuddin & Mamat, 2019). In addition, digital instruction is often aimed at the prerequisites for reading.

Different technologies and software are used in learning to read and write: computers, web-based programs, tablets, mobile applications, augmented reality mobile learning platforms, and serious games.

Specialized literacy programs for children with ASD usually take into account ASD characteristics or introduce elements of the established methods in working with this population (most frequently ABA instructional methodology)—operant conditioning, DTT, mass trial, and errorless learning technique, scaffolding, and encouraging autonomy (Gomez et al., 2018; Travers et al., 2011). In addition to these, methods generally intended for people with special educational needs (Grindle et al., 2013) and those intended for the typical population (Arciuli & Bailey, 2019) are also used.

Digital literacy programs insist on interactivity and personalization possibilities. The offered options include different difficulty levels, additional exercises, instructions, assistance or reinforcement, matching the materials with the child's interests, and adapting the feedback. Some software allows adaptations based on the frequency and proportion of each child's correct and incorrect answers, response time, or specific error pattern to provide the most appropriate learning method for a particular student (Grindle et al., 2013).

As a rule, before using the software, students prepare for using computers (following the movements on the screen from left to right and from top to bottom) and mouse (select, drag, and drop) and following computer audio instructions and language of instruction. Computer games are also sometimes used for this purpose (Serret et al., 2017).

The interface design ranges from insisting on vivid colors, an appealing environment, and cartoon characters living in different worlds to a digital whiteboard to remind the users they are being educated but in a fun way. Short computer games or animations are often used as rewards for a successfully completed task.

Learning sessions usually last for 10–20 min, and the programs have been tested in preschool and younger school children. The presence of tutors (instructors, parents), who can help students verbally, physically, or by demonstration, is recommended as support in the learning process. However, parents of children with ASD are less involved in providing instructions to their children in the school context than parent of typically developing children (Đorđević et al., 2021).

Using reading applications is most often observed as an addition to the usual literacy instruction. However, some used the opposite approach, i.e., they mainly relied on digital programs while learning to read, adding traditional learning sessions. For example, discrete-trial tabletop teaching was conducted when a child failed to complete a reading episode after several attempts. The aim of these sessions was not only reading but re-engaging the child in the program by learning essential prerequisite skills such as following the program instructions. Breaking a skill down into several smaller steps and learning those steps through DTT and related visual stimuli (e.g., picture cards) were used as a general strategy before the child would try to solve the online episode again. Also, the responses were modeled and additionally practiced using flashcards for all mistakes the program did not correct (Grindle et al., 2013).

The results obtained by applying digital technology in teaching literacy are positive. Word recognition reading takes place 8 weeks after the intervention (Grindle et al., 2013). Word- and passage-level reading accuracy improves (Arciuli & Bailey, 2019), as well as alphabet recognition, word reading, sentence reading, and ep-word segmenting (Serret et al., 2017). Furthermore, a high level of task focus and a low level of undesirable behaviors are observed (Mahayuddin & Mamat, 2019; Travers et al., 2011). Comparisons of traditional and digital teaching show that both methods improve literacy skills (Travers et al., 2011) but that there are clear differences in preferences and that students progress faster when their preferred method is used (Seok et al., 2015).

3.2.1 Minimally Verbal Children with ASD

Learning to read is even more complex in minimally verbal children with ASD. Still, Goh et al. (2013) state that reading can be a way to learn a language for some children with ASD who have little or no functional language.

Sight word recognition is most frequently used in teaching literacy to children with difficulties in understanding abstract and auditory concepts (Mandak et al., 2019; Vacca, 2007; Wang, 2021). For this purpose, Hetzroni and Shalem (2005) developed a computer program for identifying and matching words and pictures. It consists of a seven-step fading procedure that progresses from a picture of food (e.g., a bag of chips) with the written name and graphic label to a written word only. A smiley face is used as feedback. After using the program, the students were able to match the written words with food items in the classroom.

Similarly, Van der Meer et al. (2015) used graded stimulation and differential reinforcement of correct answers in four matching tasks (picture with picture, word with picture, picture with word, and word with word) in a minimally verbal child with ASD. Pictures and words were entered into an iPad. Selecting a picture or a word triggered synthesized speech (e.g., selecting a picture of a shoe was followed by "shoe" pronunciation). The student increased the number of correctly solved tasks in all four combinations.

A dynamic text differs from a static one in that it uses movement to attract students' attention. In a sample of preschool children with ASD, Mandak et al. (2019) used software functions (*Transition to Literacy—T2L*, Light et al., 2014) designed to support learning sight words that can be implemented with visual scene displays. They provide a dynamic text presentation paired with speech output when hot spot is activated. When a child touches a picture with a dynamic text function, the associated written word dynamically appears on the screen close to the selected picture and disappears after 3 s. All children successfully learned the target words.

Teachers use shared stories to involve students in the reading process by directing their attention to the text, matching the target words in the story with their meaning, and asking questions about the story. Spooner et al. (2014) used shared stories and an iPad in teaching literacy to four minimally verbal boys with ASD. The iPad was equipped with AAC and embedded text-to-speech software to encourage questions and obtain answers related to the story. Their results indicate positive effects of using an iPad together with shared stories.

SEMA-TIC is a French computer puzzle video game that aims to teach literacy skills to children with poor functional language skills and ASD. SEMA-TIC focuses on reading prerequisites such as identifying words and logograms and learning basic syntax, without focusing on phonemic awareness. It includes different logic games and exercises in an appealing virtual environment to motivate students to learn. Students move through SEMA-TIC through trial and error. The players are required to click on correct answers or drag and drop items to the correct locations. The game's difficulty increases progressively, and players can advance to the next game when they answer five out of ten multiple-choice questions and to the next set when they are successful in all ten games in one set. Feedback is given after each correct and incorrect answer and is visualized by filling a vertical color meter when the answer is correct or emptying it when the answer is incorrect. After a specific number of correct answers, 3D animation appears as reinforcement (Serret et al., 2017).

3.3 Vocabulary

Digital technology is used to expand the vocabulary of children with ASD. It has mainly been examined in preschool and younger school children. The sessions ranged from 10 to 40 min in different programs, from several times a week to daily use (Bosseler & Massaro, 2003; Khowaja et al., 2018; Khowaja & Salim, 2019; Whalen et al., 2010).

When designing the applications, the authors considered the characteristics of children with ASD, for example, simple interface design, the possibility to turn off the sound for hypersensitive children, no punishment for incorrect answers to avoid frustration, and docking used to help children with motor difficulties place the selected answer (Cunha & Barbosa, 2012). Learning and practicing are often based on DTT principles and game-based learning attributes (practice and drill, incremental learning, random item selection, showing a limited number of items) (Cunha & Barbosa, 2012; Khowaja et al., 2018; Khowaja & Salim, 2019).

Also, applications designed to improve vocabulary, as a rule, have various adaptation options, from individualizing the curriculum and goals for each child (Bosseler & Massaro, 2003; Cunha & Barbosa, 2012), adding and deleting word categories the child will learn (Husni, 2013), selecting and recording words, and choosing illustrations (Wojciechowski & Al-Musawi, 2017) to creating multiple-choice exercises according to the child's needs and characteristics (Mendonça et al., 2011).

The problem of vocabulary development in children with ASD has been approached in different ways. Khowaja et al. (2018) designed a serious game in which students first choose 1 out of 11 categories leading them to a specific word to be learned. A child can hear the pronunciation of the word by clicking on its name in the list of sounds. Furthermore, the item description can also be heard by clicking on the music icon next to the description. Once the vocabulary item is learned, the child does a short test by selecting the appropriate picture in the presence of distracting items.

Husni (2013) designed an application for fostering vocabulary development in children with ASD who live in far-off rural areas of Indonesia and cannot get direct professional help. Parents are the ones who manage the application. They add or delete categories, pictures, and sounds the child will learn. Vocabulary pictures and sounds can be downloaded from the server or an external camera.

Similarly, *VITHEA-Kids* is a platform designed to develop language and generalization skills in children with ASD. It allows caregivers to create multiple-choice exercises considering the needs and characteristics of each child. There is also a module for automatically generating exercise content (questions, stimuli, correct answers, and distractors) that makes creating exercises easier. In these exercises, a child has to provide an oral response to a stimulus (e.g., name an object in a picture or describe an activity in a video). The answer is recorded and paired with one or more correct answers. Instead of naming the object orally, the child can also click/touch the correct answer. The application gives notifications when a child selects a wrong answer, which then disappears to encourage the child to choose the correct one. An animated character (whose statements are previously recorded by a parent in audio format) provides verbal instructions and feedback on the child's response (Mendonça et al., 2011).

Let's Play is another system in which parents have a significant role. It is an assistive system for young children with ASD designed for learning the pronunciation and meaning of new words. The system combines a mobile application (it can be used on a smartwatch or smartphone) and object identifiers—small wireless sensors placed in desired places within the child's space. When the child approaches the object with the identifier while playing or moving around the house, the mobile device instantly repeats the name of the object. The child hears the systematically repeated voice of a parent naming the object. In order to establish a clear and direct association between the heard voice and the named object, the mobile device shows a picture or drawing of the object, and the child should touch the screen as a response to the heard voice and the shown picture. Parents are expected to select objects (new words), mark them with object identifiers, record the words, and choose illustrations to be shown on a mobile device (Wojciechowski & Al-Musawi, 2017).

On the other hand, *MyWord* application puts a child in a completely different position. It allows children to make a digital vocabulary containing all words important to them. It is designed so that a child first inserts personal photographs in the vocabulary format and can then add an audio recording and sounds from the

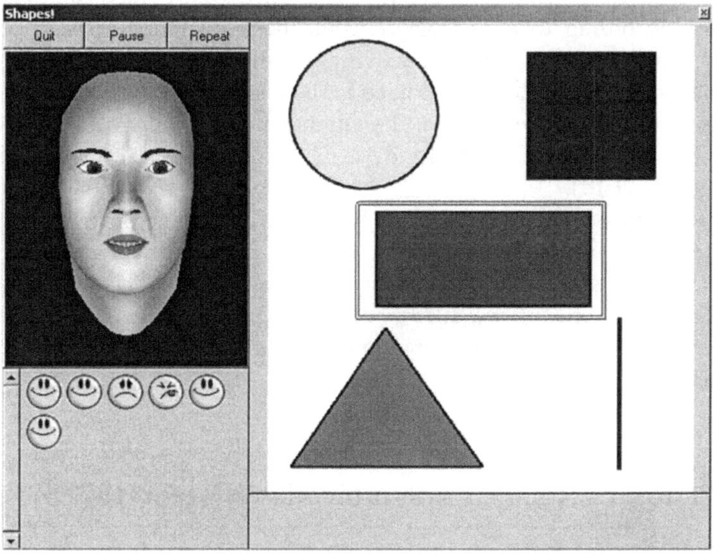

Fig. 3.1 The scene features computer-animated tutor, Baldi. In this scene, the student learns to identify shapes. For example, Baldi says "Click on the rectangle." The student chooses the appropriate shape and receives a visual feedback in the form of sticker which shows a happy or a sad face as feedback for correct or incorrect answers. The outlined region around the rectangle shows the selected shape. (Reproduced from Bosseler & Massaro, 2003)

environment, which allows the development of a personalized word catalog over time. The application is not specially designed to be an AAC or a learning tool but a simple and highly personalized application that can foster the strengths and interests of children with ASD (Wilson et al., 2018).

Using a three-dimensional computer-animated talking head (Baldi) as a tutor is an interesting approach to developing grammar and vocabulary in children with ASD (Fig. 3.1). During the program, children identify pictures and produce words. Baldi has realistic visible speech. It also has teeth, tongue, and palate to simulate the oral cavity, and tongue movements mimic the natural movements (Bosseler & Massaro, 2003).

TeachTown is a computer-assisted intervention incorporating ABA principles, designed to teach children with ASD, 2–7 years of age, social and academic skills through an online curriculum. In addition to Receptive Language, the curriculum also includes Social Understanding, Life Skills, and Academic/Cognitive Skills. The lessons use the DTT format, using the within-stimulus prompting procedure (distractors fade or are emphasized to help a child solve a task). The program gives verbal orders, and the students should click on correct answers. Multiple examples of learned concepts are used, while mass trial is not used to encourage generalization. Instead, at least two different concepts (e.g., dog and cat) are learned in the same trial set with orders being slightly different from trial to trial, so the student has to listen to the instructions for each. Furthermore, different types of pictures (photographs, clipart, drawings) are used to encourage generalization. The exercises include attempts to remember what has been learned. Short video games are used as reinforcers according to a variable schedule between the exercises. *TeachTown Connection* includes non-computer activities conducted in a natural environment to help students develop skills not included in the computer program and improve the generalization of skills learned on the computer. By structure, the activities are based on the developmental model and use the Pivotal Response Training principles (Whalen et al., 2010).

Positive results and user satisfaction have been determined in assessing the success of these programs (Husni, 2013). Progress is noted in learning new words (Bosseler & Massaro, 2003; Khowaja & Salim, 2019; Whalen et al., 2010; Wojciechowski & Al-Musawi, 2017), better engagement, focus on academic tasks, and better self-expression of personal interests and activities related to vocabulary development (Wilson et al., 2018).

3.4 Picture Exchange Communication System (PECS)

One of the researched sub-areas of using digital technology in the communication of children with ASD is augmentative and alternative communication (AAC). Nowadays, cellphones and tablets are usually used for this purpose, allowing people with ASD to communicate with the help of visual support. They compose messages by creating understandable and easy-to-use sets of pictograms. When the message is formed, the user shows it to the interlocutor and establishes communication (Gomez et al., 2018).

The most famous such tool is PECS, developed for children with limited verbal expression abilities. The idea is that the children say what they want by showing a picture. PECS has been modernized through applications for mobile devices. Children can choose from a wide range of communication options by simply touching the screen, which simplifies the process and provides various choices that were not previously available (Nkabinde, 2014).

PECS mobile application module *Autisdata* is aimed at learning functional communication. It works on the principle of a picture database in which the user can add new pictures, delete, or modify the old ones. The pictures are grouped into categories: food, drinks, activities, and objects. Autisdata has three phases adapted to the software environment. The user first has to choose the category of the desired picture. Then, a new page appears with pictures from that category. The page simulates a communication book using the same strips. After the user touches the desired picture, it is placed on the strip at the top of the page, next to a fixed sentence (e.g., "I want"). In the second phase, the user chooses a picture and drags it to the appropriate position on the strip next to the fixed sentence. The third phase stimulates the user to make short sentences and place them in the appropriate order. There are no previously placed sentences at the top of the page in this phase, but the user has to place them along with the desired picture (Oliveira et al., 2019). *PixTalk* is another smartphone application. Teachers and parents can access the website, select pictures from the online library, and download them to smartphones. Children can browse and select pictures to express their intentions, desires, and emotions (De Leo et al., 2011).

In addition to vocal phrases, picture cards, and manual signs, children with very limited or no functional speech also learn to use speech-generating devices. These are electronic devices on which a person selects a text or a picture showing a desired object or activity and thus activates a voice message (Muharib et al., 2019).

The *iCan* application uses a tablet with a built-in camera and microphone and allows the fast and simple creation of new picture cards. The cards show real objects and "say" the word when pressed. Each word category has a label, color, and image. After learning basic vocabulary, the next step is to make sentences. This is done by pressing the required picture card for a longer time (instead of dragging it, to make it easier for children with manual control difficulties). Sentences can be recorded and played later (Tang et al., 2013).

Apart from cellphones and tablets, specialized devices are also used. *Mocotos* is an augmentative communication device that supports visual communication. It is slightly bigger than a cellphone and has a touch screen. Mocotos has an installed card database. These cards include standard images used in PECS and other visual communication strategies. However, a teacher can insert other pictures or photographs. Different sounds can be added to the cards. These sounds may be recorded with a microphone or synthesized by a built-in speech-to-text function. The cards can be categorized, searched, and edited, and the number and size of the cards on the screen can be customized (Hayes et al., 2010).

3.5 Speech Intelligibility

People with ASD often have difficulty producing intelligible speech due to too fast or slow speech and atypical pitch. Through designing interactive games, Hoque et al. (2009) worked on improving speech intelligibility in students with ASD. For example, they designed a turtle race game for students who speak too fast, where one of the turtles is controlled by a child. The aim is to win the race by speaking more slowly. In addition to hearing their own speech, the children are shown a visual representation of their speech, helping them to control it (e.g., speed and loudness). The games are based on Kaypentax games (a company that designs games for people with speech impairments), using the free Scratch (scratch.mit.edu) platform, whose interface allows customization according to user preferences (changing the background, characters, and parameters of the game).

Rahman et al. (2010) designed another game for improving speech intelligibility in children with ASD. The basic idea of the game is simple—a child tries to articulate words clearly to communicate with the computer. The screen shows interesting pictures. If the children manage to say the names of the objects in the pictures loud and clear, they get points and can win the game. Children try to say words intelligibly, which helps them overcome the problems in this speech area.

Frutos et al. (2011) designed a game in which a child with ASD is encouraged to repeat the words synthesized by the system. The game has two modes: basic and advanced. In the basic mode, a child is shown randomly selected pictures along with an audio recording of the matching word. After the child repeats the word, the video signal is processed. If the word is correctly pronounced, the picture moves from the center to one of the boxes in the upper left corner of the screen. The game is successfully completed when all words are correctly pronounced and all boxes are filled with objects. The advanced mode is more interactive and consists of static images in which some parts are not colored but are marked with a small yellow star that the user has to click to get the audio output of the selected object. Once the object is selected, this mode works in the same way as the basic one, i.e., it detects the user's voice and processes the pronounced word to record and save the result. If the user pronounces the word correctly, the object will get colored. The game is successfully completed when the whole image is completely colored.

3.6 Robots

Using robots is another appealing approach to communication development. Children with ASD are very interested in robots and toy robots and can easily connect with them (Begum et al., 2016). Research in this field is still relatively scarce, and the results are inconclusive.

Srinivasan et al. (2016) used a humanoid robot called Isobot, controlled by an adult over a laptop. The children were asked to mimic the robot's motor activities (related to karate or dancing). The authors stated that the children increased their level of social verbalization during the training sessions but that they had difficulty generalizing the learned skills to a context without the robot. According to their results, the interventions conducted by people are superior in improving social verbalization during training and in other contexts.

On the other hand, Shamsuddin et al. (2012) reported that a humanoid robot NAO, which blinks, speaks, and plays music, in a simple interaction with children with ASD, attracted the children's attention, kept them involved, and thus positively influenced their communicative behavior.

3.7 Other Language Games and Applications

Applications and games have been designed, mainly for smartphones and tablets, for other areas of language development, such as the improvement of fluency, narration, understanding idioms, and learning a habitual language.

Anwar et al. (2011) designed an interactive computer game to improve speech fluency in children with ASD who have a rich vocabulary but cannot complete a sentence. The basic idea of the game is to stimulate children to say a sentence with the help of different objects shown on the screen simultaneously. An adult controls the choice of objects that appear on the screen from a different computer. For example, if we want a child to say "I am eating ice cream," the adult will choose pictures of a "person" (in this case, a child), "ice cream," and, finally, "a person eating ice cream." Once selected, the pictures are sent to the child's computer. The child is rewarded (e.g., with a cartoon or something they like) for saying a correct and complete sentence. A counter tracking the number of sentences the child can say in a specific time frame (e.g., 10 or 7 s) helps the adult decide whether the child has improved. The score is kept in a database and can be used to determine future difficulty levels. The results are also shown on the adult's computer screen, which helps them decide what sentence to generate next.

TouchStory is a software game designed to improve narration in children with ASD. The conceptual framework is set to improve narrative comprehension in children with ASD by using simple, game-like, image-based tasks that refer to primitive story components (proto-narratives—represent a single event, without being proper narratives—the precursors of narrative comprehension). The game involves arranging different parts of the story in the right order to understand the narrative better (Davis et al., 2007).

The *I Can Tell* application also allows children to compose stories together with their parents or teachers. Adults can photograph objects from the child's environment or use the existing photographs. They are then dragged to the part of the screen selected for the story and can be moved, rotated, and resized to encourage interaction or make the story more interesting. Sidebars are located on both sides of the screen so that both children and adults can use them simultaneously. All activities on the screen can be recorded together with audio files and then played when needed. This allows the child to watch previously recorded stories independently, so the adults do not need to repeat them (Wadhwa & Jianxiong, 2013).

Pistoljevic and Hulusic (2017) presented an electronic book with an integrated educational game aimed at learning basic vocabulary, foreign language words, and concepts important for starting school, such as recognizing objects, counting, recognizing colors, and answering inference questions in children with ASD 4–7 years of age. The book is bilingual (in the children's mother tongue (Bosnian/Serbian/Croatian) and English). Each scene includes three questions. The first question on each page is the easiest, requiring the children to select an answer by pointing, finding, or touching it. The second question is related to learning to count by using the scenes and objects in the book. The third question requires producing answers, making conclusions, and abstract thinking (e.g., whether someone is sad in the text the child heard).

A Chilean application is aimed at improving the understanding of idioms. The very beginning explains what idioms are (by illustrations or verbally). The user then has three options: (1) to follow the established sequences, (2) to choose the level the professional considers appropriate (easy, medium, and hard), or (3) to go directly into the evaluation mode. The idiom is represented in four ways (exact illustration, pictogram, text, and sound) in the first two options. After that, the user can select a specific idiom or follow a predetermined learning order. If the professional wants to evaluate the idioms, they first have to select the level to be evaluated. In this mode, reinforcement includes verbal praise, and if the students make a mistake, they are offered to try again (Alvarado et al., 2017).

McGonigle-Chalmers et al. (2013) created a game to examine syntactic awareness in children with ASD who have severe expressive language limitations (Fig. 3.2). The children learn to touch the words on the screen in the correct order to see the appropriate animation. The game becomes more complicated and develops from two to four sequences.

The following study is interesting because it focused on students' responsiveness. Using video self-modeling and an iPad, Hart and Whalon (2012) taught an adolescent with ASD and intellectual disability to participate in class conversation, answering the teacher's questions without additional prompts. After observing the boy, the researchers made scripts for video modeling to be learned in the following classes. The recorded responses used in editing the material were obtained with the help of verbal stimuli. The video was then edited to remove the teacher's prompts, and only the parts that showed the student answering each of the three teacher's questions were kept. The recording lasted for 1 min. At the beginning of the video, a written instruction appeared on the screen followed by audio: "(the student's name) carefully follows the lesson. He always answers the teacher's questions. See how (the student's name) answers the questions." Every day, just before the beginning of the lesson, the teacher asked the student to watch the recording at least three times (for about 3–5 min). As a result, the student increased the number of correct unprompted answers during the intervention.

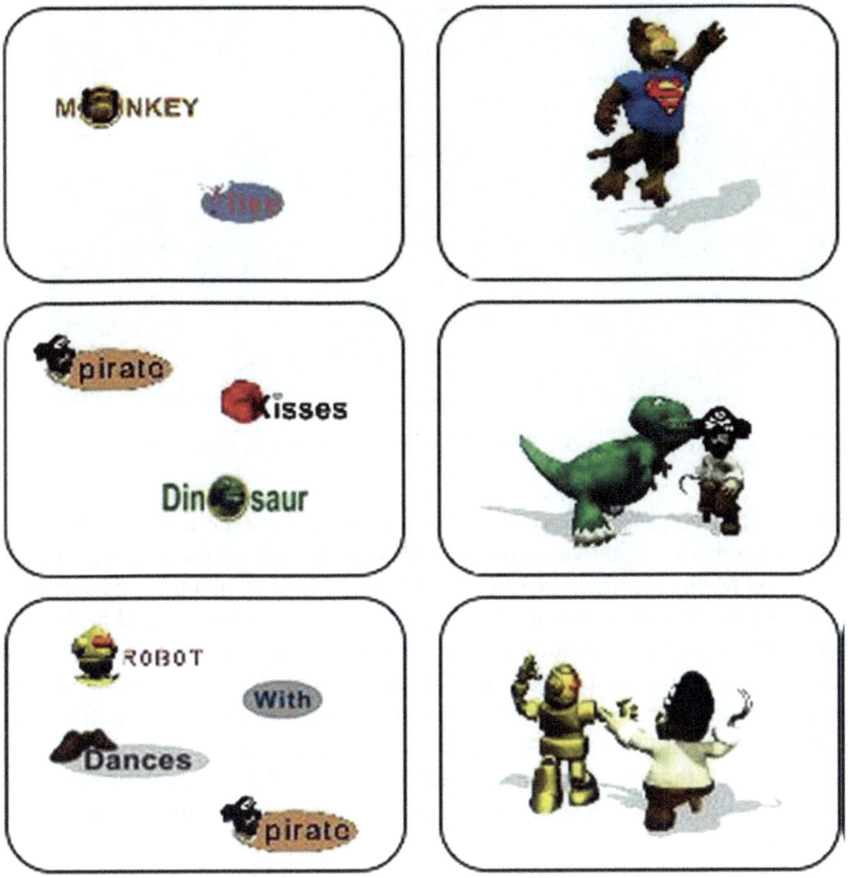

Fig. 3.2 Examples of touch screen icons in each phase of The Eventaurs along with screenshot animations after the correct response. (Reproduced from McGonigle-Chalmers et al., 2013)

3.8 Mathematics

ASD can interfere with the development of cognitive skills related to logical and mathematical thinking. Developing these skills is crucial as it enables the acquisition of knowledge needed for everyday life (Muñoz-Soto et al., 2016).

Different software applications, most often in the form of games, are used to encourage these skills. They cover various topics: from early mathematical skills and forming the concepts of numbers (Roglić et al., 2016; Tsiopela & Jimoyiannis, 2014), recognizing and writing numbers (Aziz et al., 2015), to calculation (Tashnim et al., 2017) and geometry (Santos et al., 2017). They are characterized by a simple user interface, multimodal access, the possibility to repeat operations and provide reinforcement frequently, and the possibility to store data and track user achievements.

Some math games have been developed as part of applications that cover a wider range of skills. *Fruits* (Fig. 3.3) is a serious Kinect-based game for children with

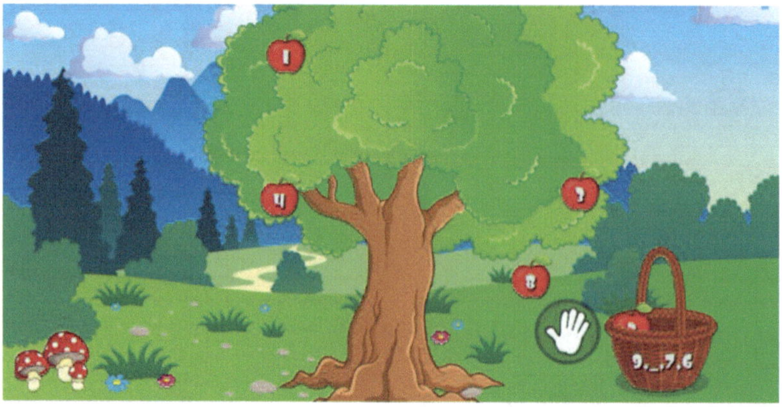

Fig. 3.3 Example for "Mathematic" task. (Reproduced from Roglić et al., 2016)

ASD aimed at the development of fine motor skills. However, it also includes tasks designed for basic cognitive skills divided into five categories, two of which are Sorting and Math exercises. *Sorting*—a child picks fruit from a tree and sorts it into appropriate baskets labeled with pictures of fruit that should be placed in them. The advanced level includes additional tasks such as sorting fruit into unlabeled baskets or choosing appropriate objects/fruit from similar ones. *Math*—an extended version of sorting fruit. In this mode, each fruit is marked by a number, and the fruit should be selected in accordance with the solution of a simple equation on the basket. At the advanced level, the children are required to continue the sequence of numbers. A teacher can track numerical scores and graphic representation of results (Roglić et al., 2016).

Pre-Vocational Skills Laboratory (PVS-Lab) is intended for older students with ASD and the development of pre-vocational skills. It is a web-based environment for students with ASD placed in a virtual classroom. The application can be accessed using a browser from any device (PC, notebook, tablet, or smartphone). The user interface is minimally designed, with a small number of buttons and almost no text, to encourage the engagement of students with severe reading and other learning disabilities. The objects are presented in one realistic 3D picture with no text or sounds included so as not to confuse the students. Classroom desks are a starting point for ten tasks related to basic skills, such as grouping items (fruit, eggs, envelopes) by number or sorting them by color, shape, or quality. By clicking on a desk, the students are transferred to a screen where they choose the task difficulty level. After completing the task, the students can repeat it to improve their performance or go back to the level selection screen and then the workshop. By clicking on the pictures on classroom walls, they can make a creative break by putting together a jigsaw puzzle. The database stores students' names, activities, difficulty levels, time spent doing the activities, and mistakes (Tsiopela & Jimoyiannis, 2014).

The aim of the *MathDS* application is to help children with learning disabilities learn to count and write numbers from one to ten. The application consists of three menus: learning, activities, and practice. In the "learning" section, the screen shows fingers with a number on each one. For example, if a child selects number one, the number and one teddy bear will appear on the next screen to help the child understand the value of number one. The "activities" section includes three activities in which children have to match numbers to the items shown to test what they have learned in the learning section. A child has to count the number of items in each box (out of the three offered) and match the box to the corresponding number shown at the bottom of the screen. The "practice" section requires a child to write numbers following the dots on the screen (Aziz et al., 2015).

Play and Learn Number (PLaN) is a touchscreen application designed to teach arithmetic and calculation to children with milder forms of ASD. It helps children remember and recognize numbers (in and out of sequence) through animated pictures. The students first learn to recognize, write down, and pair numbers and then do arithmetic tasks. Each set of tasks is followed by an evaluation set (a specific number of items appears on the screen, and the student chooses one out of four given numbers). Reinforcement (praise or short games) is provided after each successfully completed evaluation level. The children learn to recognize a number by seeing the number on the screen, hearing how it is pronounced, and seeing the corresponding number of objects. The children learn to write by connecting dots, while they pair numbers by selecting the appropriate number from an unordered set of four. The last task type in this set is puzzle-solving—the student has to fit the pieces into the written form of a number. In the arithmetic category, the children first learn the symbols (+, –). Then, with the help of mathematical symbols and objects, they learn to add and subtract. Two numbers and the result dynamically appear on the screen together with the mathematical symbol. Audio is added to the visual representation (Tashnim et al., 2017).

Digital learning environment on mathematics for autistic children (LEMA) has been designed for developing mathematical reasoning and learning geometric shapes in children with ASD 6–12 years of age. The interface is minimally designed with a few items on the screen, simplified instructions, a clear soft-colored interface, no distractors or background pictures, and buttons or icons clearly separated from other elements. LEMA provides reinforcement through visual and audio animations, and some teaching activities include feedback tutorials explaining the concept and solutions to the problems given in the example. In addition, LEMA includes alternative representations (pictures, symbols, pictograms, audio or video icons) placed next to the corresponding text to encourage understanding of symbols and contribute to the enrichment of the user's vocabulary (Santos et al., 2017).

3.9 Money

Young people with disabilities often need instruction in which academic and functional goals are merged. Functional mathematics aims to teach practical math skills that can be used in everyday life (Burton et al., 2013). With regard to that, games designed to teach students with ASD to use money have been developed.

Caria et al. (2018) presented a web-based game application designed for people with high-functioning autism to adopt the concept of money and its use in daily situations. The games include various aspects of handling money, from distinguishing bills, matching them to their names, combining them to get appropriate amounts, and calculating change to using a specific amount to buy something in a real-life situation and using a vending machine. Some elements are the same in all exercises. For example, before the game starts, the application displays a text, followed by audio, explaining what the user has to do to solve the task. Also, all games have a "Help" button that activates a video showing what needs to be done to achieve the goal. All games have smiley faces that are yellow and smiling in case of success or red and sad in case of a mistake. The games have been tested with six adolescents, and the results are positive and promising.

Hassan et al. (2011) designed a simple game based on digital storytelling to help students with ASD 9–14 years of age understand the concept of money. Furthermore, the game aims to teach these students some elements of appropriate social skills when shopping. The first part of the game focuses on identifying bills. The students are asked to click on the appropriate value of one bill shown on the screen and then choose the appropriate value from four displayed bills. The second part of the game includes four levels and focuses on money exchange. The students first choose one out of six products and buy it with one bill, while, at the fourth level, they buy products with various bill combinations. The levels in this part of the game end with exchanging polite phrases with the seller, and after the purchase, the students have to make one of the decisions: leave the store, go to another store, or return home.

iPad technology has been used in self-modeling and video prompting while teaching students with ASD to use money.

Video self-modeling is a type of video modeling in which students observe themselves correctly and independently manifesting desired behavior (Glumbić et al., 2018). It is a type of observational learning where people observe themselves performing a task at a higher level than usual. Burton et al. (2013) used video self-modeling in teaching adolescents with ASD mathematical skills. The students were given a problem story based on which they had to estimate the amount of money they needed for a specific product and the change they were supposed to get. They were allowed to watch videos on an iPad in which they could see themselves successfully solving these problems. The students could pause the videos, forward, or rewind them. Video self-modeling was systematically removed during skill maintenance sessions (the students were asked to solve new problems without the video model, while the models for previously solved problems were gradually removed), with only a slight decline in learned skills.

Video prompting refers to a video presentation of a multi-component skill where each step is recorded and explained. Students are given instructions to watch the video of one step and repeat the observed behavior before moving on to the next step. This pattern is repeated until the desired skill is completely performed (Glumbić et al., 2018). Weng and Bouck (2014) used an iPad to teach students with ASD and intellectual disability to compare prices using adapted number lines. Based on task analysis, 18 clips were recorded from the students' perspectives. The students compared the prices of the same product from different manufacturers in a simulated store. They watched video prompts before performing each step. After each video clip, they were allowed 20 s to perform the task. After that, the next clip was played regardless of whether they performed the task correctly or unsuccessfully. If video prompting alone was not enough, the most-to-least prompts system was applied.

3.10 Other Instructional Areas

Although less common, software that can be used in other teaching areas has been developed. Thus, the mobile game application FillMeApp has been designed for students with ASD as complementary material for learning parts of the human body. After applying, a student can choose whether to watch or play the game. The "play video" option launches a video related to the human body. If the user does not choose this option, the "play game" option will be activated. Instructions are given at the beginning of the game, and after the first three levels, the students are taken back to the home page, where they should choose again whether to play the game or watch the video. Teachers can log in, observe, track, and evaluate student achievement. The database stores students' attempts by game levels. Students can repeat the games as many times as they want. When summarizing positive aspects of the game, the authors emphasize that it combines the best moment for focusing attention, appealing graphics, simple tasks, video tutorials, and pleasant background music. According to teachers and parents, student motivation has significantly increased. They describe the application as easy to use, interactive, informative, and useful to students (Eder et al., 2016).

Knowledgemon Hunters is a serious game designed for children with ASD and attention deficits. Through a mobile device, the children can find virtual 3D monsters geographically distributed around the world, capture them, interact with them, and learn from them. The application is designed for mobile environments, including geolocation, camera, and gyroscope. The interface has a 3D avatar moving around virtual plans. The device can determine geographical coordinates from player movements in the real world and move the avatar. The players can see the monsters they previously caught as well as monsters and other players in the vicinity. When the player approaches the monster, it appears on the main interface so the child can catch it (Silva et al., 2017).

Sorce et al. (2018) developed an information system that allows people with ASD to access digital content related to works of art. The hardware consists of a projector and Microsoft Kinect sensors connected to a laptop. The projector is placed 1 meter from the wall, and the Kinect is behind the projector, directing the camera in the opposite direction from the projection. The interface includes an interactive avatar that appears when the user enters the Kinect field and stays in the middle of the screen, constantly repeating the user's movements. Five interactive tiles are placed around the avatar, each showing a work of art and allowing access to related content. The user can guide the avatar's hands to the tiles. Additional activation gestures are not necessary to activate the content. Once the user selects the content, multimedia is activated, displaying textual and audio-visual information about a specific work of art. Two icons appear at the end of each multimedia: one for going back to the main interface and the other for additional content helping the user understand it. Both icons are marked with familiar PECS pictures.

3.11 Tangible User Interfaces

Tangible user interfaces are an innovative instructional approach that combines digital technology and tangible objects. One of them is MicroCulture, a mixed reality learning platform where players play and learn about urban development. The system includes a computer, screen or interactive surface, web camera, and tangibles. It is based on Python and reacTIVision, free software for developing tangible interfaces. ReacTIVision uses a camera to track black and white markers, while the Python code responds to the position and orientation of multiple markers placed on the surface. The markers are printed at the top of tangibles, and each tangible represents an infrastructure that children can use to influence the development of a settlement. A web camera, placed above the game board, catches the markers on paper tangibles, while the game board is a flat television placed horizontally. A laptop launches the game, which is seen on the TV screen. The screen shows the simulated life of a world population (a Viking village). The children have to shape the settlement by arranging the infrastructure, represented by tangibles, on the screen. In this way, they can experience through play how changes in a territory affect the growing community of people and their daily lives. For example, if they place a bridge, the inhabitants will start crossing it to visit other areas and mingle with other groups. The game has been tested in 15 children with ASD 9–12 years of age. The results show that mediated play, facilitated by teachers, creates interactions that lead to conceptual thinking, cooperation, and role-play. Teachers believe that this way of work provides opportunities for discussion and research in which children are engaged through various forms of interaction. The difficulties they describe are related to finding a balance between supporting children, making them responsible, and directing them to cooperate, although this interaction often leads to conflict (Marchetti & Valente, 2016).

Sitdhisanguan et al. (2012) used similar technology to recognize shapes and colors in preschool children with ASD (Fig. 3.4). A computer screen is displayed on a semitransparent tabletop through a digital projector installed inside the table. Instead of two-dimensional shapes and a computer mouse, the system based on tangible user interfaces uses wooden blocks and toys for physical representation and

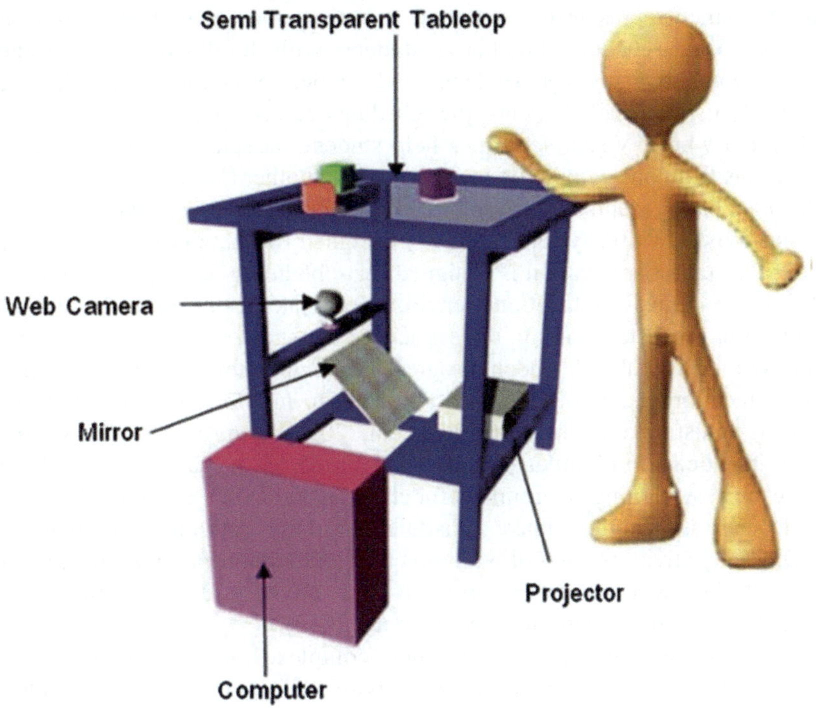

Fig. 3.4 Hardware components of the tangible user interface-based system. (Reproduced from Sitdhisanguan et al., 2012)

manipulation of teaching materials (in this case, geometric shapes and colors). Compared to conventional training, these tangible objects have the same role as picture cards in traditional teaching. When a narrative voice asks a child to choose a color or a shape that matches what is shown, they are expected to select one of the given objects (wooden blocks or toys) by taking them. To complete the task, the child has to place the chosen tangible object on the tabletop area where the picture appears. The camera placed under the surface identifies the selected tangible object. Infrared LED tubes are connected to each tangible object. Each block or toy has a unique number of tubes. From the picture identified by the camera, the child can identify the number of lighted spots and thus recognize the selected object. Touch-based systems and tangible user interfaces have proved to be easier to use and more efficient in skills acquisition than the ones based on using a mouse or non-computer training methods (e.g., instruction conducted by a therapist using cards).

3.12 Visual Schedules

Visual schedules often provide the structure needed to reduce anxiety and encourage better self-organization of time and activities in people with ASD. They include a set of symbols (words, pictures, photographs, icons) or objects attached to a surface, which represent the sequence of activities or individual steps within an activity. Visual schedules familiarize students with the description of events that await them and encourage students' independent functioning (Đorđević et al., 2019). By using visual elements, the schedules describe what will happen, in what order, and where. Visual schedules help students at school to make independent transitions from one activity or environment to another (Hirano et al., 2010). These schedules have recently been used in digital form, either as smartphone or tablet applications or within systems specially designed for that purpose. The Classroom Schedule+ tablet application is designed for scheduling activities of students with ASD in an inclusive educational environment. The designers made sure that the application promotes reading, the sequences are short, pictures and sentences are short and individualized, student progress is shown within the schedule, and audio communication channel is not used so as not to interfere with the work of other students and stigmatize the user (Fage et al., 2014). The Autisdata TEACCH module is intended for a similar purpose. It is based on the same name technique to create the best learning environment for children with ASD. This module is designed for teachers since they make schedules of daily activities for students with ASD. Each activity is marked with a picture and a description. A student uses the same interface to visualize daily routines and activities. Once completed, they are marked with a "done" button (Oliveira et al., 2019).

The vSked system is significantly more complex. It is a collaborative and interactive assistive technology for children with ASD that combines an interactive token-based reward system, choice boards, and a visual schedule integrated into a shared classroom system (Cramer et al., 2011). The system includes three different interfaces: a large touch screen that the whole class can see, a personal teacher display for administrative control, and a handheld device for each student. The large touch screen is placed in front of the class and serves as the main schedule that includes visual schedules for all students. The ongoing activity is at the top of the screen and can be activated by the teacher. This launches the activity on the student's paired device in the form of choice boards. Choice boards communicate with the big screen, enabling the students who answer correctly to be rewarded. If the students provide an incorrect answer or none at all, they get a prompt that helps them answer correctly, potentially allowing the time for teachers to help the students who need it more at that time. After successfully completing a task, each student gets a reward especially chosen for them, such as the animation of a train moving across the screen. Once the task is completed, the schedule automatically progresses. If the student has not solved a task, but the time for it is almost up, the teacher can configure the system to inform the student on the big or personal screen. Teachers can get reports on students' individual progress or a report on the achievement of the whole class in one or more tasks. The reports can be generated for different periods (daily, weekly, monthly, or yearly) (Hayes et al., 2010). The results of using vSked have shown that it improves student independence, reduces the number of teachers' prompts, and encourages consistency, predictability, and the time needed to transfer from one activity to another (Cramer et al., 2011).

Schedules have also been used for learning new skills. The My Pictures Talk application was installed on an iPad for high school students with ASD to learn how to use visual schedules with integrated video modeling to enter data, write sections with the help of graphic organizers, set the table, and solve algebra problems. When students opened the application, a visual schedule of activities would appear. A video model of the learned skill was shown by touching each picture on the schedule. The adolescents were able to switch within and between tasks independently and generalize static schedules of visual activities to new examples after the video model was removed (Spriggs et al., 2015).

Personal digital assistants (PDA) are small, mobile, handheld devices used for calculation, storing, and retrieving data. PDA devices, deigned as electronic task organizers, can be easily programmed for rather complex activity schedules, with each task being associated with an alarm as a reminder. Even cheap PDAs have additional functions that can help students with difficulty in tasks such as electronic sticky notes, address books, PDA-to-PDA message beaming, to do lists, and photo albums (Gentry et al., 2010). These devices were popular at the end of last and the beginning of this century and are the precursors of smartphones.

We can conclude that students with ASD like to use technology and that it motivates them and increases their engagement. However, although many agree that using ICT in the school context is promising, most authors who have reviewed its effectiveness are pretty reserved. Knight et al. (2013) believe practitioners should be careful when teaching academic skills to people with ASD using technology-based interventions. They can be used in learning discrete skills such as word or symbol identification. However, according to these authors, learning more complex or chained skills is questionable. Yakubova et al. (2021) report that although they can improve skills in various academic domains, augmented reality interventions do not meet the criteria that would classify them as evidence-based practice in teaching academic skills to students with ASD. Odom et al. (2015) have found positive outcomes of using technology in adolescents with ASD but point out that little is known about their possible collateral or negative effects. With regard to the use of robots in interventions, Begum et al. (2016) state that most clinicians are not convinced of their potential. Jiménez-Muñoz et al. (2022) report that video games are effective in relieving ASD symptoms, but the effect size is small.

Studies are criticized for not meeting the standards of evidence-based practices (Mazon et al., 2019) and for needing a better methodological framework to examine different approaches in a "real-life" environment such as school (Bradley & Newbutt, 2018). Furthermore, technologies are often not publicly available to practitioners (Yakubova et al., 2021), and therefore more attention should be given to adapting commercial games for therapeutic purposes (Jiménez-Muñoz et al., 2022).

However, in their meta-analysis, Sansosti et al. (2015) have found that, although moderate, the effect of computer-based interventions conducted in a school environment is the greatest in academic skills, while Steinbrenner et al. (2020) include technology-aided instruction and intervention in evidence-based practices.

References

Ain, G. I. (2018). *What is the appropriate curriculum for students with disabilities? Standards-based curriculum versus functional curriculum for students with disabilities.* Online Submission. https://files.eric.ed.gov/fulltext/ED593728.pdf

Alvarado, C., Munoz, R., Villarroel, R., Acuña, O., Barcelos, T. S., & Becerra, C. (2017, October). ValpoDijo: Developing a software that supports the teaching of chilean idioms to children with autism spectrum disorders. In *Proceedings of the Twelfth Latin American conference on learning technologies* (pp. 1–4). https://doi.org/10.1109/LACLO.2017.8120905

Anagnostopoulou, P., Lorentzou, G., & Drigas, A. (2021). ICTs in inclusive education for learning disabilities. *Research, Society and Development, 10*(9), e43410918230. https://doi.org/10.33448/rsd-v10i9.18230

Anwar, A., Rahman, M. M., Ferdous, S. M., Anik, S. A., & Ahmed, S. I. (2011, July). A computer game based approach for increasing fluency in the speech of the autistic children. In *Proceedings of the international conference on advanced learning technologies* (pp. 17–18). https://doi.org/10.1109/ICALT.2011.13

Arciuli, J., & Bailey, B. (2019). Efficacy of ABRACADABRA literacy instruction in a school setting for children with autism spectrum disorders. *Research in Developmental Disabilities, 85*, 104–115. https://doi.org/10.1016/j.ridd.2018.11.003

Aziz, N. S. A., Ahmad, W. F. W., & Zulkifli, N. J. B. (2015, April). User experience on numerical application between children with down syndrome and Autism. In *Proceedings of the international HCI and UX conference in Indonesia* (pp. 26–31). https://doi.org/10.1145/2742032.2742036

Basil, C., & Reyes, S. (2003). Acquisition of literacy skills by children with severe disability. *Child Language Teaching and Therapy, 19*(1), 27–48. https://doi.org/10.1191/0265659003ct242oa

Begum, M., Serna, R. W., & Yanco, H. A. (2016). Are robots ready to deliver autism interventions? A comprehensive review. *International Journal of Social Robotics, 8*(2), 157–181. https://doi.org/10.1007/s12369-016-0346-y

Bosseler, A., & Massaro, D. W. (2003). Development and evaluation of a computer-animated tutor for vocabulary and language learning in children with autism. *Journal of Autism and Developmental Disorders, 33*(6), 653–672. https://doi.org/10.1023/B:JADD.0000006002.82367.4f

Bradley, R., & Newbutt, N. (2018). Autism and virtual reality head-mounted displays: A state of the art systematic review. *Journal of Enabling Technologies, 12*(3), 101–113. https://doi.org/10.1108/JET-01-2018-0004

Bročin, B. (2013). *Inkluzivna edukacija*. Univerzitet u Beogradu – Fakultet za specijalnu edukaciju i rehabilitaciju. Izdavački centar (ICF).

Burton, C. E., Anderson, D. H., Prater, M. A., & Dyches, T. T. (2013). Video self-modeling on an iPad to teach functional math skills to adolescents with autism and intellectual disability. *Focus on Autism and Other Developmental Disabilities, 28*(2), 67–77. https://doi.org/10.1177/1088357613478829

Caria, S., Paternò, F., Santoro, C., & Semucci, V. (2018). The design of web games for helping young high-functioning Autistics in learning how to manage money. *Mobile Networks and Applications, 23*, 1735–1748. https://doi.org/10.1007/s11036-018-1069-0

Courtade, G., Spooner, F., Browder, D., & Jimenez, B. (2012). Seven reasons to promote standards-based instruction for students with severe disabilities: A reply to Ayres, Lowrey, Douglas, & Sievers (2011). *Education and Training in Autism and Development Disabilities, 47*(1), 3–13.

Cramer, M., Hirano, S.H., Tentori, M., Yeganyan, M.T., Hayes, G.R. (2011, May). Classroom-based assistive technology: collective use of interactive visual schedules by students with autism. In *Proceedings of the SIGCHI conference on human factors in computing systems* (pp. 1–10). https://doi.org/10.1145/1978942.1978944

Cunha, R. M., & Barbosa, S. D. J. (2012, April). Development and evaluation of a computer game for teaching vocabulary to children with autism. In *Proceedings of the international conference on web information systems and technologies* (pp. 386–392). https://doi.org/10.5220/0003940403860392

Davis, M., Otero, N., Dautenhahn, K., Nehaniv, C. L., & Powell, S. D. (2007, July). Creating a software to promote understanding about narrative in children with autism: Reflecting on the design of feedback and opportunities to reason. In *Proceedings of the international conference on development and learning* (pp. 64–69). https://doi.org/10.1109/DEVLRN.2007.4354045

De Leo, G., Gonzales, C. H., Battagiri, P., & Leroy, G. (2011). A smart-phone application and a companion website for the improvement of the communication skills of children with autism: Clinical rationale, technical development and preliminary results. *Journal of Medical Systems, 35*(4), 703–711. https://doi.org/10.1007/s10916-009-9407-1

Đorđević, M., Brojčin, B., & Glumbić, N. (2019). *Multikomponentne bihevioralne intervencije u specijalnoj edukaciji*. Univerzitet u Beogradu-Fakultet za specijalnu edukaciju i rehabilitaciju Izdavački centar (ICF).

Đorđević, M., Glumbić, N., Memisevic, H., Brojčin, B., & Krstov, A. (2021). Parent-teacher interactions, family stress, well-being, and parental depression as contributing factors to parental involvement mechanisms in education of children with autism. *International Journal of Developmental Disabilities*, 1–12. https://doi.org/10.1080/20473869.2021.1896962

Eder, M. S., Diaz, J. M. L., Madela, J. R. S., Marife, U., & Sabellano, D. D. M. (2016). Fill Me App: An interactive mobile game application for children with autism. *International Journal of Interactive Mobile Technologies, 10*(3), 59–63. https://doi.org/10.3991/ijim.v10i3.5553

Fage, C., Pommereau, L., Consel, C., Balland, E., & Sauzéon, H. (2014, October). Tablet-based activity schedule for children with autism in mainstream environment. In *Proceedings of the 16th international ACM SIGACCESS conference on Computers & accessibility* (pp. 145–152). https://doi.org/10.1145/2661334.2661369

Frutos, M., Bustos, I., Zapirain, B. G., Zorrilla, A. M. (2011, July). Computer game to learn and enhance speech problems for children with autism. In *Proceedings of the international conference on computer games: AI, animation, mobile, interactive multimedia, educational and serious games* (pp. 345–346). https://doi.org/10.1109/CGAMES.2011.6000340

Gentry, T., Wallace, J., Kvarfordt, C., & Lynch, K. B. (2010). Personal digital assistants as cognitive aids for high school students with autism: Results of a community-based trial. *Journal of Vocational Rehabilitation, 32*(2), 101–107. https://doi.org/10.3233/JVR-2010-0499

Glumbić, N., Brojčin, B., & Đorđević, M. (2018). *Specijalna edukacija zasnovana na dokazima: bihevioralne tehnike*. Univerzitet u Beogradu – Fakultet za specijalnu edukaciju i rehabilitaciju Izdavački centar (ICF).

Goh, S., Whitaker, A., Feldman, J., Cull, M. B., Hoyte, K., Algermissen, M., Maureen McSwiggan-Hardin, M., Kugelmass, D., & Peterson, B. S. (2013). Teaching non-verbal children with autistic disorder to read and write: a pilot study. *International Journal of Developmental Disabilities, 59*(2), 95–107. https://doi.org/10.1179/2047387713Y.0000000014

Gomez, J., Jaccheri, L., Torrado, J. C., & Montoro, G. (2018, June). Leo con lula, introducing global reading methods to children with ASD. In *Proceedings of the ACM conference on interaction design and children* (pp. 420–426). https://doi.org/10.1145/3202185.3202765

Grindle, C. F., Hughes, J. C., Saville, M., Huxley, K., & Hastings, R. P. (2013). Teaching early reading skills to children with autism using MimioSprout early reading. *Behavioral Interventions, 28*(3), 203–224. https://doi.org/10.1002/bin.1364

Grynszpan, O., Weiss, P. L., Perez-Diaz, F., & Gal, E. (2014). Innovative technology-based interventions for autism spectrum disorders: A meta-analysis. *Autism, 18*(4), 346–361. https://doi.org/10.1177/1362361313476767

Hart, J. E., & Whalon, K. J. (2012). Using video self-modeling via iPads to increase academic responding of an adolescent with autism spectrum disorder and intellectual disability. *Education and Training in Autism and Developmental Disabilities, 47*(4), 438–446.

Hassan, A. Z., Zahed, B. T., Zohora, F. T., Moosa, J. M., Salam, T., Rahman, M. M., Ferdous, H. S., & Ahmed, S. I. (2011, December). Developing the concept of money by interactive computer

games for autistic children. In *Proceedings of the IEEE international symposium on multimedia* (pp. 559–564). https://doi.org/10.1109/ISM.2011.99
Hayes, G. R., Hirano, S., Marcu, G., Monibi, M., Nguyen, D. H., & Yeganyan, M. (2010). Interactive visual supports for children with autism. *Personal and Ubiquitous Computing, 14*(7), 663–680. https://doi.org/10.1007/s00779-010-0294-8
Hetzroni, O. E., & Shalem, U. (2005). From logos to orthographic symbols: A multilevel fading computer program for teaching nonverbal children with autism. *Focus on Autism and Other Developmental Disabilities, 20*(4), 201–212. https://doi.org/10.1177/10883576050200040201
Hirano, S. H., Yeganyan, M. T., Marcu, G., Nguyen, D. H., Boyd, L. A., & Hayes, G. R. (2010, April). vSked: Evaluation of a system to support classroom activities for children with autism. In *Proceedings of the SIGCHI conference on human factors in computing systems* (pp. 1633–1642). https://doi.org/10.1145/1753326.1753569
Hong, E. R., Gong, L. Y., Ninci, J., Morin, K., Davis, J. L., Kawaminami, S., Shi, Y., & Noro, F. (2017). A meta-analysis of single-case research on the use of tablet-mediated interventions for persons with ASD. *Research in Developmental Disabilities, 70*, 198–214. https://doi.org/10.1016/j.ridd.2017.09.013
Hoque, M. E., Lane, J. K., El Kaliouby, R., Goodwin, M., & Picard, R. W. (2009, September). Exploring speech therapy games with children on the autism spectrum. In *Proceedings of Conference of the International Speech Communication Association*, INTERSPEECH (pp. 1–4).
Husni, E. (2013). Mobile applications BIUTIS: Let's study vocabulary learning as a media for children with autism. *Procedia Technology, 11*, 1147–1155. https://doi.org/10.1016/j.protcy.2013.12.307
Jiménez-Muñoz, L., Peñuelas-Calvo, I., Calvo-Rivera, P., Díaz-Oliván, I., Moreno, M., Baca-García, E., & Porras-Segovia, A. (2022). Video games for the treatment of autism spectrum disorder: A systematic review. *Journal of Autism and Developmental Disorders, 52*(1), 169–188. https://doi.org/10.1007/s10803-021-04934-9
Jones, C. R. G., Happé, F., Golden, H., Marsden, A. J. S., Tregay, J., Simonoff, E., Pickles, A., Baird, G., & Charman, T. (2009). Reading and arithmetic in adolescents with autism spectrum disorders: Peaks and dips in attainment. *Neuropsychology, 23*(6), 718–728. https://doi.org/10.1037/a0016360
Kagohara, D. M., van der Meer, L., Ramdoss, S., O'Reilly, M. F., Lancioni, G. E., Davis, T. N., Rispoli, M., Lang, R., Marschik, P. B., Sutherland, D., Green, V. A., & Sigafoos, J. (2013). Using iPods® and iPads® in teaching programs for individuals with developmental disabilities: A systematic review. *Research in Developmental Disabilities, 34*(1), 147–156. https://doi.org/10.1016/j.ridd.2012.07.027
Khowaja, K., & Salim, S. S. (2019). Serious game for children with autism to learn vocabulary: An experimental evaluation. *International Journal of Human Computer Interaction, 35*(1), 1–26. https://doi.org/10.1080/10447318.2017.1420006
Khowaja, K., Al-Thani, D., & Salim, S. S. (2018, October). Vocabulary learning of children with autism spectrum disorder (ASD): From the development to an evaluation of serious game prototype. In *Proceedings of the European conference on games-based learning* (pp. 288–298).
Knight, V., McKissick, B. R., & Saunders, A. (2013). A review of technology-based interventions to teach academic skills to students with autism spectrum disorder. *Journal of Autism and Developmental Disorders, 43*(11), 2628–2648. https://doi.org/10.1007/s10803-013-1814-y
Light, J., McNaughton, D., Jakobs, T., & Hershberger, D. (2014). *Investigating AAC technologies to support the transition from graphic symbols to literacy*. RERC on AAC: Rehabilitation Engineering Research Center on Augmentative and Alternative Communication. Retrieved from, https://rerc-aac.psu.edu/research/r2-investigating-aac-technologies-to-support-the-transition-from-graphic-symbols-to-literacy/
Mahayuddin, Z. R., & Mamat, N. (2019). Implementing augmented reality (AR) on phonics-based literacy among children with autism. *International Journal on Advanced Science, Engineering and Information Technology, 9*(6), 2176–2181. https://doi.org/10.18517/ijaseit.9.6.6833

Mandak, K., Light, J., & McNaughton, D. (2019). Digital books with dynamic text and speech output: Effects on sight word reading for preschoolers with autism spectrum disorder. *Journal of Autism and Developmental Disorders, 49*(3), 1193–1204. https://doi.org/10.1007/s10803-018-3817-1

Marchetti, E., & Valente, A. (2016). What a tangible digital installation for museums can offer to autistic children and their teachers. *International Journal of Game-Based Learning (IJGBL), 6*(2), 29–45. https://doi.org/10.4018/IJGBL.2016040103

Mazon, C., Fage, C., & Sauzéon, H. (2019). Effectiveness and usability of technology-based interventions for children and adolescents with ASD: A systematic review of reliability, consistency, generalization and durability related to the effects of intervention. *Computers in Human Behavior, 93*, 235–251. https://doi.org/10.1016/j.chb.2018.12.001

McGonigle-Chalmers, M., Alderson-Day, B., Fleming, J., & Monsen, K. (2013). Profound expressive language impairment in low functioning children with autism: An investigation of syntactic awareness using a computerised learning task. *Journal of Autism and Developmental Disorders, 43*(9), 2062–2081. https://doi.org/10.1007/s10803-012-1753-z

Mendonça, V., Coheur, L., & Sardinha, A. (2011, March). VITHEA-Kids: A platform for improving language skills of children with Autism spectrum disorder. In *Proceedings of the International ACM SIGACCESS conference on computers and accessibility* (pp. 345–346). https://doi.org/10.1145/2700648.2811371

Muharib, R., Correa, V. I., Wood, C. L., & Haughney, K. L. (2019). Effects of functional communication training using GoTalk NowTM iPad® application on challenging behavior of children with autism spectrum disorder. *Journal of Special Education Technology, 34*(2), 71–79. https://doi.org/10.1177/0162643418783479

Munoz-Soto, R., Becerra, C., Noël, R., Barcelos, T., Villarroel, R., Kreisel, S., & Camblor, M. (2016, October). Proyect@ matemáticas: A learning object for supporting the practitioners in autism spectrum disorders. In *Proceedings of the 11th Latin American conference on learning objects and technology* (pp. 1–6). https://doi.org/10.1109/LACLO.2016.7751760

Nation, K., Clarke, P., Wright, B., & Williams, C. (2006). Patterns of reading ability in children with autism spectrum disorder. *Journal of Autism and Developmental Disorders, 36*(7), 911–919. https://doi.org/10.1007/s10803-006-0130-1

Nkabinde, Z. P. (2014). Information and computer technology for individuals with autism. In N. R. Silton (Ed.), *Innovative technologies to benefit children on the Autism spectrum* (pp. 71–85). IGI Global. https://doi.org/10.4018/978-1-4666-5792-2.ch005

Odom, S. L., Thompson, J. L., Hedges, S., Boyd, B. A., Dykstra, J. R., Duda, M. A., Szidon, K. L., Smith, L. E., & Bord, A. (2015). Technology-aided interventions and instruction for adolescents with autism spectrum disorder. *Journal of Autism and Developmental Disorders, 45*(12), 3805–3819. https://doi.org/10.1007/s10803-014-2320-6

Oliveira, M. S., Pereira, C. P., de Santana, K. C., & Rossinholli, K. O. C. (2019, May). Autisdata: Software to help the development of people with ASD based on TEACCH and PECS Methodologies. *In Proceedings of the international conference on computer supported education* (pp. 331–338). https://doi.org/10.5220/0007716303310338

Pistoljevic, N., & Hulusic, V. (2017, September). An interactive E-book with an educational game for children with developmental disorders: A pilot user study. In *Proceedings of the international conference on virtual Worlds and games for serious applications* (pp. 87–93). https://doi.org/10.1109/VS-GAMES.2017.8056575

Ploog, B. O., Scharf, A., Nelson, D., & Brooks, P. J. (2013). Use of computer-assisted technologies (CAT) to enhance social, communicative, and language development in children with autism spectrum disorders. *Journal of Autism and Developmental Disorders, 43*(2), 301–322. https://doi.org/10.1007/s10803-012-1571-3

Rahman, M. M., Ferdous, S. M. & Ahmed, S. I. (2010, December). Increasing intelligibility in the speech of the autistic children by an interactive computer game. In *Proceedings of the IEEE International Symposium on Multimedia* (pp. 383–387). https://doi.org/10.1109/ISM.2010.64

Rahman, M. R., Naha, S., Roy, P. C., Ahmed, I., Samrose, S., Rahman, M. M., Ahmed, S. I. (2011, March). A-class: A classroom software with the support for diversity in aptitudes of autistic children. In *Proceedings of the IEEE symposium on computers and informatics* (pp. 727–731). https://doi.org/10.1109/ISCI.2011.5959007

Ramdoss, S., Mulloy, A., Lang, R., O'Reilly, M., Sigafoos, J., Lancioni, G., Didden, R., & El Zein, F. (2011). Use of computer-based interventions to improve literacy skills in students with autism spectrum disorders: A systematic review. *Research in Autism Spectrum Disorders, 5*(4), 1306–1318. https://doi.org/10.1016/j.rasd.2011.03.004

Rasche, N., Pourcho, J., Wei, S., Qian, C. Z., & Chen, V. Y. (2013, July). Literacy LABELS: Emergent literacy application design for children with autism. In *Posters on the ACM SIGGRAPH*. Article No.: 24. https://doi.org/10.1145/2503385.2503411

Roglić, M., Bobić, V., Djurić-Jovičić, M., Djordjević, M., Dragašević, N., & Nikolić, B. (2016, November). Serious gaming based on Kinect technology for autistic children in Serbia. In *Proceedings of the 13th symposium on neural networks and applications (neurel)* (pp. 1–4). https://doi.org/10.1109/NEUREL.2016.7800105

Sansosti, F. J., Doolan, M. L., Remaklus, B., Krupko, A., & Sansosti, J. M. (2015). Computer-assisted interventions for students with autism spectrum disorders within school-based contexts: A quantitative meta-analysis of single-subject research. *Review Journal of Autism and Developmental Disorders, 2*(2), 128–140. https://doi.org/10.1007/s40489-014-0042-5

Santos, M. I., Breda, A., & Almeida, A. M. (2017). Design approach of mathematics learning activities in a digital environment for children with autism spectrum disorders. *Educational Technology Research and Development, 65*(5), 1305–1323. https://doi.org/10.1007/s11423-017-9525-2

Seok, S., DaCosta, B., & Yu, B. M. (2015). Spelling practice intervention: A comparison of tablet PC and picture cards as spelling practice methods for students with developmental disabilities. *Education and Training in Autism and Developmental Disabilities, 50*(1), 84–94. https://www.jstor.org/stable/24827503

Serret, S., Hun, S., Thümmler, S., Pierron, P., Santos, A., Bourgeois, J., & Askenazy, F. (2017). Teaching literacy skills to French minimally verbal school-aged children with autism spectrum disorders with the serious game SEMA-TIC: An exploratory study. *Frontiers in Psychology, 8*, 1523. https://doi.org/10.3389/fpsyg.2017.01523

Shamsuddin, S., Yussof, H., Ismail, L. I., Mohamed, S., Hanapiah, F. A., & Zahari, N. I. (2012). Humanoid robot NAO interacting with autistic children of moderately impaired intelligence to augment communication skills. *Procedia Engineering, 41*, 1533–1538. https://doi.org/10.1016/j.proeng.2012.07.346

Silva, S. D., Neto, F. M. M., de Lima, R. M., de Macêdo, F. T., Santo, J. R. S., & Silva, W. L. N. (2017, November). Knowledgemon hunter: A serious game with geolocation to support learning of children with autism and learning difficulties. In *Proceedings of the 19th symposium on virtual and augmented reality (SVR)* (pp. 293–296). https://doi.org/10.1109/SVR.2017.45

Sitdhisanguan, K., Chotikakamthorn, N., Dechaboon, A., & Out, P. (2012). Using tangible user interfaces in computer-based training systems for low-functioning autistic children. *Personal and Ubiquitous Computing, 16*(2), 143–155. https://doi.org/10.1007/s00779-011-0382-4

Sorce, S., Gentile, V., Oliveto, D., Barraco, R., Malizia, A., & Gentile, A. (2018, June). Exploring usability and accessibility of avatar-based touchless gestural interfaces for autistic people. In *Proceedings of the 7th ACM International Symposium on Pervasive Displays* (pp. 1–2). https://doi.org/10.1145/3205873.3210705

Spooner, F., Ahlgrim-Delzell, L., Kemp-Inman, A., & Wood, L. A. (2014). Using an iPad2® with systematic instruction to teach shared stories for elementary-aged students with autism. *Research and Practice for Persons with Severe Disabilities, 39*(1), 30–46. https://doi.org/10.1177/1540796914534631

Spriggs, A. D., Knight, V., & Sherrow, L. (2015). Talking picture schedules: Embedding video models into visual activity schedules to increase independence for students with ASD. *Journal of Autism and Developmental Disorders, 45*(12), 3846–3861. https://doi.org/10.1007/s10803-014-2315-3

Srinivasan, S. M., Eigsti, I. M., Gifford, T., & Bhat, A. N. (2016). The effects of embodied rhythm and robotic interventions on the spontaneous and responsive verbal communication skills of children with Autism Spectrum Disorder (ASD): A further outcome of a pilot randomized controlled trial. *Research in Autism Spectrum Disorders, 27*, 73–87. https://doi.org/10.1016/j.rasd.2016.04.001

Steinbrenner, J. R., Hume, K., Odom, S. L., Morin, K. L., Nowell, S. W., Tomaszewski, B., Szendrey, S., McIntyre, N. S., Yücesoy-Özkan, S., & Savage, M. N. (2020). *Evidence-based practices for children, youth, and young adults with Autism*. The University of North Carolina at Chapel Hill, Frank Porter Graham Child Development Institute, National Clearinghouse on Autism Evidence and Practice Review Team.

Tang, H. H., Jheng, C. M., Chien, M. E., Lin, N. M., & Chen, M. Y. (2013, March). iCAN: A tablet-based pedagogical system for improving the user experience of children with autism in the learning process. In *Proceedings of International Conference on Orange Technologies* (pp. 177–180). https://doi.org/10.1109/ICOT.2013.6521186

Tashnim, A., Nowshin, S., Akter, F., & Das, A. K. (2017, October). Interactive interface design for learning numeracy and calculation for children with autism. In *Proceedings of the 9th international conference on information technology and electrical engineering* (pp. 1–6). https://doi.org/10.1109/ICITEED.2017.8250507

Travers, J. C., Higgins, K., Pierce, T., Boone, R., Miller, S., & Tandy, R. (2011). Emergent literacy skills of preschool students with autism: A comparison of teacher-led and computer-assisted instruction. *Education and Training in Autism and Developmental Disabilities, 46*(3), 326–338. https://www.jstor.org/stable/23880589

Tsiopela, D., & Jimoyiannis, A. (2014). Pre-vocational skills laboratory: Development and investigation of a web-based environment for students with autism. *Procedia Computer Science, 27*, 207–217. https://doi.org/10.1016/j.procs.2014.02.024

Vacca, J. S. (2007). Autistic children can be taught to read. *International Journal of Special Education, 22*(3), 54–61.

Valencia, K., Rusu, C., Quiñones, D., & Jamet, E. (2019). The impact of technology on people with autism spectrum disorder: A systematic literature review. *Sensors, 19*(20), 4485. https://doi.org/10.3390/s19204485

Van der Meer, L., Achmadi, D., Cooijmans, M., Didden, R., Lancioni, G. E., O'Reilly, M. F., Roche, L., Stevens, M., Carnett, A., Hodis, F., Green, V. A., Sutherland, D., Lang, R., Rispoli, M., Marschik, P. B., & Sigafoos, J. (2015). An iPad-based intervention for teaching picture and word matching to a student with ASD and severe communication impairment. *Journal of Developmental and Physical Disabilities, 27*(1), 67–78. https://doi.org/10.1007/s10882-014-9401-5

Wadhwa, B., & Jianxiong, C. C. (2013, September). Collaborative tablet applications to enhance language skills of children with autism spectrum disorder. In *Proceedings of the Asia Pacific conference on computer human interaction* (pp. 39–44). https://doi.org/10.1145/2525194.2525297

Wang, Z. (2021). Evaluation of different teaching strategies in sight words instruction of Chinese children with autism: Text-picture matching, picture-embedded, and word tracing. *Advances in Educational Technology and Psychology, 5*(9), 8–21. https://doi.org/10.23977/aetp.2021.59002

Weng, P. L., & Bouck, E. C. (2014). Using video prompting via iPads to teach price comparison to adolescents with autism. *Research in Autism Spectrum Disorders, 8*(10), 1405–1415. https://doi.org/10.1016/j.rasd.2014.06.014

Whalen, C., Moss, D., Ilan, A. B., Vaupel, M., Fielding, P., Macdonald, K., Cernich, S., & Symon, J. (2010). Efficacy of TeachTown: Basics computer-assisted intervention for the intensive comprehensive autism program in Los Angeles Unified School District. *Autism, 14*(3), 179–197. https://doi.org/10.1177/1362361310363282

Wilson, C., Brereton, M., Ploderer, B., Sitbon, L. (2018, June). MyWord: Enhancing engagement, interaction and self-expression with minimally-verbal children on the autism spectrum through

a personal audio-visual dictionary. In *Proceedings of the ACM conference on interaction design and children* (pp. 106–118). https://doi.org/10.1145/3202185.3202755
Wojciechowski, A., & Al-Musawi, R. (2017). Assistive technology application for enhancing social and language skills of young children with autism. *Multimedia Tools and Applications, 76*(4), 5419–5439. https://doi.org/10.1007/s11042-016-3995-9
Wright, J. C., Knight, V. F., & Barton, E. E. (2020). A review of video modeling to teach STEM to students with autism and intellectual disability. *Research in Autism Spectrum Disorders, 70*, 101476. https://doi.org/10.1016/j.rasd.2019.101476
Yakubova, G., Defayette, M. A., Chen, B. B., & Proulx, A. L. (2021). The use of augmented reality interventions to provide academic instruction for children with autism, intellectual, and developmental disabilities: An evidence-based systematic review. *Review Journal of Autism and Developmental Disorders*, 1–17. https://doi.org/10.1007/s40489-021-00287-2

Chapter 4
Leisure Activities

4.1 Leisure Activities: History and Concept

Leisure activities are a significant segment of a person's life. Historically, understanding and doing leisure activities depended on social circumstances, divisions, and relations. The roots of defining leisure date back to ancient Greek philosophers who believed that the essence of "good life" was leisure time when a person could search for the truth, engage in oratory, music, etc. (Juniu, 2000; Mowatt, 2018; Veal, 2004). However, only the upper class could enjoy leisure activities in ancient times. This stratification trend continued throughout history, so the clergy, nobility, and, later, all free citizens could use leisure time. The next important factor for the modern definition of leisure was the Industrial Revolution when leisure time lost its previously acquired reputation and was not viewed favorably compared to work participation (Juniu, 2000; Mommaas, 1997). The third significant factor for the modern definition of leisure was the strengthened left wing around World War I, which initiated public dialogues about working conditions and leisure time. Furthermore, it contributed to the establishment of different organizations which advocated the clear separation of leisure time and work and the right to use that time for entertainment, emancipation, and recreation (Mommaas, 1997). These social reforms resulted in the universal Declaration of Human Rights adopted by the UN General Assembly in 1948 (UN, 1948). Article 24 of this Declaration emphasizes every person's right to rest and leisure.

Further changes in the conceptualization of leisure time, its organization, and related experiences were caused by technological development, especially Internet discovery (Bryce, 2001; Gershuny, 2003; López Sintas et al., 2015). Before the Internet, leisure usually referred to leisure at home (e.g., time for reading a book, listening to music, handcrafts, etc.) or out of home (e.g., going to the cinema, to a cafe, for a walk, to the park, etc.). However, technology created opportunities for virtual leisure available anywhere (e.g., outside, at work, at home, etc.) and anytime

N. Glumbić et al., *Digital Inclusion of Individuals with Autism Spectrum Disorder*, Autism and Child Psychopathology Series,
https://doi.org/10.1007/978-3-031-12037-4_4

(López Sintas et al., 2015). Thus, we can say that technological development contributed to the development of a new trend described as "online leisure," "cyber leisure," or "E-leisure" (Arora, 2011; Cheng & Yang, 2010; Nimrod & Adoni, 2012). The Internet and technologies provide a wide range of leisure activities, such as playing games, browsing, online chatting, listening to music, watching films (Žumárová, 2015), shopping (Díaz et al., 2017), etc.

Although first empirical research on leisure time appeared in the 1920s, greater scientific interest in studying leisure activities appeared in the 1940s (Liu et al., 2008), which resulted in numerous publications on leisure activities and the "birth" of leisure studies at different faculties around the world (Godbey, 2000; Roberts, 2018). Nowadays, leisure studies are characterized by fragmentation and pluralism, i.e., diverse methodological designs, inconsistent terminology, and reference to many principles and theories (Henderson, 2010).

Different theoretical and methodological viewpoints have led to numerous definitions of leisure. Leisure has usually been perceived in three ways (Fig. 4.1). The concept of leisure as time refers to understanding leisure as an amount of time not used for obligations and work, i.e., as the remaining time free from any work and compulsory activities. On the other hand, leisure as activities implies freedom to choose and perform desired activities without any obligation or coercion (Ropke & Godskesen, 2007). These dimensions are interrelated, making it even more difficult to define leisure. Ropke and Godskesen (2007) indicate that if individuals have more time free from other activities, they will have more opportunities to choose freely. According to Mannell and Kleiber (1997), leisure as time and leisure as activities are objective, while leisure as state of mind is subjective and refers to an individual's mental experience while participating in leisure activities, i.e., while using leisure time.

Although different people experience leisure differently and link it to various times and contexts, Watkins and Bond (2007) state that we can relate most experiences to four dimensions—leisure as achieving fulfillment, escaping pressure, exercising choice, and passing the time. López Sintas et al. (2015) point out that freedom

Fig. 4.1 Three ways of perceiving leisure

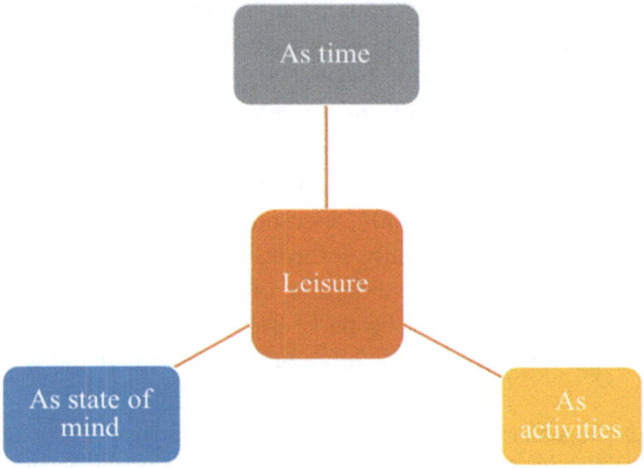

of choice is the most significant for leisure activities and that the choice refers to not only the desired activity but also the time, space, and company. Some authors distinguish between serious leisure (e.g., hobbies, amateur activities, etc.) and casual leisure (e.g., play, passive entertainment, active entertainment, conversation, etc.), pointing out that feelings such as "satisfaction" and "rewardingness" are associated with serious leisure, while casual leisure is associated with "pleasure" and "enjoyment" (Stebbins, 1997, 1982). In trying to define leisure, the World Health Organization (2001) equates it with recreation and play, providing a list of activities which an individual can do for pleasure—unstructured or structured play, sports activities, going to cultural and entertainment venues, reading, sightseeing, traveling, etc. Since this chapter deals with people with ASD, we were also interested in how these people understand and define leisure. They perceive meaningful leisure time as a time during which a person feels comfortable and productive, which contributes to the quality of life, and during which a person can pursue hobbies and interests. With regard to leisure time intensity, people with ASD believe that they need to find a balance in pursuing hobbies (neither too much nor too little), i.e., that as long as pursuing special interests and hobbies contributes to self-development and increased community participation, it can last long or until the person gets tired (Rosqvist, 2017).

Researchers agree that participation in leisure activities is related to better subjective well-being in typically developing people of different ages (Brajša-Žganec et al., 2011; Kuykendall et al., 2020; Liu, 2014; Newman et al., 2014; Simone et al., 2013; Schulz et al., 2018; Wiese et al., 2018) and that the controlled use of the Internet and technology in leisure activities can contribute to the quality of life (Leung & Lee, 2005).

4.2 Participation of People with ASD in Leisure Activities

Research studies show that people with ASD are less frequently employed (Shattuck et al., 2012; Taylor & Seltzer, 2012), i.e., they have significantly more free time for leisure activities. Although the results of numerous studies point out the significance of leisure activities for the quality of life in people with ASD (Billstedt et al., 2011; Bishop-Fitzpatrick et al., 2017; Chiang & Wineman, 2014; García-Villamisar & Dattilo, 2010; Hesselmark et al., 2014), their socio-emotional cognition (Garcia-Villamisar & Dattilo, 2011), reduction of maladaptive behaviors (O'Brien, 2010), and mental health (Bohnert et al., 2016), they still participate in leisure activities less frequently (Hilton et al., 2020; Hochhauser & Engel-Yeger, 2010; LaVesser & Berg, 2011; Ratcliff et al., 2018; Stacey et al., 2018; Taheri et al., 2016; Tint et al., 2017; Venkatesan, 2005). The most commonly stated reason is the lack of a repertoire of leisure skills that would allow for a constructive organization of leisure time (Solish et al., 2010). The factors of the lower participation rate in leisure activities are usually divided into those referring to the characteristics of autism (e.g., difficulties in social interaction, level of internalizing behavior, disruptive behavior, sensory specificities, motor difficulties, etc.) and environmental factors (e.g., climate, family finances, having adequate equipment and requisites, environmental attitudes, number of available services, mother's involvement, lack of technological solutions, etc.) (Coussens et al., 2020; Hochhauser & Engel-Yeger, 2010; Howel & Pierson, 2010; LaVesser & Berg, 2011; Marques et al., 2020; Obrusnikova & Cavalier, 2011; Obrusnikova & Miccinello, 2012; Orsmond et al., 2004; Shattuck et al., 2011). These two groups of factors are interrelated. Thus, for example, an obstacle for people with autism to participate in leisure activities can also be that the environment does not recognize their interests and preferences. This obstacle, and consequent inadequate options for leisure activities, can also be partly caused by ASD characteristics (e.g., limited interests, resistance to change, stereotyped activities, communication difficulties, etc.) (McCarron, 2018).

Based on the review of previous studies on leisure activities in people with ASD, Ratcliff et al. (2018) found the following categories of leisure activities: physical activities (e.g., participating in individual or group sports activities, physical exercise, cycling, etc.), recreational activities (e.g., watching TV, playing computer games, talking on the phone, using some technological devices, etc.), social activities (e.g., participating in the activities of some clubs, organizations, etc.), jobs and chores (e.g., babysitting, lawn mowing, etc.), and skill-based activities (e.g., attending lessons in singing, musical instruments, playing, etc.). Some authors also add self-improvement activities that include reading, writing, going shopping, participating in religious activities, etc. (Eversole et al., 2015; King et al., 2006). Others divide all mentioned activities into two categories—formal (e.g., participating in clubs and organizations, taking dancing, language, painting, playing lessons, participating in religious activities, etc.) and informal (e.g., collecting favorite items, playing computer games, talking on the phone, watching TV, preparing food, etc.) (Eversole et al., 2015; King et al., 2006). Regardless of the existing divisions, leisure activities are considered less structured activities that require daily living skills and skills related to communication and social skills (Turygin & Matson, 2014).

Research on how satisfied people with ASD are with their leisure activities is scarce. According to Stacey et al. (2018), adults with ASD are less satisfied with leisure activities in the following areas—social, relaxation, physiological, and aesthetic.

Although most typically developing people develop leisure skills spontaneously, people with ASD require structured teaching in this area. McCarron (2018) points out the following steps in encouraging people with ASD to participate in leisure activities: (1) finding potential activities of interest for people with ASD (usually through techniques of expanding their existing interests); (2) determining preferred leisure activities; (3) selecting a repertoire of leisure activities; (4) teaching skills to people with ASD they need to participate in selected and preferred leisure activities; and (5) raising the level of autonomy and independence in participating in leisure activities. Furthermore, Coyne et al. (1999) suggest that exposure to a wide range of different leisure activities may expand the interests of people with ASD. When developing skills relevant to leisure activities in people with ASD, several things should be kept in mind: the skills and activities need to be clear and understandable for these people (with a clear beginning and end, predictable steps, accompanying visual and other stimuli, etc.); the used materials should be reactive (so that people with ASD can have some feedback when using them, e.g., light, sound, touch, etc.); and participating in these activities should provide a sense of comfort but also active engagement (Coyne et al., 1999). Dattilo and Schlein (1994) emphasize that, when offering and choosing leisure activities, they should be age-appropriate, a person should be able to perform them (they should be available in the person's environment), and they should enable involvement in community activities and interaction with the environment.

The literature describes many different ways to empower leisure skills, some of which are backward chaining (Edwards et al., 2017), constant time delay and simultaneous prompting (Kurt & Tekin-Iftar, 2008; Yılmaz et al., 2005), most-to-least prompting (Vuran, 2008), finding university volunteers to keep company and provide individualized support to people with ASD participating in leisure activities (Nieto et al., 2015), using printed visual schedules with pictures (Becerra et al., 2020; Cuhadar & Diken, 2011), second-order lag schedule (Ivy et al., 2019), and client-centered goal-directed approach (Ullenhag et al., 2020).

4.3 The Role of Technology in the Leisure Time of People with Autism

Technology is undoubtedly very significant in the leisure time of people with ASD. The presence of technology in the literature within this field can be observed through at least three research approaches (Fig. 4.2).

The first approach focuses on how, to what extent, and with what pleasure people with ASD use technological resources during their leisure time. The second area of the literature deals with scientists' attempts to improve the digital skills of people with ASD necessary for organized and independent performance of desired leisure activities. Finally, the third approach involves using digital technology as a tool for teaching or empowering leisure skills (not necessarily related to technology).

4.3.1 Technology as a Medium of Leisure: Screen Media Use and Leisure Time

The significance of technology in leisure time is also confirmed by the fact that digital activities are very often among the highly preferred leisure activities of children and adults with ASD. Some research studies show that when trying to determine the preferences of people with ASD, excluding technological devices from the offered items, these people almost always choose food over items symbolizing leisure activities (Fahmie et al., 2015). On the other hand, with the introduction of technological

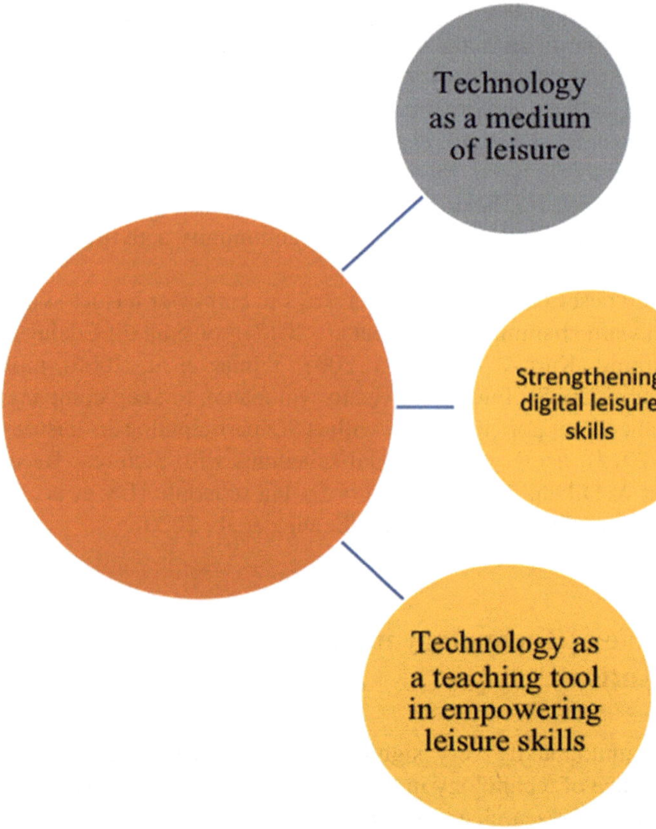

Fig. 4.2 One of the possible ways to observe the presence of technology in the literature on leisure activities in people with ASD

items, the preferences change to some extent, since, for some participants, digital leisure activities replace edible items as the first choice, i.e., preferences for leisure activities increase in general (Conine & Vollmer, 2019; Slanzi et al., 2019). Mineo et al. (2008) show that not all technological devices are equally preferred in people with ASD, i.e., that these people have different levels of preferences for various types of electronic screen media. For example, people with ASD show a slightly greater preference for videos in which they can see themselves and for VR scenarios.

By surveying children and young people with ASD, Brewster and Coleyshaw (2011) discovered that younger participants had a greater tendency to participate in out-of-home leisure activities with their families (e.g., bowling, swimming, etc.), while older children more frequently engaged in leisure activities at home (e.g., the Internet). Both groups of children reported that their feeling of insecurity and other people's hostility had adverse effects on their participation in out-of-home leisure activities. Shane and Albert (2008) obtained somewhat different results indicating that children with ASD generally, regardless of age, choose DVD and video games more than any other leisure activities. This research showed that over 90% of the participants had a home collection of favorite movies on DVD and over 60% had a collection of favorite computer games. By analyzing the content of videos and games, the authors concluded that children with ASD preferred animated activities to the ones with real human characters. Interestingly, the characters in DVDs and video games were the same ones the children generally liked to watch on TV (e.g., Winnie the Pooh) (Shane & Albert, 2008).

Simpson et al. (2018) confirmed previous findings and pointed out that in two age groups of participants (5 and 9–10 years of age), watching TV and DVDs and playing video games were the most common leisure activities. Orsmond and Kuo (2011) obtained similar results in a sample of 12- and 21-year-old participants, indicating that the most common leisure activities included watching TV (these people spent 2.27 h a day on this activity), computer activities (on average 1.65 h a day), and physical activities (about 1.21 h a day). Kuo et al. (2014) pointed out that adolescents with ASD were most interested in watching cartoons and playing action video games during the day (e.g., games that require physical skills and coordination and games that involve shooting, killing, etc.). Half of them played games alone, while a quarter played with peers.

Watching TV and listening to music are among the most common leisure activities of adults with ASD (Stacey et al., 2018). They are more likely to participate in recreational than social leisure activities weekly, which makes them different from typically developing adults (Bishop-Fitzpatrick et al., 2017; Orsmond et al., 2004).

The role of technology in the leisure activities of children and adults with ASD cannot be determined only from its incidence and intensity but also from the feeling of satisfaction and enjoyment while using it. By analyzing the literature dated between 2000 and 2013, Askari et al. (2015) found that most research studies focusing on leisure activities in children with ASD were quantitative, mainly dealing with participation frequency and diversity of leisure activities. On the other hand, few studies examined the qualitative aspects, such as the participants' subjective feelings while participating in leisure activities, satisfaction, or enjoyment. This literature review showed that children with ASD participated to a lesser extent and in a smaller number of leisure activities in all contexts—home, out-of-school setting, and social events. Eversole et al. (2015) pointed out that the studies on leisure activities in people with ASD unfairly neglected the aspect of enjoyment. They indicated that, although more abstract and subjective, this concept was a significant determinant of participation that should be further studied since knowing the activities people with ASD enjoyed could be the basis for planning further intervention steps. Comparing typically developing participants and children with ASD in how much they enjoyed leisure activities, the authors of different studies showed that children with ASD enjoyed different categories of leisure activities to a similar extent as their typically developing peers (Eversole et al., 2015; Hilton et al., 2008; Potvin et al., 2013). Also, it was determined that there were apparent differences in formal leisure activities (Eversole et al., 2015; Hilton et al., 2008, 2016; Hochhauser & Engel-Yeger, 2010), social activities in which people with ASD showed a lower level of enjoyment (Chevallier et al., 2011), and swimming in which people with ASD

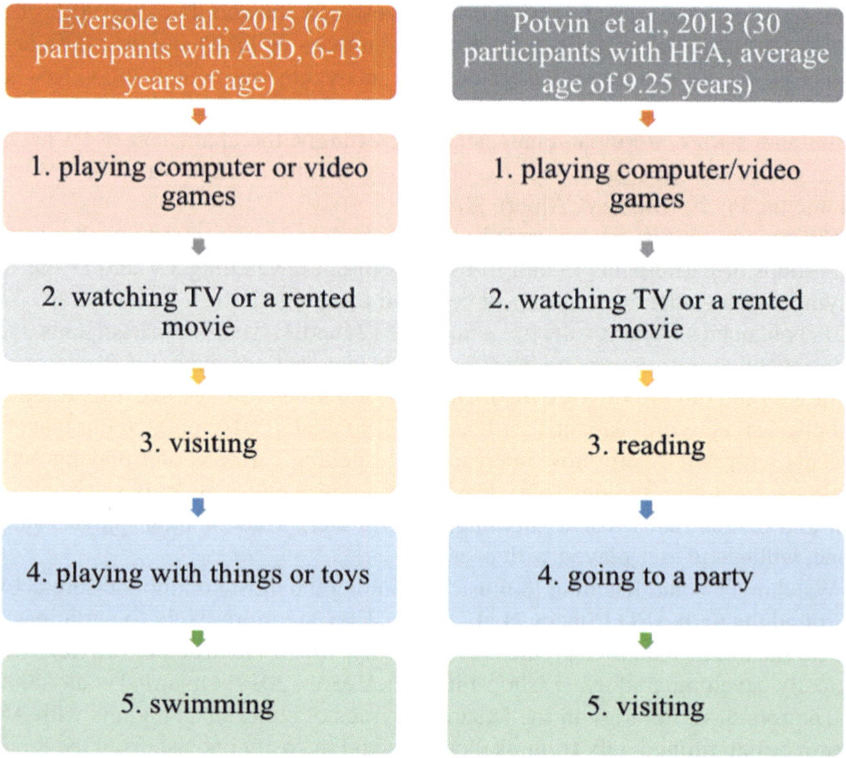

Fig. 4.3 An example of the top five leisure activities that people with ASD enjoy the most according to research by Eversole et al. (2015) and Potvin et al. (2013)

showed a higher level of enjoyment than their peers (Hilton et al., 2016). An example of the top five leisure activities in which children with ASD enjoy the most is shown in Fig. 4.3.

Other studies also confirm the significance of technology in the leisure activities of people with ASD. Thus, for example, in a research study that used a self-report technique in young people with ASD (8–15 years of age), more than half of the participants stated that they most enjoyed the activities related to technology and electronics (e.g., watching YouTube; playing games on a computer, iPad, and Xbox; etc.) (Clark & Adams, 2020).

4.3.2 Empowering Digital Leisure Skills

The use of technological devices implies having specific procedural skills and knowledge—e.g., starting a computer, opening or closing a particular program, starting a program, pausing or rewinding, searching for words, etc. Although people with autism have certain competence in these skills, it is noticeable that usually 50% of the participants, or less, use them successfully depending on the specific skill (Shane & Albert, 2008).

Surfing the Internet is a common way of spending leisure time in many typically developing people of different ages (Buse, 2009; Genoe et al., 2018). Some people with autism also tend to browse their favorite websites (Brewster & Coleyshaw, 2011; Shane & Albert, 2008). Shane and Albert (2008) indicate that the websites children with ASD visit can be divided into two categories—websites with animated video characters and websites with information about their (limited) interests (e.g., railways, elevators, etc.). However, not all people with autism are successful in browsing the web. Some need support. Jerome et al. (2007) examined to what extent three adults with ASD and a comorbid intellectual disability could be taught to access age-appropriate websites (specifically online games and musical websites) through errorless learning and backward chaining. Accessing the desired website was broken down into 12 steps using task analysis. The results showed that the applied techniques increased the number of independent steps in starting the computer and accessing the website.

People with ASD tend to play video games often (Eversole et al., 2015; Potvin et al., 2013). According to one research, children with ASD play video games six days a week, i.e., about 12 h a week, and the games they most frequently choose are Mario game, LEGO game, Angry Birds, Pokémon, or Minecraft (Finke et al., 2015). Mazurek and Wenstrup (2012) warn that children with ASD are more prone to problematic behavior when playing video games than typically developing children. This is manifested in problems when they stop playing, feeling bored without the games, tendency to spend their whole free time playing games, etc. Adolescents with ASD play video games because they allow them to make friends or meet other people. Also, the games calm them down and help them feel better, while at the same time they provide a challenge, raise motivation, and give them opportunities to feel success (Finke et al., 2018). Adults with ASD also often spend time playing computer games, most commonly stating the following reasons: stress relief, mental stimulation, creativity, and opportunities for social interaction (Mazurek et al., 2015). However, some individuals need teaching to be successful in these games. Blum-Dimaya et al. (2010) examined the effects of visual scheduling and simultaneous video modeling on teaching four children with ASD to play Guitar Hero IITM (Fig. 4.4). The activity of playing guitar in the video game was broken down into 26 steps. The teaching process included physical stimuli that were removed over time and edible reinforcers that the students selected before each session. All participants successfully mastered all steps in playing the mentioned game and performed the acquired steps for 30 days after the training.

Spriggs (2011, 2016) showed that, by using video modeling and observational learning, four students with ASD successfully learned how to play at least one of the following games: Nintendo Wii Video Game (an interactive wireless console), Nintendo DS (a portable handheld game console), Power-Joy Plug and Play Video Game (games played on TV), and V-Flash Scooby Doo. By comparing these two procedures, we can see that video modeling is much more efficient. However, peer

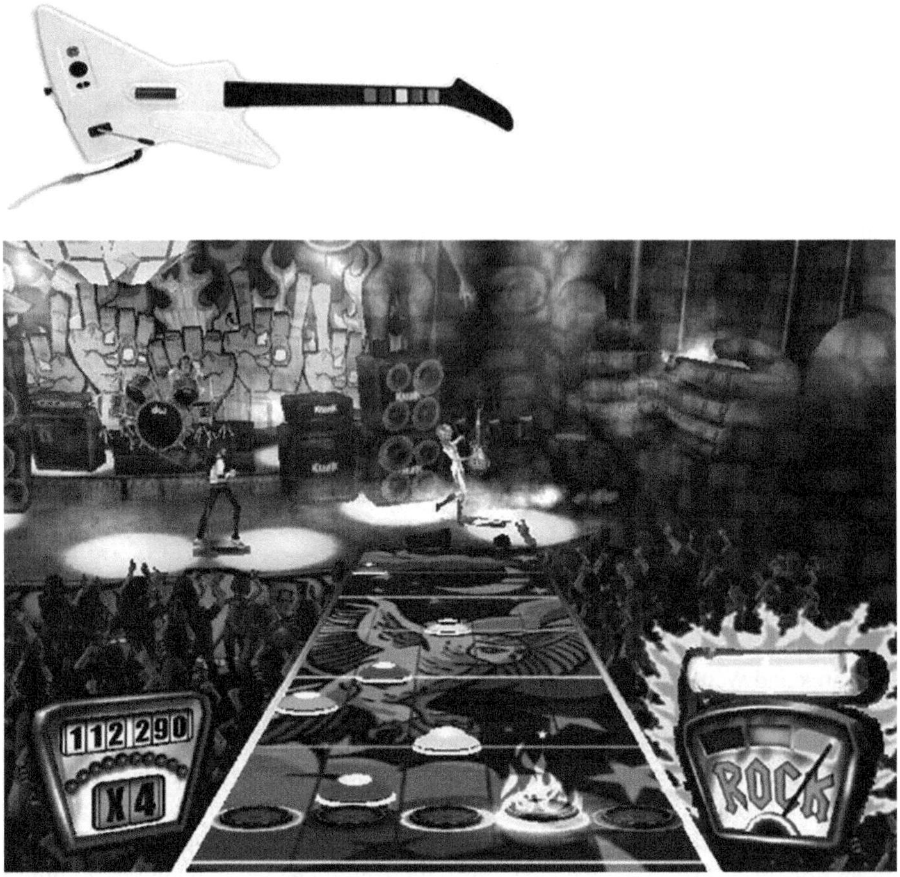

Fig. 4.4 Guitar as a game controller with a screenshot of the game. (Reproduced from Blum-Dimaya et al., 2010)

observation was also useful in mastering individual steps in the games. Kurnaz and Yanardag (2018) found that video self-modeling was also efficient in teaching four children with ASD to play active video games from the Microsoft XBOX Adventures package.

Many people like photography and use their free time for that purpose. People with ASD can also be interested in this activity but may lack the necessary knowledge and skills. Edrisinha et al. (2011) presented the results of using video prompting in teaching four adults to pursue a hobby of digital photography and printing photographs. The whole activity was broken down into 11 steps (from turning on the camera to getting a photo from a printer). The results showed that the participants successfully mastered all steps and enjoyed sharing their albums with other people from their environment. The albums mainly included photographs of flowers, cars, and people, and their quality improved over time. Tsai (2019) obtained similar results in a sample of eight children with ASD who were taught the same skill but by using different techniques and a different number of steps. Teaching students to take photographs by a digital camera was performed by verbal instructions, modeling, rehearsal, and feedback. The results showed that all participants fulfilled the learning criterion, i.e., they successfully completed all steps twice in a row with support, and six students fulfilled the mastery criterion. The participants who did not fully master digital photography had difficulties with a step called "identify a target scene," which involved independent verbalizing or showing what the person wanted to photograph. These participants needed prompting in the form of questions or guidance regarding this step.

Since Dattilo and Schlein (1994) believed that one of the reasons for the inadequate involvement of people with developmental disabilities in leisure activities was the prejudice of professionals or parents that these people cannot master or learn leisure skills, the obtained results can be used to contradict them.

4.3.3 Technology as a Teaching Tool in Empowering Leisure Skills

Bearing in mind the presence of technology and digital devices in our lives, their accessibility, their portability, and the tendency of people with ASD to use or select screen media devices, it is natural that their functions multiply and that they can also be used in teaching people with ASD. Another reason for using technology in teaching is that many devices or applications provide visual support, which is considered significant in educating people with ASD. Also, the existing scientifically confirmed teaching techniques can be combined quite well with technological devices, which may expand their existing potentials (Stromer et al., 2006).

The literature review showed that digital (computer or electronic) activity schedules, video modeling, and video prompting are the most frequently applied techniques (combined with other behavioral strategies) in teaching leisure skills to people with ASD.

4.3.3.1 Using Digital Activity Schedules to Teach Leisure Skills to Children and Adults with ASD

Kelly et al. (2013) conducted a research study to examine how a digital schedule on an iPad can be successfully used to structure leisure activities. The sample included four school-age children with ASD experienced in using an iPad but with no experience in using digital schedules. Teaching children to independently use schedules on an iPad, i.e., independently participate in leisure activities, was accompanied by using the following behavioral techniques—manual prompts, progressive time delay procedures, and reinforcement. The intervention was organized through nine levels, and at each level, the number of prompts was reduced, i.e., an adult was at a greater distance. At the last level, adults and reinforcement were absent, and the child independently used an iPad and schedules for organizing and participating in leisure activities. Each activity was timed and had a limited duration. After the intervention, all four participants increased the percentage of successfully completed steps within leisure activity schedules. Also, there was an increase in appropriate behaviors related to using the schedules and performing leisure activities. It was determined that the obtained results persisted 2 weeks, 1 month, and 3 months after the intervention, accompanied by a high percentage of generalization.

Nepo et al. (2020) conducted two mini studies within one research in six adults with ASD with the aim to examine the effects of training in using iPad applications that the participants preferred and that they could use in their free time (e.g., listening to music on an iPad; putting together digital jigsaw puzzles; playing a digital memory game; etc.). They also wanted to evaluate the effect of training in using digital visual schedules to organize leisure time. Both studies included a baseline, training with gradually reduced prompts (full physical, gestural, and verbal), and generalization tests. During the instruction in using digital visual schedules, the participants were expected to master the following steps: checking the digital schedule application on an iPad; opening the application which was first on schedule; exiting and closing the application after hearing time expiration sound alarm; and checking and opening the activity next on the schedule. The results indicated that all participants increased their independence in doing leisure activities on an iPad after the most-to-least prompting procedure. They also increased the duration of leisure activities. On the other hand, instruction in using digital schedules had positive effects in two participants who fully mastered schedule navigation and participation in leisure activities as guided by the digital schedule. Difficulties in digital schedules were partly overcome by using an alternative printed visual schedule. The participants found it confusing that they had to leave the digital schedule application to start a leisure activity and then go back to the application after the activity. These results suggest that the development of digital applications should take into account their compatibility with individual abilities (e.g., motor skills) and their design simplicity that minimizes the barriers.

In a similar study, Brodhead et al. (2018) showed that digital schedules could improve the use of various iPad applications during leisure time in three boys with ASD. Before using digital schedules, the boys repeatedly used the same application. The participants were offered seven applications during the intervention, six of which were different games, and the seventh was YouTube. The results showed that all participants expanded their choice of leisure activities (to four applications) and the number of independently completed steps within each activity. Unfortunately, when they stopped using digital schedules, the participants returned to their old habits. However, when the schedules were re-introduced, the number of independently and successfully used applications increased to four per user.

In addition, Hill et al. (2013) point out that iPad2® can be used to teach leisure, age-appropriate activities to adults with ASD with comorbid conditions and that it can contribute to raising these people's independence in everyday life.

One group of research studies emphasized the significance of combining technological devices (such as digital schedules) with independent decision and choice making, developing schedules, and self-managing tasks for successfully practicing leisure skills. Douglas and Uphold (2014) confirmed that high school students with intellectual disability, among whom there were students with ASD, could be trained to photograph the schedule steps, use the application to self-manage task directives, and then independently follow the scheduled steps. It has often been pointed out that people with ASD prefer passive leisure activities and that digital schedules are frequently used to improve online leisure activities. Uphold et al. (2014) went one step further in their research to show that adults with disabilities, including people with ASD, were able to create, i.e., program their own fitness schedule (by choosing individual exercises) on iPod touch® by using the constant time delay technique. The mentioned studies indicate that using technological devices in practicing leisure skills also improves self-management, self-monitoring, and self-evaluation skills.

4.3.3.2 Using Video Prompting and Video Modeling to Teach Leisure Skills to Children and Adults with ASD

Cannella-Malone et al. (2016) examined the effects of video prompting on teaching leisure skills. The sample included nine participants with severe developmental disabilities, five of whom were diagnosed with ASD. The researchers evaluated each participant's preferences for specific leisure activities before the intervention. After that, they analyzed individual steps of 14 preferred activities (e.g., setting up and knocking down lines of dominos, painting one's own nails, taking a picture of oneself using an iPad, etc.). The number of steps differed between different activities and ranged from 7 to 66. A video with verbal instructions was recorded for each activity and each individual step. The intervention involved playing videos of individual steps and then providing 30 s for the participants to perform the activity they watched on the video. If the participant failed, the recording was repeated. After another failure, a teacher would demonstrate the activity after playing the video. If the participants made mistakes, the teacher applied the following prompts: full physical, partial physical, and gestural. The results showed that five participants fully mastered the steps of their leisure activities and three participants had mixed responses, while the intervention had no effect on one participant's leisure skills.

Armendariz and Hahs (2019) examined how video prompting can be applied in teaching play and social initiation skills during leisure time in three minimally verbal children with ASD, 2–9 years of age. After the parents assessed three preferred activities for each participant, one was selected for intervention (marble run, Legos, and crafting). Video prompting was organized in two differing phases. In the first phase, teachers provided students with necessary materials after watching the recorded steps, while in the second phase, the participants took the missing piece (e.g., a Lego) on their own. If necessary, other prompts were provided during both phases (e.g., gestural, physical). Although the chosen activities differed in content and the number of steps, the authors indicated that two participants successfully mastered all leisure activity steps, while one participant mastered social initiation skills. The authors also point out that it is never too early to provide support within leisure skills.

Some researchers examined the efficacy of video prompting on a single leisure activity. Those were usually the activities shown in other studies to be the preferred ones or the ones people with ASD particularly enjoyed. Thus, for example, Yanardag et al. (2012) examined how this technique can be used to teach pool skills (water games) in three children with ASD. The selected games were broken down into smaller steps, for which videos were recorded and later played on a laptop that was positioned on the edge of the pool. The participants performed the activities after watching the recordings. After a 12-week intervention, the participants improved not only pool skills but also motor performance. Gies (2012) showed that video prompting could successfully be applied in teenagers with ASD for learning Cupid Shuffle dance as a fun leisure activity. It is interesting that, after the intervention, the participants learned the dance moves and improved motor performance, but also stated that the experience made them feel great and that they enjoyed themselves, had fun, and looked forward to every subsequent session.

References

Armendariz, V., & Hahs, A. D. (2019). Teaching leisure activities with social initiations through video prompting. *Journal of Behavioral Education*. https://doi.org/10.1007/s10864-019-09320-1

Arora, P. (2011). Online social sites as virtual parks: An investigation into leisure online and offline. *The Information Society, 27*(2), 113–120.

Askari, S., Anaby, D., Bergthorson, M., Majnemer, A., Elsabbagh, M., & Zwaigenbaum, L. (2015). Participation of children and youth with autism spectrum disorder: A scoping review. *Review Journal of Autism and Developmental Disorders, 2*(1), 103–114. https://doi.org/10.1007/s40489-014-0040-7

Becerra, L. A., Higbee, T. S., Vieira, M. C., Pellegrino, A. J., & Hobson, K. (2020). The effect of photographic activity schedules on moderate-to-vigorous physical activity in children with autism spectrum disorder. *Journal of Applied Behavior Analysis*. https://doi.org/10.1002/jaba.796

Billstedt, E., Gillberg, I. C., & Gillberg, C. (2011). Aspects of quality of life in adults diagnosed with autism in childhood. *Autism, 15*(1), 7–20. https://doi.org/10.1177/1362361309346066

Bishop-Fitzpatrick, L., Smith DaWalt, L., Greenberg, J. S., & Mailick, M. R. (2017). Participation in recreational activities buffers the impact of perceived stress on quality of life in adults with autism spectrum disorder. *Autism Research, 10*(5), 973–982. https://doi.org/10.1002/aur.1753

Blum-Dimaya, A., Reeve, S. A., Reeve, K. F., & Hoch, H. (2010). Teaching children with autism to play a video game using activity schedules and game-embedded simultaneous video modeling. *Education and Treatment of Children, 33*(3), 351–370. https://doi.org/10.1353/etc.0.0103

Bohnert, A., Lieb, R., & Arola, N. (2016). More than leisure: Organized activity participation and socio-emotional adjustment among adolescents with autism spectrum disorder. *Journal of Autism and Developmental Disorders, 49*(7), 2637–2652. https://doi.org/10.1007/s10803-016-2783-8

Brajša-Žganec, A., Merkaš, M., & Šverko, I. (2011). Quality of life and leisure activities: How do leisure activities contribute to subjective well-being? *Social Indicators Research, 102*(1), 81–91. https://doi.org/10.1007/s11205-010-9724-2

Brewster, S., & Coleyshaw, L. (2011). Participation or exclusion? Perspectives of pupils with autistic spectrum disorders on their participation in leisure activities. *British Journal of Learning Disabilities, 39*(4), 284–291. https://doi.org/10.1111/j.1468-3156.2010.00665.x

Brodhead, M. T., Courtney, W. T., & Thaxton, J. R. (2018). Using activity schedules to promote varied application use in children with autism. *Journal of Applied Behavior Analysis, 51*(1), 80–86. https://doi.org/10.1002/jaba.435

Bryce, J. (2001). The technological transformation of leisure. *Social Science Computer Review, 19*(1), 7–16.

Buse, C. E. (2009). When you retire, does everything become leisure? Information and communication technology use and the work/leisure boundary in retirement. *New Media & Society, 11*(7), 1143–1161. https://doi.org/10.1177/1461444809342052

Cannella-Malone, H. I., Miller, O., Schaefer, J. M., Jimenez, E. D., Page, E. J., & Sabielny, L. M. (2016). Using video prompting to teach leisure skills to students with significant disabilities. *Exceptional Children, 82*(4), 463–478. https://doi.org/10.1177/0014402915598778

Cheng, C., & Yang, X. (2010). Study of online leisure activities – Exemplified by shopping online without initial intention. *Second International Conference on Communication Systems, Networks and Applications*. https://doi.org/10.1109/iccsna.2010.5588674

Chevallier, C., Grezes, J., Molesworth, C., Berthoz, S., & Happe, F. (2011). Brief report: Selective social anhedonia in high functioning autism. *Journal of Autism and Developmental Disorders, 42*, 1504–1509. https://doi.org/10.1007/s10803-011-1364-0

Chiang, H. M., & Wineman, I. (2014). Factors associated with quality of life in individuals with autism spectrum disorders: A review of literature. *Research in Autism Spectrum Disorders, 8*(8), 974–986. https://doi.org/10.1016/j.rasd.2014.05.003

Clark, M., & Adams, D. (2020). The self-identified positive attributes and favourite activities of children on the autism spectrum. *Research in Autism Spectrum Disorders, 72*, 101512. https://doi.org/10.1016/j.rasd.2020.101512

Conine, D. E., & Vollmer, T. R. (2019). Relative preferences for edible and leisure stimuli in children with autism. *Journal of Applied Behavior Analysis*. Advance online publication. https://doi.org/10.1002/jaba.525

Coussens, M., Van Driessen, E., De Baets, S., Van Regenmortel, J., Desoete, A., Oostra, A., Vanderstraeten, G., Waelvelde, H., & Van de Velde, D. (2020). Parents' perspectives on participation of young children with attention deficit hyperactivity disorder, developmental coordination disorder, and/or autism spectrum disorder: A systematic scoping review. *Child: Care, Health and Development, 46*(2), 232–243. https://doi.org/10.1111/cch.12735

Coyne, P., Nyberg, C., & Vandenburg, M. L. (1999). *Developing leisure time skills for persons with autism: A practical approach for home, school and community*. Future Horizons, Incorporated.

Cuhadar, S., & Diken, I. H. (2011). Effectiveness of instruction performed through activity schedules on leisure skills of children with autism. *Education and Training in Autism and Developmental Disabilities*, 386–398. https://www.jstor.org/stable/23880593

Dattilo, J., & Schlein, S. J. (1994). Understanding leisure services for individuals with mental retardation. *Mental Retardation, 32*, 53–59.

Díaz, A., Gómez, M., & Molina, A. (2017). A comparison of online and offline consumer behaviour: An empirical study on a cinema shopping context. *Journal of Retailing and Consumer Services, 38*, 44–50. https://doi.org/10.1016/j.jretconser.2017.05.003

Douglas, K. H., & Uphold, N. M. (2014). iPad® or iPod Touch®: Evaluating self-created electronic photographic activity schedules and student preferences. *Journal of Special Education Technology, 29*(3), 1–14. https://doi.org/10.1177/016264341402900301

Edrisinha, C., O'Reilly, M. F., Choi, H. Y., Sigafoos, J., & Lancioni, G. E. (2011). "Say cheese": Teaching photography skills to adults with developmental disabilities. *Research in Developmental Disabilities, 32*(2), 636–642. https://doi.org/10.1016/j.ridd.2010.12.006

Edwards, C. K., Landa, R. K., Frampton, S. E., & Shillingsburg, M. A. (2017). Increasing functional leisure engagement for children with autism using backward chaining. *Behavior Modification, 42*(1), 9–33. https://doi.org/10.1177/0145445517699929

Eversole, M., Collins, D. M., Karmarkar, A., Colton, L., Quinn, J. P., Karsbaek, R., Johnson, J. R., Callier, P., & Hilton, C. L. (2015). Leisure activity enjoyment of children with autism spectrum disorders. *Journal of Autism and Developmental Disorders, 46*(1), 10–20. https://doi.org/10.1007/s10803-015-2529-z

Fahmie, T. A., Iwata, B. A., & Jann, K. E. (2015). Comparison of edible and leisure reinforcers. *Journal of Applied Behavior Analysis, 48*, 331–343. https://doi.org/10.1002/jaba.200

Finke, E. H., Hickerson, B., & McLaughlin, E. (2015). Parental intention to support video game play by children with autism spectrum disorder: An application of the theory of planned behavior. *Language, Speech, and Hearing Services in Schools, 46*(2), 154. https://doi.org/10.1044/2015_lshss-13-0080

Finke, E. H., Hickerson, B. D., & Kremkow, J. M. (2018). "To be quite honest, if it wasn't for videogames I wouldn't have a social life at all": Motivations of young adults with autism spectrum disorder for playing videogames as leisure. *American Journal of Speech-Language Pathology, 27*(2), 672–689. https://doi.org/10.1044/2017_AJSLP-17-0073

García-Villamisar, D. A., & Dattilo, J. (2010). Effects of a leisure programme on quality of life and stress of individuals with ASD. *Journal of Intellectual Disability Research, 54*(7), 611–619. https://doi.org/10.1111/j.1365-2788.2010.01289.x

Garcia-Villamisar, D., & Dattilo, J. (2011). Social and clinical effects of a leisure program on adults with autism spectrum disorder. *Research in Autism Spectrum Disorders, 5*(1), 246–253. https://doi.org/10.1016/j.rasd.2010.04.006

Genoe, R., Kulczycki, C., Marston, H., Freeman, S., Musselwhite, C., & Rutherford, H. (2018). E-leisure and older adults: Findings from an international exploratory study. *Therapeutic Recreation Journal, 52*(1), 1–18. https://doi.org/10.18666/TRJ-2018-V52-I1-8417

Gershuny, J. (2003). Web use and net nerds: A neofunctionalist analysis of the impact of information technology in the home. *Social Forces, 82*, 141–168. https://doi.org/10.1353/sof.2003.0086

Gies, M. (2012). *The use of video prompting on the acquisition, maintenance, and generalization of a line dance by adolescents with autism spectrum disorders*. Doctoral dissertation, The Ohio State University.

Godbey, G. (2000). The future of leisure studies. *Journal of Leisure Research, 32*(1), 37–41. https://doi.org/10.1080/00222216.2000.11949883

Henderson, K. A. (2010). Leisure studies in the 21st century: The sky is falling? *Leisure Sciences, 32*(4), 391–400. https://doi.org/10.1080/01490400.2010.488614

Hesselmark, E., Plenty, S., & Bejerot, S. (2014). Group cognitive behavioural therapy and group recreational activity for adults with autism spectrum disorders: A preliminary randomized controlled trial. *Autism, 18*(6), 672–683. https://doi.org/10.1177/1362361313493681

Hill, D. A., Belcher, L., Brigman, H. E., Renner, S., & Stephens, B. (2013). The Apple iPad™ as an innovative employment support for young adults with autism spectrum disorder and other developmental disabilities. *Journal of Applied Rehabilitation Counseling, 44*(1), 28–37. https://doi.org/10.1891/0047-2220.44.1.28

Hilton, C. L., Crouch, M. C., & Israel, H. (2008). Out-of-school participation patterns in children with high-functioning autism spectrum disorders. *American Journal of Occupational Therapy, 62*, 554–563. https://doi.org/10.5014/ajot.62.5.554

Hilton, C., Eversole, M., & Collins, D. (2016). Enjoyment of leisure activities experienced by children with autism spectrum disorders. *American Journal of Occupational Therapy, 70*(4_Supplement_1), 7011505095p1. https://doi.org/10.5014/ajot.2016.70S1-RP401B

Hilton, C. L., Ratcliff, K., & Hong, I. (2020). Participation difficulties in autism spectrum disorders and intellectual disabilities: Findings from the 2011 survey of pathway to diagnosis and services. *Journal of Autism and Developmental Disorders*. https://doi.org/10.1007/s10803-020-04591-4

Hochhauser, M., & Engel-Yeger, B. (2010). Sensory processing abilities and their relation to participation in leisure activities among children with high-functioning autism spectrum disorder (HFASD). *Research in Autism Spectrum Disorders, 4*(4), 746–754. https://doi.org/10.1016/j.rasd.2010.01.015

Howel, E., & Pierson, M. (2010). Parents' perspectives on the participation of their children with autism in Sunday school. *Journal of Religion, Disability & Health, 14*(2), 153–166.

Ivy, J. W., Payne, J., & Neef, N. A. (2019). Increasing across-session variability of leisure activity selection for children with autism. *Behavior Analysis: Research and Practice, 19*(3), 261–272. https://doi.org/10.1037/bar0000132

Jerome, J., Frantino, E. P., & Sturmey, P. (2007). The effects of errorless learning and backward chaining on the acquisition of internet skills in adults with developmental disabilities. *Journal of Applied Behavior Analysis, 40*(1), 185–189. https://doi.org/10.1901/jaba.2007.41-06

Juniu, S. (2000). Downshifting: Regaining the essence of leisure. *Journal of Leisure Research, 32*(1), 69–73. https://doi.org/10.1080/00222216.2000.11949888

Kelly A., Carlile Sharon A., Reeve Kenneth F., Reeve Ruth M., DeBar (2013). Using Activity Schedules on the iPod touch to Teach Leisure Skills to Children with Autism. *Education and Treatment of Children, 36*(2), 33–57. https://doi.org/10.1353/etc.2013.0015

King, G. A., Law, M., King, S., Hurley, P., Hanna, S., Kertoy, M., & Rosenbaum, P. (2006). Measuring children's participation in recreation and leisure activities: Construct validation of the CAPE and PAC. *Child: Care, Health and Development, 33*(1), 28–39. https://doi.org/10.1111/j.1365-2214.2006.00613.x

Kuo, M. H., Orsmond, G. I., Coster, W. J., & Cohn, E. S. (2014). Media use among adolescents with autism spectrum disorder. *Autism: The International Journal of Research and Practice, 18*(8), 914–923. https://doi.org/10.1177/1362361313497832

Kurnaz, E., & Yanardag, M. (2018). The effectiveness of video self-modeling in teaching active video game skills to children with autism spectrum disorder. *Journal of Developmental and Physical Disabilities, 30*(4), 455–469. https://doi.org/10.1007/s10882-018-9596-y

Kurt, O., & Tekin-Iftar, E. (2008). A comparison of constant time delay and simultaneous prompting within embedded instruction on teaching leisure skills to children with autism. *Topics in Early Childhood Special Education, 28*(1), 53–64. https://doi.org/10.1177/0271121408316046

Kuykendall, L., Lei, X., Zhu, Z., & Hu, X. (2020). Leisure choices and employee well-being: Comparing need fulfillment and well-being during TV and other leisure activities. *Applied Psychology. Health and Well-Being, 12*(2), 532–558. https://doi.org/10.1111/aphw.12196

LaVesser, P., & Berg, C. (2011). Participation patterns in preschool children with an autism spectrum disorder. *OTJR: Occupation, Participation and Health, 31*(1), 33–39. https://doi.org/10.3928/15394492-20100823-01

Leung, L., & Lee, P. S. (2005). Multiple determinants of life quality: The roles of Internet activities, use of new media, social support, and leisure activities. *Telematics and Informatics, 22*(3), 161–180. https://doi.org/10.1016/j.tele.2004.04.003

Liu, H. (2014). Personality, leisure satisfaction, and subjective well-being of serious leisure participants. *Social Behavior and Personality: An International Journal, 42*(7), 1117–1125. https://doi.org/10.2224/sbp.2014.42.7.1117

Liu, H., Yeh, C. K., Chick, G. E., & Zinn, H. C. (2008). An exploration of meanings of leisure: A Chinese perspective. *Leisure Sciences, 30*(5), 482–488. https://doi.org/10.1080/01490400802353257

López Sintas, J., Rojas de Francisco, L., & García Álvarez, E. (2015). The nature of leisure revisited: An interpretation of digital leisure. *Journal of Leisure Research, 47*, 79–101.

Mannell, R. C., & Kleiber, D. A. (1997). *A social psychology of leisure*. Venture.

Marques, J. S., Regalado, I. C. R., Galvão, É. R. V. P., Ferreira, H. N. C., Longo, E., & Lindquist, A. R. R. (2020). Participation in leisure activities from the perception of children with disabilities and their families in Brazil. *Journal of Rehabilitation Medicine*. https://doi.org/10.2340/16501977-2768

Mazurek, M. O., & Wenstrup, C. (2012). Television, video game and social media use among children with ASD and typically developing siblings. *Journal of Autism and Developmental Disorders, 43*(6), 1258–1271. https://doi.org/10.1007/s10803-012-1659-9

Mazurek, M. O., Engelhardt, C. R., & Clark, K. E. (2015). Video games from the perspective of adults with autism spectrum disorder. *Computers in Human Behavior, 51*, 122–130. https://doi.org/10.1016/j.chb.2015.04.062

McCarron, M. (2018). Clinical corner: Leisure skills for adults with autism. *Science in Autism Treatment, 15*(2), 19–26.

Mineo, B. A., Ziegler, W., Gill, S., & Salkin, D. (2008). Engagement with electronic screen media among students with autism spectrum disorders. *Journal of Autism and Developmental Disorders, 39*(1), 172–187. https://doi.org/10.1007/s10803-008-0616-0

Mommaas, H. (1997). European leisure studies at the crossroads? A history of leisure research in Europe. *Leisure Sciences, 19*(4), 241–254. https://doi.org/10.1080/01490409709512253

Mowatt, R. A. (2018). A people's history of leisure studies: Leisure, the tool of racecraft. *Leisure Sciences, 40*(7), 663–674. https://doi.org/10.1080/01490400.2018.1534622

Nepo, K., Tincani, M., & Axelrod, S. (2020). Teaching mobile device-based leisure to adults with autism spectrum disorder and intellectual disability. *Focus on Autism and Other Developmental Disabilities*, 108835762094350. https://doi.org/10.1177/1088357620943500

Newman, D. B., Tay, L., & Diener, E. (2014). Leisure and subjective well-being: A model of psychological mechanisms as mediating factors. *Journal of Happiness Studies, 15*(3), 555–578. https://doi.org/10.1007/s10902-013-9435-x

Nieto, C., Murillo, E., Belinchón, M., Giménez, A., Saldaña, D., Martínez, M. Á., & Frontera, M. (2015). Supporting people with autism spectrum disorders in leisure time: Impact of an University Volunteer Program, and related factors. *Anales de Psicología/Annals of Psychology, 31*(1), 145–154. https://doi.org/10.6018/analesps.31.1.166591

Nimrod, G., & Adoni, H. (2012). Conceptualizing e-leisure. *Loisir et Société/Society and Leisure, 35*(1), 31–56. https://doi.org/10.1080/07053436.2012.10707834

O'Brien, K. (2010). Recreation and children with autism: A critical appraisal of the topic. *Journal of Occupational Therapy, Schools, & Early Intervention, 3*(1), 61–75. https://doi.org/10.1080/19411241003684159

Obrusnikova, I., & Cavalier, A. (2011). Perceived barriers and facilitators of participation in after-school physical activity by children with autism spectrum disorders. *Journal of Developmental and Physical Disabilities, 23*, 195–211. https://doi.org/10.1007/s10882-010-9215-z

Obrusnikova, I., & Miccinello, D. (2012). Parent perceptions of factors influencing after-school physical activity of children with autism spectrum disorders. *Adapted Physical Activity Quarterly, 29*, 63–80. https://doi.org/10.1123/apaq.29.1.63

Orsmond, G. I., & Kuo, H. Y. (2011). The daily lives of adolescents with an autism spectrum disorder: Discretionary time use and activity partners. *Autism, 15*(5), 579–599. https://doi.org/10.1177/1362361310386503

Orsmond, G. I., Krauss, M. W., & Seltzer, M. M. (2004). Peer relationships and social and recreational activities among adolescents and adults with autism. *Journal of Autism and Developmental Disorders, 34*(3), 245–256. https://doi.org/10.1023/b:jadd.0000029547.96610.df

Potvin, M. C., Snider, L., Prelock, P., Kehayia, E., & Wood-Dauphinee, S. (2013). Recreational participation of children with high functioning autism. *Journal of Autism and Developmental Disorders, 43*, 445–457. https://doi.org/10.1007/s10803-012-1589-6

Ratcliff, K., Hong, I., & Hilton, C. (2018). Leisure participation patterns for school age youth with autism spectrum disorders: Findings from the 2016 national survey of children's health. *Journal of Autism and Developmental Disorders, 48*(11), 3783–3793. https://doi.org/10.1007/s10803-018-3643-5

Roberts, K. (2018). Writing about leisure. *World Leisure Journal, 60*(1), 3–13. https://doi.org/10.1080/16078055.2016.1261645

Ropke, I., & Godskesen, M. (2007). Leisure activities, time and environment. *International Journal of Innovation and Sustainable Development, 2*(2), 155. https://doi.org/10.1504/ijisd.2007.016931

Rosqvist, H. B. (2017). Exploring meanings of leisure among people with autism: "To have some fun on your own". *Research and Practice in Intellectual and Developmental Disabilities, 5*(1), 39–46. https://doi.org/10.1080/23297018.2017.1324737

Schulz, P., Schulte, J., Raube, S., Disouky, H., & Kandler, C. (2018). The role of leisure interest and engagement for subjective well-being. *Journal of Happiness Studies, 19*(4), 1135–1150. https://doi.org/10.1007/s10902-017-9863-0

Shane, H. C., & Albert, P. D. (2008). Electronic screen media for persons with autism spectrum disorders: Results of a survey. *Journal of Autism and Developmental Disorders, 38*(8), 1499–1508. https://doi.org/10.1007/s10803-007-0527-5

Shattuck, P., Orsmond, G., Wagner, M., & Cooper, B. (2011). Participation in social activities among adolescents with an autism spectrum disorder. *PLoS One, 6*(11), e27176. https://doi.org/10.1371/journal.pone.0027176

Shattuck, P. T., Narendorf, S. C., Cooper, B., Sterzing, P. R., Wagner, M., & Taylor, J. L. (2012). Postsecondary education and employment among youth with an autism spectrum disorder. *Pediatrics, 129*(6), 1042–1049. https://doi.org/10.1542/peds.2011-2864

Simone, P. M., & Haas, A. L. (2013). Frailty, leisure activity and functional status in older adults: Relationship with subjective well being. *Clinical Gerontologist, 36*(4), 275–293. https://doi.org/10.1080/07317115.2013.788114

Simpson, K., Keen, D., Adams, D., Alston-Knox, C., & Roberts, J. (2018). Participation of children on the autism spectrum in home, school, and community. *Child: Care, Health and Development, 44*(1), 99–107. https://doi.org/10.1111/cch.12483

Slanzi, C. M., Graziano, M., D'Angelo, G., Vollmer, T. R., & Conine, D. E. (2019). Relative preferences for edible and leisure stimuli in children with autism: A replication in Italy. *Journal of Applied Behavior Analysis*. https://doi.org/10.1002/jaba.666

Solish, A., Perry, A., & Minnes, P. (2010). Participation of children with and without disabilities in social, recreational and lei- sure activities. *Journal of Applied Research in Intellectual Disabilities, 23*, 226–236. https://doi.org/10.1111/j.1468-3148.2009.00525.x

Spriggs, A. D. (2011). *Video modeling and observational learning to teach recreation and leisure skills to students with autism*. Doctoral dissertation, University of Georgia.

Spriggs, A. D., Gast, D. L., & Knight, V. F. (2016). Video modeling and observational learning to teach gaming access to students with ASD. *Journal of Autism and Developmental Disorders, 46*(9), 2845–2858. https://doi.org/10.1007/s10803-016-2824-3

Stacey, T. L., Froude, E. H., Trollor, J., & Foley, K. R. (2018). Leisure participation and satisfaction in autistic adults and neurotypical adults. *Autism*, 136236131879127. https://doi.org/10.1177/1362361318791275

Stebbins, R. A. (1982). Serious leisure: A conceptual statement. *The Pacific Sociological Review, 25*(2), 251–272.

Stebbins, R. A. (1997). Casual leisure: A conceptual statement. *Leisure Studies, 16*(1), 17–25. https://doi.org/10.1080/026143697375485

Stromer, R., Kimball, J. W., Kinney, E. M., & Taylor, B. A. (2006). Activity schedules, computer technology, and teaching children with autism spectrum disorders. *Focus on Autism and Other Developmental Disabilities, 21*(1), 14–24. https://doi.org/10.1177/10883576060210010301

Taheri, A., Perry, A., & Minnes, P. (2016). Examining the social participation of children and adolescents with intellectual disabilities and autism spectrum disorder in relation to peers. *Journal of Intellectual Disability Research, 60*(5), 435–443. https://doi.org/10.1111/jir.12289

Taylor, J. L., & Seltzer, M. M. (2012). Developing a vocational index for adults with autism spectrum disorders. *Journal of Autism and Developmental Disorders, 42*(12), 2669–2679. https://doi.org/10.1007/s10803-012-1524-x

Tint, A., Maughan, A. L., & Weiss, J. A. (2017). Community participation of youth with intellectual disability and autism spectrum disorder. *Journal of Intellectual Disability Research, 61*(2), 168–180. https://doi.org/10.1111/jir.12311

Tsai, A. (2019). *Teaching the leisure skill of photography to children with autism spectrum disorder*. CMC Senior Theses.

Turygin, N. C., & Matson, J. L. (2014). Adaptive behavior, life skills, and leisure skills training for adolescents and adults with autism spectrum disorders. In *Adolescents and adults with autism spectrum disorders* (pp. 131–160). Springer.

Ullenhag, A., Granlund, M., Almqvist, L., & Krumlinde-Sundholm, L. (2020). A strength-based intervention to increase participation in leisure activities in children with neuropsychiatric disabilities: A pilot study. *Occupational Therapy International*. https://doi.org/10.1155/2020/1358707

UN General Assembly. (1948). *Universal declaration of human rights* (217 [III] A). Paris.

Uphold, N. M., Douglas, K. H., & Loseke, D. L. (2014). Effects of using an iPod app to manage recreation tasks. *Career Development and Transition for Exceptional Individuals, 39*(2), 88–98. https://doi.org/10.1177/2165143414548572

Veal, A. J. (2004). A brief history of work and its relationship to leisure. *Work and Leisure*, 15–33.

Venkatesan, S. (2005). Activity log of preschool children with developmental disabilities and autism spectrum disorders. *Asia Pacific Disability Rehabilitation Journal, 16*(1), 68–76.

Vuran, S. (2008). Empowering leisure skills in adults with autism: An experimental investigation through the most to least prompting procedure. *International Journal of Special Education, 23*(1), 174–181.

Watkins, M., & Bond, C. (2007). Ways of experiencing leisure. *Leisure Sciences, 29*(3), 287–307. https://doi.org/10.1080/01490400701259985

Wiese, C. W., Kuykendall, L., & Tay, L. (2018). Get active? A meta-analysis of leisure-time physical activity and subjective well-being. *The Journal of Positive Psychology, 13*(1), 57–66. https://doi.org/10.1080/17439760.2017.1374436

World Health Organization. (2001). *ICF: International Classification of Functioning, Disability and Health*. World Health Organization.

Yanardag, M., Akmanoglu, N., & Yilmaz, I. (2012). The effectiveness of video prompting on teaching aquatic play skills for children with autism. *Disability and Rehabilitation, 35*(1), 47–56. https://doi.org/10.3109/09638288.2012.687030

Yılmaz, I., Birkan, B., Konukman, F., & Erkan, M. (2005). Using a constant time delay procedure to teach aquatic play skills to children with autism. *Education and Training in Developmental Disabilities*, 171–182.

Žumárová, M. (2015). Computers and children's leisure time. *Procedia-Social and Behavioral Sciences, 176*, 779–786. https://doi.org/10.1016/j.sbspro.2015.01.540

Chapter 5
Community Living

5.1 Community Living: Conceptual Definition

For people with disabilities, community living is both a goal to be pursued and a way to achieve many others (Myers et al., 1998). The phrase "community living" has been used in the literature since the late 1950s to denote a movement that emerged as an alternative to the institutional care of people with disabilities. Twenty years later, community living became a replacement for institutional living, and this term was closely linked to the deinstitutionalization movement (Mansell, 2006). Bearing in mind the changes in the meaning of this phrase over time, it is not surprising that the concept of community living is nowadays closely related to social inclusion.

According to Simplican et al. (2015), social inclusion includes two domains—interpersonal relationships and community participation (Fig. 5.1). Interpersonal relationships can be viewed through formal and informal or family and intimate relationships. Although community participation is frequently mentioned and researched in people with disabilities, the literature is inconsistent regarding its conceptualization, definition, and operationalization.

The International Classification of Functioning, Disability and Health (ICF) (WHO, 2001) defines community participation as the participation of individuals in social activities in their community through interacting with others. ICF (WHO, 2001) mentions four domains of community participation—(1) domestic life, (2) interpersonal life, (3) major life activities, and (4) community, civic, and social life (Fig. 5.2).

According to a different approach, community living involves participating in various categories of activities in three forms—mainstream, segregated activities (most often in segregated centers or groups for people with disabilities), and semi-segregated (e.g., participating in activities within community facilities with the help

N. Glumbić et al., *Digital Inclusion of Individuals with Autism Spectrum Disorder*, Autism and Child Psychopathology Series,
https://doi.org/10.1007/978-3-031-12037-4_5

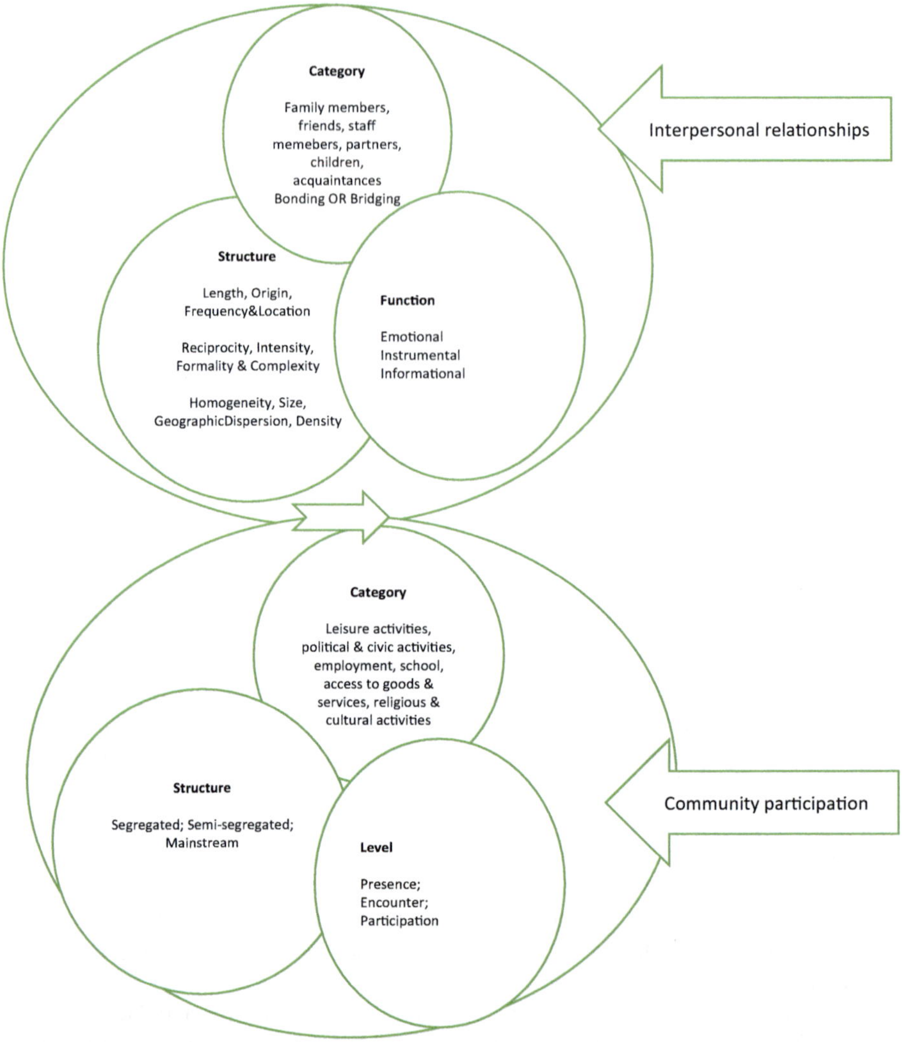

Fig. 5.1 Social inclusion model. (Adapted from Simplican et al., 2015)

of paid staff or family members or within segregated facilities but with the help of volunteers or other community representatives). Levels of participation vary and range from physical presence without contact with other people, through short encounters, to full cooperation and participation (Simplican et al., 2015).

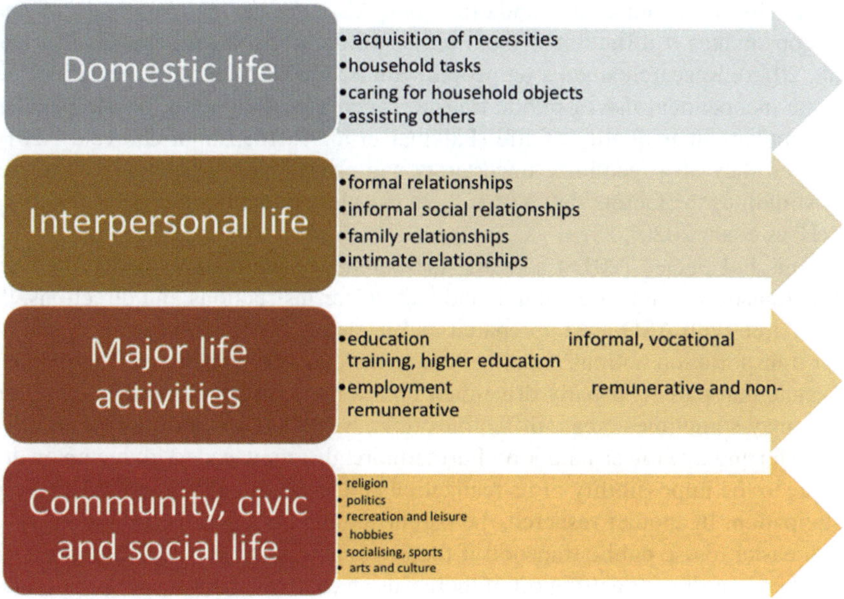

Fig. 5.2 Graphic representation of community participation according to ICF

Chang et al. (2013) believe that community participation should be observed separately from family and institutional housing activities, i.e., from domestic roles. When discussing community involvement, Chang et al. (2013) mention that these activities must be "intrinsically social," not necessarily involving physical presence in the community but also remote access. These authors relate community participation with nondomestic roles, i.e., roles of workers, friends, neighbors, etc.

5.2 Participation in Community Living of People with ASD

Various research studies indicate that most adults with ASD live with their parents or are in care (Billstedt et al., 2005; Gray et al., 2014).

Regarding their participation in daily community activities, adults with ASD most frequently participate in day programs or sheltered workshops. Also, it is noticeable that they tend to participate in activities organized by other people in the community instead of taking the initiative (Gray et al., 2014). Over 80% of adults with ASD are not independent in moving through the community. In other words, these people rely on the transportation organized by their parents or other adults in their environment since their independent walks are hindered by the inability to estimate distances and understand directions. Also, not having clear maps of roads and stops makes it difficult for them to use public transport independently (Deka et al., 2016). Research studies on people with ASD show that these people believe that the independent use of public transport increases their sense of independence and improves their quality of life (Falkmer et al., 2015; Lubin & Feeley, 2016). However, they also recognize uncertainty and crowds accompanied by other sensory stimuli as the factors that bother them in public transport and affect their anxiety (Haas et al., 2020).

Lubin and Feeley (2016) add that the parents of children with ASD feel that public transport is not safe enough and lacks clear instructions and directions, that the children with ASD are unprepared and inadequately trained to use it, and that other transportation options are either unavailable or very expensive. These authors also state that parents usually drive their children to various community activities, which may sometimes create difficulties (e.g., being late to work, losing their job, or transferring to a lower-paid job). Furthermore, this may lead to giving up on driving due to the impossibility of its realization and, consequently, the child's reduced participation. In another research, the parents pointed out that their children would find it easier to use public transport if there was less noise, if the children had support when boarding or getting off, if there was an easier way for them to ask for help through easily accessible buttons or visual aids, and, finally, if that routine was entirely predictable for them (Lim et al., 2021).

On the other hand, when the parents were interviewed about their children's ability to drive, they expressed concern, fear, and doubt that their children with ASD could drive independently (Cox et al., 2012). Daly et al. (2014) examined the experiences of drivers with ASD. They found that these people got a driving license significantly later than their peers, drove less frequently, had more rigid driving rules (e.g., not driving at night or in heavy traffic), and were more often involved in traffic accidents.

When transitioning from adolescence to adulthood, young people with ASD face another significant factor that hinders their community participation—the end of schooling (accompanied by numerous structured activities and contents) (Myers et al., 2015).

Examining the predictors of community participation in adults with ASD, Chan et al. (2020) emphasized communication skills, daily living skills, access to public transport, and access to religious communities as four significant involvement factors. This study showed that community size, population, and development were not predictors of participation.

5.3 The Role of Technology in Community Living of People with Autism

Digital technology is considered the main facilitator in social inclusion and community living in people with disabilities. However, research results indicate that, although some efforts have been made to develop various technological devices,

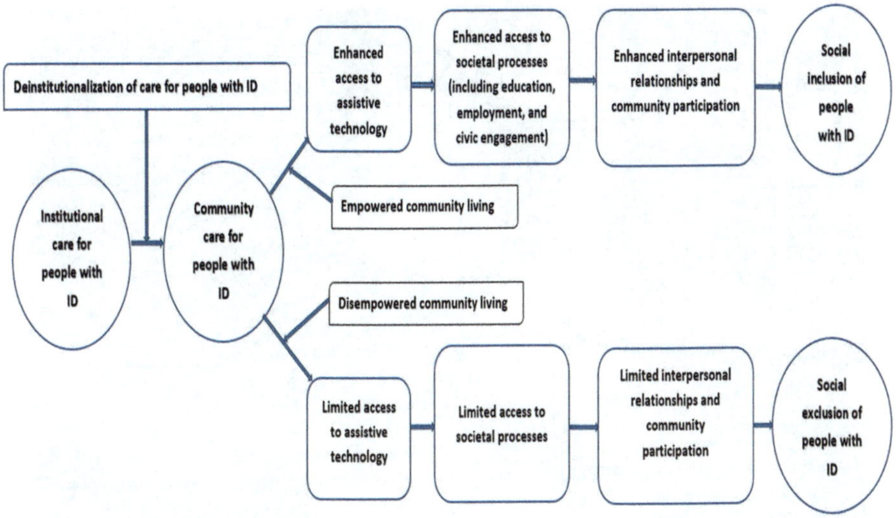

Fig. 5.3 Access to technologies and community living transformations for people with intellectual disability. (Reproduced from Owuor et al., 2017)

there is no significant progress in achieving full implementation of technological advances. Manzoor and Vimarlund (2018) believe that the characteristics of the labor market, social market, and political sphere should be considered in addition to the development of technological devices.

Similarly, Owuor et al. (2017) analyzed the role of technology in the lives of people with intellectual disability. They found that technology was a significant aspect of normalization in these people's lives, allowing them to interact with people from their environment, access services, and be more mobile and independent (Fig. 5.3).

Parsons et al. (2016) point out several factors that could contribute to the greater use of technological advances in the lives of people with ASD. These factors include greater accessibility, universal design, and conducting participatory research that would provide answers to what devices, programs, and applications people with ASD need and what they consider useful and important for improving their community participation.

5.4 Use of Technology to Improve Access to Goods and Services for People with ASD

Technological devices that include visual schedules can be very useful for developing community skills in people with ASD. One research study shows that, by using an iPhone and digital self-managed activity schedule, people with ASD can master

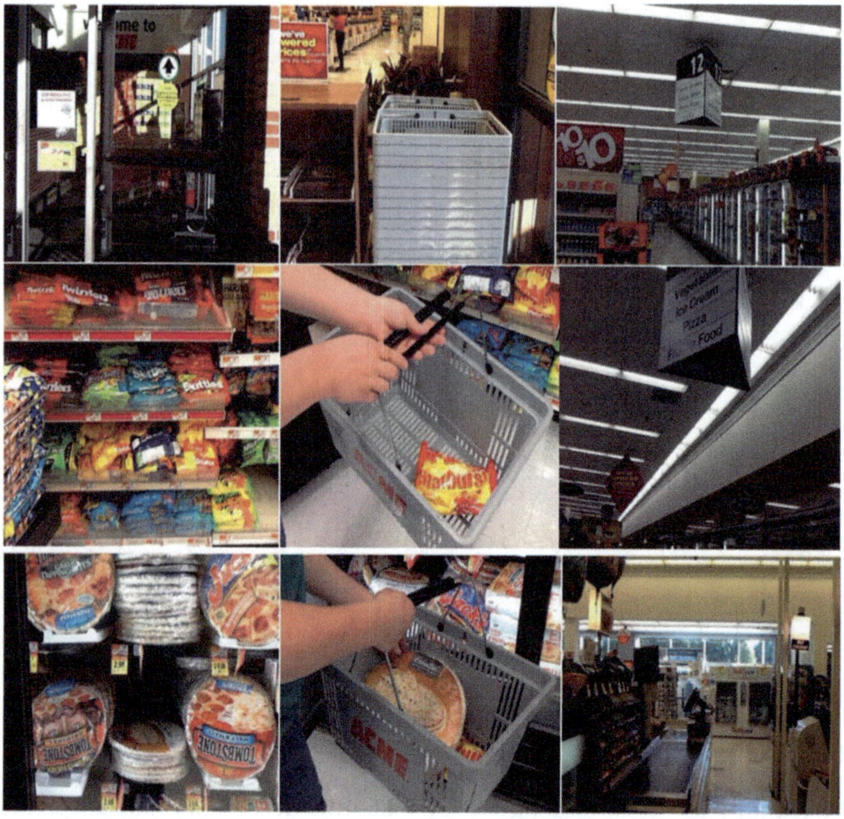

Fig. 5.4 Example of visual and video prompts that can be used in teaching grocery shopping skills to people with ASD. (Reproduced from Burckley et al., 2015)

all the steps of buying goods in a bakery (e.g., from taking a tray, choosing food, paying, to leaving the bakery) and use the acquired skills in their community over time (Cheung et al., 2016).

Similar research used an iPad with visual cues and video prompting to improve grocery shopping skills in young people with ASD and intellectual disability (from entering the store, taking a basket, choosing groceries, to going to the checkout). Realistic photographs and videos of all nine grocery shopping steps were made for the purpose of this research and inserted into an iPad (Fig. 5.4). The training and generalization tests were performed in an actual store in the community. Burckley et al. (2015) pointed out that an iPad with inserted prompts could be considered an important tool in teaching community skills to people with ASD.

Weng and Bouck (2014) used an iPad with visual cues and video prompting to test its effectiveness in teaching three adolescents with ASD to compare prices when shopping. The research was conducted with three participants in two different settings—a classroom and actual grocery stores. The task of comparing prices was broken down into 18 steps, and a video was recorded for each step. The participants watched the videos on an iPad. They practiced with 34 products previously estimated to be frequently purchased. Three different brands with different prices were prepared for each product. Also, this research used an 18″ × 2″, paper-based, horizontal number line, containing the numbers 0–19 arranged from left to right. This line was plastic-coated, and the users could write on it with a marker and wipe it. The participants were expected to watch the videos before each step (e.g., observing the numbers on prices before decimals; finding the price of the first product on the number line; rounding that amount; repeating these steps for the second and third product; choosing the product with the lowest price; putting that product in the basket; erasing previously drawn circles). If, after ten trials, the participant did not benefit from watching the videos, the following prompts were hierarchically introduced—hand-over-hand assistance with verbal cues, a model with verbal cues, gesture with verbal cues, and verbal cues only. The results indicated that this teaching method had positive outcomes for two participants. Weng and Bouck (2014) suggested that future research should focus on teaching people with ASD to buy a product based on its quality, amount, or personal preference.

Lamash et al. (2017) pointed out that virtual reality (VR) could be used to improve skills at a supermarket. Their research included 56 adolescents with ASD (33 of whom were involved in the intervention) and used the Virtual Action Planning Supermarket (VAP-S) program. This program involves using a laptop or a desktop and requires the use of keyboard arrows and a mouse. Lamash et al. (2017) showed that VR technology could improve metacognitive strategies in grocery shopping in young people with ASD, such as making a shopping list, sorting groceries by category, comparing prices, paying, and faster and more skilled shopping.

In the virtual practice of shopping skills, Thomsen and Adjorlu (2021) suggested using virtual shopping lists along with virtual baskets, fruit and vegetable scales, and virtual money. They also propose including teachers who can use head-mounted display-based technology to express emotions, use gestures, or take on different roles in the same virtual environment depending on the needs of a person with ASD involved in the shopping process. Other authors also reported the positive effects of head-mounted display-based VR on shopping skills (Adjorlu et al., 2017; Adjorlu & Serafin, 2018).

Young people with ASD need training in the community skills related to going to cafes, bars, and clubs, which also develop adequate social skills in these people. VR technology has very frequently been used for these purposes. Parsons et al. (2004) included 12 teenagers with ASD in their research on using simple VR technology to practice skills, such as sitting at a table in a café, ordering food and drinks, and paying a check. The participants were expected to answer questions asked by a computer and use a mouse and a joystick for interaction and navigation. Although it was expected that these people's problems in executive functions would adversely affect their skills in a virtual café, that did not happen. It was assumed that virtual environment, clear instructions, and a predetermined sequence of steps contributed to the success of people with ASD in these tasks. Furthermore, it was encouraging that most people with ASD understood the relation between the virtual environment and the real world and, at the same time, differentiated between reality and representation. This was shown in their comments on the similarities and differences between videos of an actual and virtual bar in the VR game.

Subsequently, Mitchell et al. (2006) aimed to examine whether a VR café could also be used to improve social understanding and judgment outside a virtual environment. Their research included six people with ASD 14–16 years of age. Over 6 weeks, Mitchell et al. (2006) taught people with ASD to find a free seat with the help of a VR café (in situations when the tables were not occupied, partially occupied, or completely occupied). Then, they checked to what extent the acquired knowledge could be applied to the videos of cafes and buses. The results showed that, over time, the participants improved their skills in the VR café tasks and generalized the acquired skills to other contexts. However, this study did not answer whether the acquired skills were permanent and whether the participants could use the improved social understanding skills from the VR café in real life.

5.5 Using Technology to Improve Community Mobility

The ability to move independently from one location to another can, in people with ASD, be considered a prerequisite for their community participation. Josman et al. (2008) believe that crossing the street is the first precondition of independent moving through the environment. These authors also state that the previously used methods of teaching this skill to children with ASD were usually considered unsuccessful since they were implemented in a classroom and not in the natural context. To overcome the existing drawbacks, Josman et al. (2008) used a street-crossing desktop virtual environment with PECS symbols in 12 participants (six of whom were diagnosed with ASD with moderate and severe symptoms) to develop their street-crossing skills. A participant, who appeared in the program as an avatar, was supposed to decide when it was safe to cross a four-lane street, where there were a traffic light and a pedestrian crossing. The program included nine difficulty levels. Success at one level meant going on to the next, and vice versa, failure at a current level returned the participant to the previous one. The results showed that five participants learned how to use the simulation program and three improved their street-crossing skills, i.e., after the completed training, they stopped at pedestrian crossings, looked left and right before crossing the street, and waited for the green light, which they had not done before. Interestingly, the participants' age and the severity of ASD were not related to their success in using this computer program.

Saiano et al. (2015) went one step further, examining whether virtual environments and natural interfaces could be successfully used to teach people with ASD how to cross a street in order to reach their destination—a pharmacy or a police station. This research included seven participants, 19–44 years of age, who used Microsoft Kinect for interacting with a virtual standard urban environment. The results showed that this method was effective in teaching people with ASD to follow street signs and arrive at their destination by crossing the street at a pedestrian crossing. Saiano et al. (2015) did not directly examine whether this training influenced the participants' skills, but they asked the parents whether they had noticed an improvement in their child's ability to move through the environment. The parents reported that their children's street-crossing skills had improved.

Goldsmith (2008) included five participants with ASD, 9–15 years of age, in the research on the effects of a VR program for developing street-crossing skills. Before the training, the participants were tested in a natural environment. After that, verbal instructions, modeling, and feedback were used to introduce VR equipment (a joystick) to the participants so that they could learn how to use it before the training phase. After the preparatory phases and the baseline, they moved on to the training phase, in which four versions of virtual space were used. Depending on the difficulty level, these virtual space versions included traffic lanes, parking places, pedestrian crossings, sidewalks, traffic signs, moving cars, distractors, and sound stimuli (e.g., a horn). The results showed that all five participants mastered crossing the street even with various distractors. However, the generalization of acquired skills in the natural context was not equal in all participants. Goldsmith (2008) believed that the reasons for somewhat weaker generalization could be found in the fact that the virtual environment differed from natural (e.g., in appearance and content), that it included unexpected stimuli, and that potential dangers were more emphasized in the virtual environment.

The results of other studies showed that immersive VR also positively affected teaching people with ASD to cross a street (Alharbi et al., 2020; Dixon et al., 2020; Tzanavari et al., 2015).

Honsberger (2015) examined to what extent video modeling with in situ video prompting feedback could be an effective strategy in teaching five people with ASD (6–21 years of age) to walk safely across a parking lot. The video presented an adult who performed the target behavior and provided short, slow, and clear explanations of the performed activities for each step (walking to the front of the car; walking in front of the parked car; walking between parked cars; looking right and left; going to the destination). After watching the video, the participants with ASD performed the steps accompanied by a teacher. In case of performing a step incorrectly, the teacher physically directed the participant to the video scene that was done wrong or skipped. The results indicated that two out of five participants fully mastered all steps after watching the video just once. The remaining three participants required slightly more practice, but they also learned all the skills needed to walk safely across a parking lot. The main limitation of this study was that generalization was not tested, i.e., it remained unclear whether the participants would walk across some other parking lots successfully.

In addition to the street-crossing skill, reading symbols and maps is also important for moving safely around the environment and finding destinations. McKissick et al. (2013) conducted a research study on using computer-assisted explicit instruction to teach three people with ASD to read food, toilet, and exit symbols on three maps (school, shopping mall, and park). This research used slides with audio and visual stimuli (Fig. 5.5). After hearing "Your turn," the participants were expected to choose and press the required symbol (indicated by an arrow) from three different

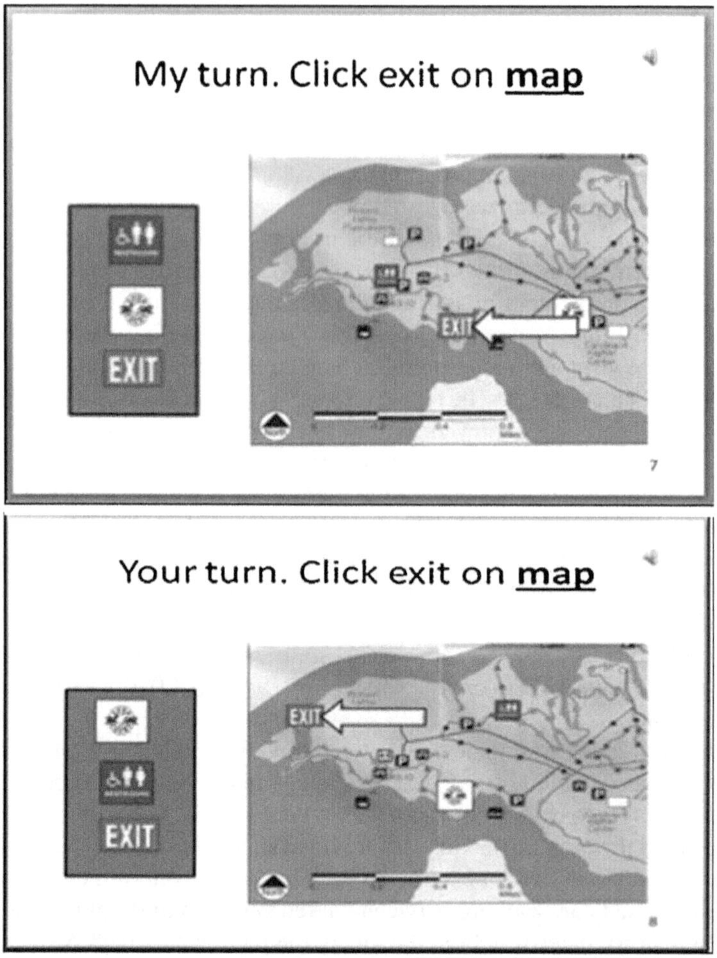

Fig. 5.5 Example of slides with text and sound icons. (Reproduced from McKissick et al., 2013)

symbols on a map. The symbols were in different places on different slides. Then, the arrow stopped appearing, and only the verbal stimulus remained. Two out of three participants made significant progress in understanding and following symbols on a map, while the third showed minimal changes. The first two participants were also able to generalize the acquired skills to unfamiliar maps.

Training people with ASD to drive independently would undoubtedly contribute to easier access to various services. However, the usual driver training methods do not mainly achieve the expected results in people with ASD. Therefore, to overcome this difficulty, VR-based driving simulator programs are often designed to improve the driving skills of people with ASD. VR technology is considered appropriate for driver training since it provides safety and security to the program user. Furthermore, this type of intervention is motivating for people with ASD as they are believed to show a preference for technology. Also, VR technology makes it possible to gather a lot of information about the user's behavior during virtual driving, which is considered significant for predicting real situations in traffic. Bian et al. (2013) created a driving simulation program and tested it in 12 young people with ASD. Within this program, the participants were expected to virtually drive a vehicle without making mistakes and by paying attention to important objects in the environment (e.g., traffic lights, pedestrians, traffic signs, etc.). Although the results were obtained from a small sample, the authors considered them very encouraging.

Zhang et al. (2014) pointed out that a driving simulator should completely suit the user, i.e., that the driving task should be neither too easy nor too difficult, but in accordance with the driver's condition and characteristics. Thus, these authors used a VR-based driving simulator in seven teenagers with ASD, 13–17 years of age, to monitor their success and level of engagement in driving tasks. They collected this data from professionals' observations that reported whether participants expressed engagement, enjoyment, anxiety, and boredom while doing different tasks.

After that, these researchers pointed out that data on the reactions and possible anxiety of people with ASD while driving should not be collected solely on the basis of therapists' and observers' remarks but also with the help of specific devices. Thus, in their following research, Bian et al. (2015) tested the accuracy and precision of the CorrelationAttributeEval algorithm in detecting affective and physiological characteristics of drivers with ASD during driving simulation (Bian et al., 2015). Bian et al. (2015) believe that precise identification of affective factors in people with ASD is very significant, if not crucial, for creating an adequate intervention aiming to improve driving skills in these people.

Bian et al. (2016) upgraded this simulator, making it fully adaptable to each user with flexibility in changing the parameters of driving (responsiveness of brake pedal, of accelerator pedal, and of the steering wheel) and the environment (intensity of light in the environment, speed of agent vehicles) and, at the same time, monitoring the driver's physiological indicators (photoplethysmogram, galvanic skin response, and respiration).

Finally, Wade et al. (2016) used this upgraded VR-based driving simulator in 20 young people with ASD over 6 weeks. They concluded that this type of driver training could be effective, i.e., that the participants had a significantly smaller number of errors in the post-test. However, they did not examine whether these results could be generalized to real driving situations and all people with ASD.

Since public transport is considered a more economical and safer option, many authors studied the possibility of creating and using applications that would enable people with ASD to use public transport independently. Rezae et al. (2019) started a process of developing a mobile application that included the following steps—gathering information on the needs of people with ASD in public transport and designing a mobile application that would satisfy the needs of people with ASD through an imaginary character with ASD and the route it should follow. This process resulted in the OrienTrip application that enabled better public transport planning regarding the person's current location, desired destination, time, cost, and traffic jams. This application could guide a passenger with ASD step by step from

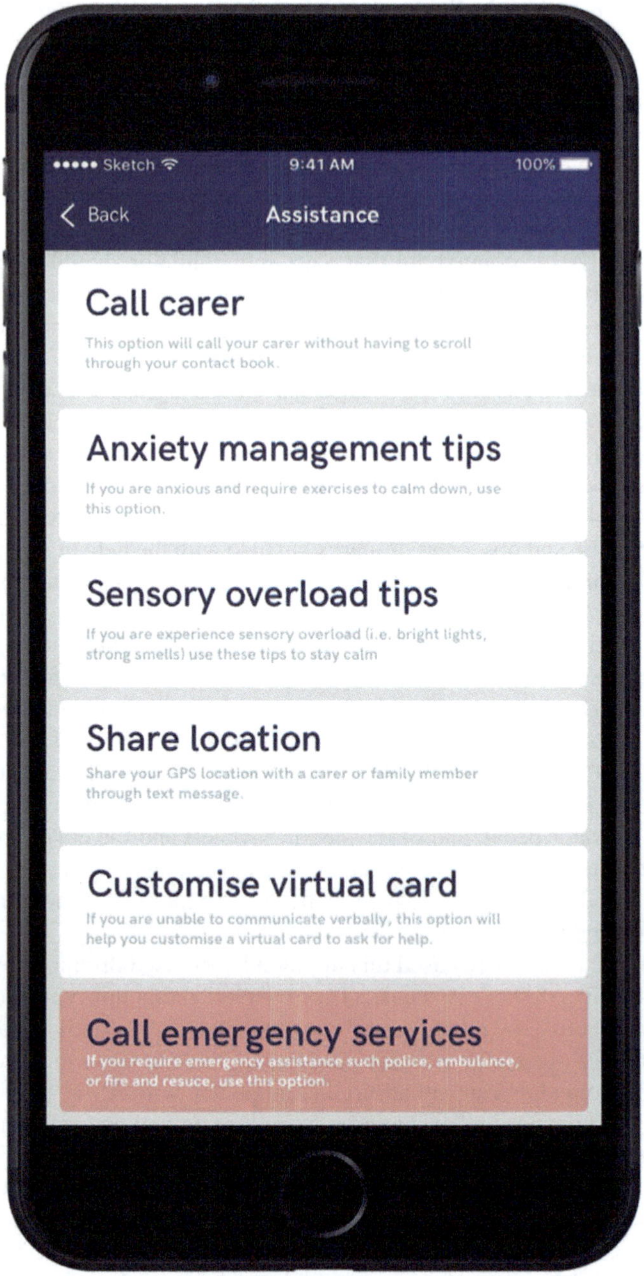

Fig. 5.6 Options offered by the OrienTrip application. (Reproduced from Rezae et al., 2020)

the beginning to the end of the transit. Also, this application allows people with ASD to easily contact a person and share their location without leaving the application (Fig. 5.6).

Rezae et al. (2020) used OrienTrip in 16 people with ASD and 22 professionals. The results showed that both groups agreed that using public transport was easier with the help of this application.

Playing VR serious games with clear instructions can also enhance the skills needed for independent use of public transport in people with ASD (Bernardes et al., 2015). Furthermore, VR technology is considered helpful in preparing people with ASD to travel by plane (Miller et al., 2020; Soccini et al., 2020).

Access to tourist attractions is often closely related to traveling. Transportation problems can adversely affect the tourism of people with ASD. However, tourist visits can also be hindered by these people's resistance to change, fear of the unknown, insufficient information about the sensory characteristics of the location, etc. With regard to that, and in order to relieve the stress of people with ASD while traveling, Cena et al. (2020) developed the Personalized Interactive Urban Maps for Autism (PIUMA), a map of tourist locations that people with ASD can choose according to their preferences or avoid according to their aversions. In addition to the information about the location, distance, and ways of reaching a place, this application also provides numerical data—from one to five—about the intensity of lighting, the average number of visitors at a specific time, level of noise, present and dominant odors, and temperature.

5.6 The Role of Technology in Interpersonal Relationships of People with ASD

Community living also includes occasional interactions with various service providers. Due to difficulties in social communication, people with ASD can face great challenges in making contacts, asking for help, or requesting additional information in their community. These skills are usually practiced through frequent role-play or repeated reading of social stories. However, McCleery et al. (2020) believe that these traditional techniques have drawbacks, especially when preparing people with ASD to contact police officers. These contacts are often sudden, unplanned, and highly stressful. McCleery et al. (2020) believe the wireless immersive VR technology can be very useful in preparing people with ASD to interact with police officers. Their research included 60 verbal participants with ASD, 12–38 years of age. The aim was to examine to what extent VR technology was safe in teaching people with ASD to contact police officers, i.e., whether it contributed to their anxiety and sensory hypersensitivity. The participants were divided into two groups—one group was involved in one 45-min session, while the other group attended three sessions during which they talked to virtual police officers. The Floreo Police Safety Module VR tool was used in this research. It uses an application that links an iPhone in a lightweight headset worn by the participant to an iPad held by the intervention provider via wireless Internet connection. The rate of mild adverse effects reported in the first session decreased in the subsequent two sessions. Only one participant left the study because he experienced dizziness, shivers, and nausea while using this VR tool. The results showed that this technology was safe, applicable, and with no adverse effects in verbal participants with ASD. Furthermore, the participants' experiences indicated that this approach was useful, that they felt more ready to meet with police officers, and that they found the activity interesting and realistic. Also, the participants gave guidelines for improving the program, indicating that various types of meetings with police officers should be included (since the existing scenario included just one), that voices should vary (in pitch and tone), that additional characters should be introduced, etc.

Apart from service providers, we also have daily contact with various shop assistants. Shopping requires specific communication skills as well. Some authors point out that video-based instruction can be successfully used to improve the interpersonal skills of people with ASD in shopping situations (e.g., greeting a shop assistant back; responding to a shop assistant's greeting with a smile; saying "Thank you" when done with shopping; or responding to questions such as "Do you need a bag? Would you like anything else? Is that all?") (Alcantara, 1994; Haring et al., 1987; Yakubova & Taber-Doughty, 2013).

In order to improve interpersonal interactions in people with ASD in shopping situations, Wahlbrink (2017) used an iPhone with the List Recorder application (an application with numerous sound recording, listening, and pausing options used to direct the participants to forthcoming steps) and wireless earphones (that allowed the participant to hear the sequence of steps). The training took place in an actual store (Dunkin Donuts), and the generalization process was tested in three Starbucks coffee shops. The intervention aimed to improve the following skills: greeting the shop assistant, ordering (requesting) goods, short communication while paying, and saying goodbye and thanking. All three participants improved their interpersonal shopping skills and generalized them successfully to a new environment. The limitations referred to the participants sometimes turning off the iPhone or putting it into a pocket and then needing more time to get back to the application and the list of steps. Also, the earphones occasionally fell out of the participants' ears, and putting them back slowed them down or distracted them.

Since interpersonal activities within a community are both formal and informal, Boyd et al. (2015) examined to what extent technology could be used to improve membership, partnership, and friendship in school-age children with ASD. The research included eight students with ASD within the ABAB design. The participants were divided into pairs. Each pair played Lego, traditional bricks (during the first and the third weeks), and Zody's World, collaborative iPad game (during the second and fourth weeks), three times a week, sharing one iPod and one set of bricks. Boyd et al. (2015) believed that playing collaborative video games could contribute to the physical closeness between people with ASD and other players and improve their interaction initiative, collaborative behavior, and sharing joy. The authors explained these results by stating that the iPad size indicated the inevitable closeness and sharing, that clear roles at different levels helped the players achieve interactions, and that turn-taking in alternately pressing two keys, or synchronization of movements in situations when they were expected to press two keys simultaneously, strengthened cooperation and partnership. Hourcade et al. (2012) also reported the positive outcomes of collaborative applications (for drawing, creating music, solving visual puzzles, and emotion modeling) on a multi-touch tablet and their influence on improving social interactions between students with ASD.

In addition to collaborative desktop games, virtual environments alone can be a space for making friends for some young people with ASD. Rizzo et al. (2012) mention The Lab, a technology club for young people with autism, as a place that will gather adolescents interested in computers and games and create an opportunity for them to socialize. Rizzo et al. (2012) point out that this club requires one room with high-speed Internet and LAN network that can support up to 20 participants and that uses some of the following software—Minecraft, RPG Maker, Game Maker, CuteHTML, and Comic Life. Donahoo and Steele (2013) used The Lab concept in their research on adolescents, 10–16 years of age, with high-functioning autism. The participants came to The Lab, where they worked on developing various applications once a week throughout one school year, with the help of a mentor, but with no structured units, tasks, or expectations in terms of assessment. The participants were very happy to attend these meetings and reported that they liked to come, socialize, and work on developing the game they created. Donahoo and Steele (2013) also pointed out the challenges they encountered, which included funding the activities in the lab and the problem with waiting lists of interested people and their parents. Ng (2017) also indicated that The Lab could be a good opportunity for young people with ASD to socialize and communicate. In this research, 16 young people came to The Lab once a week for 12 weeks with their own laptops. Their task was to form groups and create an online world within Minecraft—a 3D sandbox simulation game. It turned out that the participants communicated with each other in weekly gatherings more than usual, i.e., that network sociality fully functioned since the participants communicated with each other about their needs and completed activities. It is also interesting that although they shared physical space, these participants tended to communicate online (instead of talking to each other directly) even when sitting in close proximity. Addressing these specificities, Ng (2017) used the phrase "the physicality of technology," pointing out that online socializing helped people with ASD not to worry about whether they should adhere to the general rules of face-to-face communication, i.e., that such contacts were quite relaxing for them. Being physically distant from the place of gatherings, some people cannot participate in The Lab. Therefore, certain authors developed the Online Lab concept. Schutt (2018) used the WordPress platform for Online Lab in his research, within which 13 participants uploaded or downloaded various attachments. The results showed that some young people with ASD enjoyed participating in this technology club through remote access and that it contributed to strengthening their relationships with other people.

References

Adjorlu, A., & Serafin, S. (2018). Head-mounted display-based virtual reality as a tool to teach money skills to adolescents diagnosed with autism spectrum disorder. In *Interactivity, game creation, design, learning, and innovation* (pp. 450–461). Springer. https://doi.org/10.1007/978-3-030-06134-0_48

Adjorlu, A., Hoeg, E. R., Mangano, L., & Serafin, S. (2017). Daily living skills training in Virtual Reality to help children with autism spectrum disorder in a real shopping scenario. In *2017 IEEE international symposium on mixed and augmented reality (ISMAR-Adjunct)*. https://doi.org/10.1109/ismar-adjunct.2017.93

Alcantara, P. R. (1994). Effects of videotape instructional package on purchasing skills of children with autism. *Exceptional Children, 61*(1), 40–55. https://doi.org/10.1177/001440299406100105

Alharbi, A., Aloufi, S., Assar, R., & Meccawy, M. (2020). Virtual Reality street-crossing training for children with autism in Arabic language. In *2020 international conference on innovation and intelligence for informatics, computing and technologies (3ICT)* (pp. 1–6). IEEE.

Bernardes, M., Barros, F., Simoes, M., & Castelo-Branco, M. (2015). A serious game with virtual reality for travel training with autism spectrum disorder. In *2015 international conference on virtual rehabilitation (ICVR)* (pp. 127–128). IEEE.

Bian, D., Wade, J. W., Zhang, L., Bekele, E., Swanson, A., Crittendon, J. A., Sarkar, M., Warren, Z., & Sarkar, N. (2013). A novel virtual reality driving environment for autism intervention. In M. Antona & C. Stephanidis (Eds.), *International conference on universal access in human-computer interaction* (pp. 474–483). Springer. https://doi.org/10.1007/978-3-319-20684-4_66

Bian, D., Wade, J., Swanson, A., Warren, Z., & Sarkar, N. (2015). Physiology-based affect recognition during driving in virtual environment for autism intervention. In *International conference on physiological computing systems* (Vol. 2, pp. 137–145). SCITEPRESS.

Bian, D., Wade, J., Warren, Z., & Sarkar, N. (2016). Online engagement detection and task adaptation in a Virtual Reality based driving simulator for autism intervention. In M. Antona & C. Stephanidis (Eds.), *Universal access in human-computer interaction. Users and context diversity* (UAHCI 2016. Lecture Notes in Computer Science) (Vol. 9739). Springer. https://doi.org/10.1007/978-3-319-40238-3_51

Billstedt, E., Gillberg, C., & Gillberg, C. (2005). Autism after adolescence: Population-based 13- to 22-year follow-up study of 120 individuals with autism diagnosed in childhood. *Journal of Autism and Developmental Disorders, 35*(3), 351–360. https://doi.org/10.1007/s10803-005-3302-5

Boyd, L. E., Ringland, K. E., Haimson, O. L., Fernandez, H., Bistarkey, M., & Hayes, G. R. (2015). Evaluating a collaborative iPad game's impact on social relationships for children with autism spectrum disorder. *ACM Transactions on Accessible Computing (TACCESS), 7*(1), 1–18. https://doi.org/10.1145/2751564

Burckley, E., Tincani, M., & Guld Fisher, A. (2015). An iPad™-based picture and video activity schedule increases community shopping skills of a young adult with autism spectrum disorder and intellectual disability. *Developmental Neurorehabilitation, 18*(2), 131–136. https://doi.org/10.3109/17518423.2014.945045

Cena, F., Mauro, N., Ardissono, L., Mattutino, C., Rapp, A., Cocomazzi, S., Brighenti, S., & Keller, R. (2020). *Adjunct publication of the 28th ACM conference on user modeling, adaptation and personalization* (pp. 347–351). https://doi.org/10.1145/3386392.3399280

Chan, D. V., Klinger, M. R., Adkisson, K. A., & Klinger, L. G. (2020). Examining environmental predictors of community participation for adults with autism spectrum disorder using geographic information systems (GIS). *Journal of Autism and Developmental Disorders*, 1–7. https://doi.org/10.1007/s10803-020-04660-8

Chang, F.-H., Coster, W. J., & Helfrich, C. A. (2013). Community participation measures for people with disabilities: A systematic review of content from an international classification of functioning, disability and health perspective. *Archives of Physical Medicine and Rehabilitation, 94*(4), 771–781. https://doi.org/10.1016/j.apmr.2012.10.031

Cheung, Y., Schulze, K. A., Leaf, J. B., & Rudrud, E. (2016). Teaching community skills to two young children with autism using a digital self-managed activity schedule. *Exceptionality, 24*(4), 241–250. https://doi.org/10.1080/09362835.2016.1215654

Cox, N. B., Reeve, R. E., Cox, S. M., & Cox, D. J. (2012). Brief report: Driving and young adults with ASD: Parents' experiences. *Journal of Autism and Developmental Disorders, 42*(10), 2257–2262. https://doi.org/10.1007/s10803-012-1470-7

Daly, B. P., Nicholls, E. G., Patrick, K. E., Brinckman, D. D., & Schultheis, M. T. (2014). Driving behaviors in adults with autism spectrum disorders. *Journal of Autism and Developmental Disorders, 44*(12), 3119–3128. https://doi.org/10.1007/s10803-014-2166-y

Deka, D., Feeley, C., & Lubin, A. (2016). Travel patterns, needs, and barriers of adults with autism spectrum disorder. *Transportation Research Record: Journal of the Transportation Research Board, 2542*(1), 9–16. https://doi.org/10.3141/2542-02

Dixon, D. R., Miyake, C. J., Nohelty, K., Novack, M. N., & Granpeesheh, D. (2020). Evaluation of an immersive virtual reality safety training used to teach pedestrian skills to children with autism spectrum disorder. *Behavior Analysis in Practice, 13*(3), 631–640. https://doi.org/10.1007/s40617-019-00401-1

Donahoo, D., & Steele, E. (2013). *Evaluation of The Lab: A technology club for young people with Asperger's Syndrome*. Young and Well Cooperative Research Centre.

Falkmer, M., Barnett, T., Horlin, C., Falkmer, O., Siljehav, J., Fristedt, S., Lee, H., Derserri, C., Wretstrand, A., & Falkmer, T. (2015). Viewpoints of adults with and without Autism Spectrum Disorders on public transport. *Transportation Research Part A: Policy and Practice, 80*, 163–183. https://doi.org/10.1016/j.tra.2015.07.019

Goldsmith, T. R. (2008). *Using virtual reality enhanced behavioral skills training to teach street-crossing skills to children and adolescents with Autism Spectrum Disorders*. Western Michigan University.

Gray, K. M., Keating, C. M., Taffe, J. R., Brereton, A. V., Einfeld, S. L., Reardon, T. C., & Tonge, B. J. (2014). Adult outcomes in autism: Community inclusion and living skills. *Journal of Autism and Developmental Disorders, 44*(12), 3006–3015. https://doi.org/10.1007/s10803-014-2159-x

Haas, K., Wilson, N. J., Cordier, R., Vaz, S., & Chung-yeung Lee, H. (2020). *The experiences of young autistic adults in using metropolitan public transport*. Cooperative Research Centre for Living with Autism.

Haring, T. G., Kennedy, C. H., Adams, M. J., & Pitts-Conway, V. (1987). Teaching generalization of purchasing skills across community settings to autistic youth using videotape modeling. *Journal of Applied Behavior Analysis, 20*(1), 89–96. https://doi.org/10.1901/jaba.1987.20-89

Honsberger, T. (2015). *Teaching individuals with autism spectrum disorder safe pedestrian skills using video modeling with in situ video prompting*. Florida Atlantic University.

Hourcade, J. P., Bullock-Rest, N. E., & Hansen, T. E. (2012). Multitouch tablet applications and activities to enhance the social skills of children with autism spectrum disorders. *Personal and Ubiquitous Computing, 16*(2), 157–168. https://doi.org/10.1007/s00779-011-0383-3

Josman, N., Ben-Chaim, H. M., Friedrich, S., & Weiss, P. L. (2008). Effectiveness of virtual reality for teaching street-crossing skills to children and adolescents with autism. *International Journal on Disability and Human Development, 7*(1), 49–56. https://doi.org/10.1515/ijdhd.2008.7.1.49

Lamash, L., Klinger, E., & Josman, N. (2017). Using a virtual supermarket to promote independent functioning among adolescents with Autism Spectrum Disorder. In *2017 international conference on virtual rehabilitation (ICVR)* (pp. 1–7). IEEE. https://doi.org/10.1109/icvr.2017.8007467

Lim, P. Y., Kong, P., Cornet, H., & Frenkler, F. (2021). Facilitating independent commuting among individuals with autism – A design study in Singapore. *Journal of Transport & Health, 21*, 101022. https://doi.org/10.1016/j.jth.2021.101022

Lubin, A., & Feeley, C. (2016). Transportation issues of adults on the autism spectrum. *Transportation Research Record: Journal of the Transportation Research Board, 2542*(1), 1–8. https://doi.org/10.3141/2542-01

Mansell, J. (2006). Deinstitutionalisation and community living: Progress, problems and priorities. *Journal of Intellectual and Developmental Disability, 31*(2), 65–76. https://doi.org/10.1080/13668250600686726

Manzoor, M., & Vimarlund, V. (2018). Digital technologies for social inclusion of individuals with disabilities. *Health and Technology, 8*(5), 377–390. https://doi.org/10.1007/s12553-018-0239-1

McCleery, J. P., Zitter, A., Solórzano, R., Turnacioglu, S., Miller, J. S., Ravindran, V., & Parish-Morris, J. (2020). Safety and feasibility of an immersive virtual reality intervention program for teaching police interaction skills to adolescents and adults with autism. *Autism Research, 13*(8), 1418–1424. https://doi.org/10.1002/aur.2352

McKissick, B. R., Spooner, F., Wood, C. L., & Diegelmann, K. M. (2013). Effects of computer-assisted explicit instruction on map-reading skills for students with autism. *Research in Autism Spectrum Disorders, 7*(12), 1653–1662. https://doi.org/10.1016/j.rasd.2013.09.013

Miller, I. T., Wiederhold, B. K., Miller, C. S., & Wiederhold, M. D. (2020). Virtual reality air travel training with children on the autism spectrum: A preliminary report. *Cyberpsychology, Behavior, and Social Networking, 23*(1), 10–15. https://doi.org/10.1089/cyber.2019.0093

Mitchell, P., Parsons, S., & Leonard, A. (2006). Using virtual environments for teaching social understanding to 6 adolescents with autistic spectrum disorders. *Journal of Autism and Developmental Disorders, 37*(3), 589–600. https://doi.org/10.1007/s10803-006-0189-8

Myers, F., Ager, A., Kerr, P., & Myles, S. (1998). Outside looking in? Studies of the community integration of people with learning disabilities. *Disability and Society, 13*, 389–413. https://doi.org/10.1080/09687599826704

Myers, E., Davis, B. E., Stobbe, G., & Bjornson, K. (2015). Community and social participation among individuals with autism spectrum disorder transitioning to adulthood. *Journal of Autism and Developmental Disorders, 45*(8), 2373–2381. https://doi.org/10.1007/s10803-015-2403-z

Ng, L. E. (2017). Technology as an extension of the self: Socialising through technology for young people with autism. In *International conference of design, user experience, and usability* (pp. 393–402). Springer. https://doi.org/10.1007/978-3-319-58640-3_28

Owuor, J., Larkan, F., & MacLachlan, M. (2017). Leaving no-one behind: Using assistive technology to enhance community living for people with intellectual disability. *Disability and Rehabilitation: Assistive Technology, 12*(5), 426–428. https://doi.org/10.1080/17483107.2017.1312572

Parsons, S., Mitchell, P., & Leonard, A. (2004). The use and understanding of virtual environments by adolescents with autistic spectrum disorders. *Journal of Autism and Developmental Disorders, 34*, 449–466. https://doi.org/10.1023/B:JADD.0000037421.98517.8d

Parsons, S., Yuill, N., Good, J., Brosnan, M., Austin, L., Singleton, C., & Bossavit, B. (2016). What technology for autism needs to be invented? Idea generation from the autism community via the ASCmeI. T. app. In *International conference on computers helping people with special needs* (pp. 343–350). Springer. https://doi.org/10.1007/978-3-319-41267-2_49

Rezae, M., McMeekin, D., Tan, T., Krishna, A., Lee, H., & Falkmer, T. (2019). Public transport planning tool for users on the autism spectrum: From concept to prototype. *Disability and Rehabilitation: Assistive Technology*, 1–11. https://doi.org/10.1080/17483107.2019.1646818

Rezae, M., McMeekin, D., Tan, T., Krishna, A., & Lee, H. (2020). Evaluating the effectiveness of an autism-specific public transport app for individuals on the autism spectrum: A pilot study. *Disability and Rehabilitation: Assistive Technology*, 1–16. https://doi.org/10.1080/17483107.2020.1785563

Rizzo, A., Schutt, S., & Linegar, D. (2012). Imagine that: Creating a 'third space' for young people with high-functioning autism through the use of technology in a social setting. In *Proceedings of the 24th Australian computer-human interaction conference* (pp. 513–516).

Saiano, M., Pellegrino, L., Casadio, M., Summa, S., Garbarino, E., Rossi, V., Dall'Agata, D., & Sanguineti, V. (2015). Natural interfaces and virtual environments for the acquisition of street crossing and path following skills in adults with Autism Spectrum Disorders: A feasibility study. *Journal of Neuroengineering and Rehabilitation, 12*(1), 1–13. https://doi.org/10.1186/s12984-015-0010-z

Schutt, S. (2018). The Online Lab: Piloting video-based digital participation for isolated young people with high functioning autism. *The Journal of Community Informatics, 14*(1). https://doi.org/10.15353/joci.v14i1.3406

Simplican, S. C., Leader, G., Kosciulek, J., & Leahy, M. (2015). Defining social inclusion of people with intellectual and developmental disabilities: An ecological model of social networks and community participation. *Research in Developmental Disabilities, 38*, 18–29. https://doi.org/10.1016/j.ridd.2014.10.008

Soccini, A. M., Cuccurullo, S. A. G., & Cena, F. (2020). Virtual Reality experiential training for individuals with autism: The airport scenario. In *International conference on virtual reality and augmented reality* (pp. 234–239). Springer. https://doi.org/10.1007/978-3-030-62655-6_16

Thomsen, L. A., & Adjorlu, A. (2021). A collaborative Virtual Reality supermarket training application to teach shopping skills to young individuals with autism spectrum disorder. In *2021 IEEE conference on virtual reality and 3D user interfaces abstracts and workshops (VRW)* (pp. 50–55). IEEE. https://doi.org/10.1109/VRW52623.2021.00015

Tzanavari, A., Charalambous-Darden, N., Herakleous, K., & Poullis, C. (2015). Effectiveness of an Immersive Virtual Environment (CAVE) for teaching pedestrian crossing to children with PDD-NOS. In *2015 IEEE 15th international conference on advanced learning technologies* (pp. 423–427). IEEE.

Wade, J., Zhang, L., Bian, D., Fan, J., Swanson, A., Weitlauf, A., Sarkar, M., Warren, Z., & Sarkar, N. (2016). A gaze-contingent adaptive virtual reality driving environment for intervention in individuals with autism spectrum disorders. *ACM Transactions on Interactive Intelligent Systems (TiiS), 6*(1), 1–23. https://doi.org/10.1145/2892636

Wahlbrink, L. L. (2017). *Use of an iPhone to enhance interpersonal daily living skills in the community for adolescents with autism spectrum disorder*. Doctoral dissertation, Florida Atlantic University.

Weng, P.-L., & Bouck, E. C. (2014). Using video prompting via iPads to teach price comparison to adolescents with autism. *Research in Autism Spectrum Disorders, 8*(10), 1405–1415. https://doi.org/10.1016/j.rasd.2014.06.014

World Health Organization (WHO). (2001). *International classification of functioning, disability and health*. WHO.

Yakubova, G., & Taber-Doughty, T. (2013). Effects of video modeling and verbal prompting on social skills embedded within a purchasing activity for students with special education. *Journal of Special Education Technology, 28*(1), 35–47. https://doi.org/10.1177/016264341302800104

Zhang, L., Wade, J. W., Bian, D., Swanson, A., Warren, Z., & Sarkar, N. (2014). Data fusion for difficulty adjustment in an adaptive virtual reality game system for autism intervention. In *International conference on human-computer interaction* (pp. 648–652). Springer.

Chapter 6
Daily Living

6.1 Introduction

DLS are an adaptive behavior category that includes three main areas: personal, domestic, and community. Personal skills include eating, getting dressed, personal hygiene, and healthcare. Domestic skills are related to household chores, such as preparing food and cleaning. Community skills focus on out-of-home functioning and activities such as managing money, transportation, safety, rights, responsibilities, etc. (Sparrow et al., 2016). These are routine self-care activities that most people perform daily without the help of others (Tsikinas et al., 2017). They provide independence at home, at school, and in a community and are usually acquired at a certain developmental age (e.g., most children 8–10 years old can bathe on their own). DLS usually require teaching, practicing, and feedback before they can be performed independently. Mastering and independence in performing these skills are a basis for achieving important goals in adulthood, such as keeping a job and living independently (Duncan et al., 2018, 2021).

People with ASD have significantly worse DLS than expected regarding their cognitive abilities and chronological age, and they can have deficits even if they do not have intellectual disability (Alvares et al., 2020; Duncan & Bishop, 2015; Kanne et al., 2011). Although DLS develop in adolescence in people with ASD (Bal et al., 2015), they often plateau or become worse in adulthood, especially after finishing school (Clarke et al., 2021) or in their late 20s (Smith et al., 2012).

According to Pérez-Fuster et al. (2019), acquiring DLS is a priority in educating people with ASD, especially those with intellectual disability, for at least three reasons: self-confidence and self-esteem, reducing dependence on others, and increasing the chances of getting and keeping a job. Better developed DLS in people with ASD are associated with more positive outcomes in employment, independent living, and friendship (Duncan et al., 2018).

N. Glumbić et al., *Digital Inclusion of Individuals with Autism Spectrum Disorder*, Autism and Child Psychopathology Series,
https://doi.org/10.1007/978-3-031-12037-4_6

Digital technology can help people with ASD learn DLS. For example, the meta-analysis of Karami et al. (2021) shows that, in people with ASD, instruction based on virtual reality has the strongest effect in teaching DLS (compared to cognitive skills, emotion regulation and recognition skills, social and communication skills) and that these effects are not achieved by conventional teaching. Thus, they encourage professionals to use this technology to teach DLS. Digital technology can improve the ways in which people with ASD practice these skills. It also allows them to use touch screens, sensors, cameras, and visual and audio cues to recognize the activity they need to perform and automatically get the next one (Baragash et al., 2020). Digital technology encourages independence in the learning process and increases the control an individual has over this process.

The following pages are dedicated to games, applications, and video-based instruction used to improve DLS in people with ASD.

6.2 Personal Skills

Developed hygiene habits are of great importance because of their short- and long-term benefits. They are key to full integration into modern society and improving social relations (Hayes & Hosaflook, 2013). In addition to causing physical discomfort, poor personal hygiene skills can also cause long-term health problems, negatively affect self-confidence and social acceptance, and increase dependence on others (Kang & Chang, 2019). Although relatively rare in terms of their significance, some games and applications have been developed specifically for this DLS area.

Aurasma is a free application that provides users with an augmented reality experience by pairing a visual marker created by the user with launching digital content (picture, video, and/or audio material). The application uses a camera to identify the marker for launching a video. Cihak et al. (2016) used this application to launch a toothbrushing video model. A static image of five-step task analysis, placed horizontally next to a sink, was used as a marker. The video model was a video of a 7-year-old girl brushing her teeth. The video was made from the child's perspective. When the picture was scanned by an iPod camera, the video automatically started and continuously displayed all task analysis steps accompanied by narration. The video was placed under the image-reinforcer to create an augmented reality experience. Three elementary students with ASD participated in the study. They were first presented with everything they needed to brush their teeth. Then they got a verbal prompt to perform the task. The teacher would say, "[student's name] scan the picture and brush your teeth," pointing to a static image of brushing teeth. If the students did not independently start the first step within 5 s, or if they did not finish the step within 10 s, the teacher helped them by using the least prompts system. All participants learned to brush their teeth independently and maintained this skill for 9 weeks after the intervention.

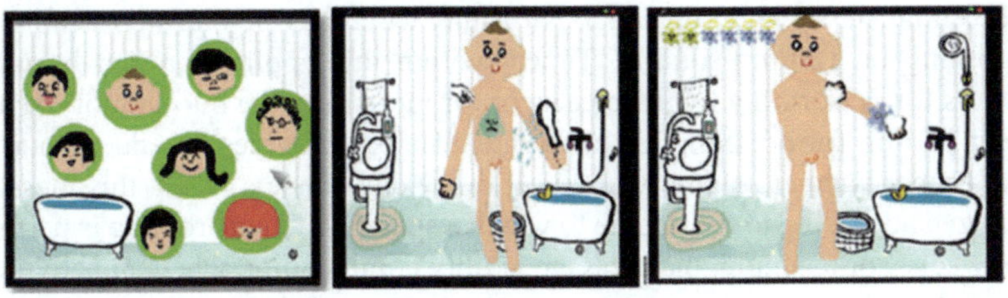

Fig. 6.1 Scenes from the video game "Take a Show-er"—selecting a role, wetting the body, and applying the shampoo. (Reproduced from Kang & Chang, 2019)

Take a Show-er is a one-player video game that teaches children with ASD to take a shower (Fig. 6.1). The game is based on Kinect motion recognition technology according to 25 steps identified as important when performing this skill. It starts with a child choosing a favorite cartoon model by holding the hand over the selected model on the screen for 3 s. The child's body movements control the model's movements, including undressing, taking a hand shower, and turning the water on/off. To make the game more fun, a water fairy is used as a visual sign that moves around the model's body parts, directing the child to make them wet. For example, to prompt the child to wet the chest, the fairy stops at the chest of the cartoon model. Points are awarded when the child points the hand shower precisely at the water fairy. Similarly, an animated germ demon marks the model's body parts that need to be washed. The result is generated based on how many body parts of the model the child washes by using a wand that is activated by performing showering movements in front of the Kinect camera. Reinforcement is provided by a cute small animal that appears on the screen and praises the child (e.g., "You're great!") when the action is performed correctly. In addition, the face of the germ demon turns sad before disappearing when that body part is washed. Kang and Chang (2019) evaluated the effectiveness of this game in four boys and two girls with ASD 9–12 years of age. The students played the game twice a week at school for 11 weeks and then independently took a shower at home. The parents monitored the showering process but gave no verbal instructions nor intervened in any other way. The children's achievements in task correctness increased as soon as the game was introduced, and all participants acquired and maintained the skills for independently taking a shower.

HygieneHelper is a cellphone application that supports young people with ASD in learning and maintaining healthy hygiene. It includes a multimedia module for learning; an interactive, customizable interface for tracking progress in hygiene routines; and reinforcement and feedback from a virtual trainer. Educational modules provide information on various hygiene-related topics, such as washing hands, brushing teeth, getting dressed, wearing clothes to suit weather conditions, using deodorants, etc. Student access to different content is recorded for later analysis by researchers, parents, teachers, or students themselves. HygieneHelper offers two sample routines—morning and evening. Customizing these routines enables meeting the users' needs and providing appropriate details in these activities. For example, some young people with ASD may need routines that involve detailed toothbrushing steps, while for others, brushing teeth may be one step within a longer morning or evening routine. Timers within this application can be used as reminders for performing hygiene tasks or for measuring the duration of the activities (e.g., 3 min for brushing teeth). HygieneHelper provides an educational message a teacher wants to share with a user every day. Once a week, this message is customized according to the degree to which a specific hygiene routine is performed in that week. For example, the message is fully commending when all activities are performed, and when most routines are performed, the message encourages the users to improve their achievements. The application can be configured to alert a parent or a teacher if some data is not recorded or if the threshold of performing an activity is not reached (Hayes & Hosaflook, 2013).

De Urturi et al. (2011) presented a system of games for tablets and cellphones for first aid education in people with ASD. The application includes three sets of minigames. In the first set, the players are expected to arrange image sequences by touching them in the correct order, related to different first aid aspects (e.g., what to do when you cut yourself or when you want to call a doctor). A short explanation accompanies all images. The player needs to solve as many sequences as possible in a limited time. If the pictures are arranged in the right order, the user continues the game with more difficult sequences and gets the result at the end. It is possible to choose whether the tasks will have a time limit. A user report is generated after the activity is completed. The report states correct and incorrect sequences, the time needed to complete each, etc. The second set of games involves pairing pictures and medical specialists based on uniform colors and body parts they specialize in. In the third set, the player needs to seek help in a hospital, recognize hospital signs, and talk to specialists.

6.3 Domestic Skills

Mistakes are common when learning DLS in the traditional way, which can lead to injuries. Games based on real stories or scenarios provide an authentic but safe environment for children with ASD (Rias & Dehkordi, 2013). Using real stories in games helps children match their play experiences with real-life situations. Thus, several games have been designed for acquiring DLS in a virtual home environment. Although various technologies have been used, they all involve moving around different spaces at home.

Charitos et al. (2000) used virtual reality to design a virtual five-room house. The scenario begins with an avatar arriving home. Children use the avatar to perform different activities in specific rooms. For example, they wash their hands in the bathroom, set the table in the kitchen, get dressed in the parents' room, help clean the living room, and make the bed in the children's room. If a child does not know how to perform an activity, they can choose the animation mode in which a virtual character demonstrates how to do it.

Chang et al. (2012) developed a flash-based situated game based on real stories to teach children with ASD to perform daily activities. The game includes an activity generation mechanism that measures the difficulty of activities and automatically generates personalized quests for children. The database contains 11 activities performed in 4 rooms in an apartment. For example, a task can involve a child helping the mother clear the table after breakfast and wash a fork in the sink. The screen shows the activity description and a dining room where some objects are moveable (e.g., a fork, a spoon). Children can directly move the objects around the room. When they want to move an object to another room, they have to place it in a specific area on the screen.

A serious game connecting a home and school environment takes place in three virtual rooms of an apartment where different objects are randomly arranged. A child's task is to pack them in a school bag according to the daily schedule at a specific time. Once the players select the game level (they choose from ten levels of various difficulties), the augmented reality camera is activated, and the player has to physically move around the environment looking for objects. When they find an object, the players have to point the camera at it, select, and drag it through 3D space into the bag (Aziz et al., 2021).

Another three-dimensional game taking place from the player's perspective is placed in a typical Singaporean apartment. The game is intended for learning to turn off a clock alarm, brush teeth, and make a drink. It uses the Leap Motion sensor, a device designed to detect the position of a user's hand and fingers. The sensor is equipped with two cameras and three infrared light-emitting diodes (LED). Compared to Microsoft Kinect, the advantage of this sensor is that it can track more delicate hand and finger movements. It can display players' movements when taking objects such as toothbrushes, cups, etc. However, its limitation is that it can only detect simple finger movements and positions in a limited field covered by the sensor (Chung et al., 2021).

Chong et al. (2021) designed a three-dimensional game for tablets and computers to improve a domestic skill that also improves potential vocational skills. The game is intended to teach children with ASD to clean horizontal surfaces. A real cleaning cloth with a built-in optical sensor is used, which allows the game to detect the cloth movements while a player is cleaning. A player can choose 1 out of 12 scenarios in a work or home environment, which differ according to the characteristics of the surfaces to be wiped (size, color, shape, height, and roughness). The initial position of a virtual hand is always in the far corner of the cleaning surface to make it easier for a player to plan the path for cleaning the whole surface. The virtual hand is metal so that children are not afraid of a realistic floating hand. Textual instructions appear throughout the game to lead the player through activities that need to be performed. The instructions appear for about 2 s, then slide down the page, and disappear.

6.4 Community Skills

6.4.1 Shopping

With virtual supermarket serious games, children with ASD can learn and practice their shopping skills in a safe and controlled environment guided by a teacher or parent. They can learn to recognize different products, link them to textual information on a shopping list, and look for various items in appropriate store sections (Goh et al., 2021).

ShopAut 2.0 is a three-dimensional game conceptually based on conventional 3D games and intended for children and teenagers with ASD to practice shopping skills. A player can choose from three modes based on the DSM-5 classification of ASD severity. The game includes ten levels with different missions of increasing difficulty. Players get a medal after completing a level, which allows them to advance to the next level. New challenges are introduced after every three levels. They refer to the number and type of tasks on a shopping list, unexpected events, sound distractors, the complexity of money transactions, and interactions with avatars. The game facilitator provides support during the game, depending on the missions and the game difficulty. For example, at the first few levels, where the main task is to buy specific products, the third game mode directs the player to the desired path with the help of arrows and lights, and visual and audio signals are used when necessary to attract the player's attention. In addition, the shopping list contains appropriate pictures, and the products are highlighted with lights of various colors to facilitate their identification. Instructions are given in written, visual, and audio messages. These characteristics allow the game to adapt to the player without disturbing the course of the game and prevent the feeling of failure or frustration in children (Vallefuoco et al., 2022).

ParaShop is an augmented reality mobile application for Android and iOS devices, which helps people with ASD go through different stages of supermarket shopping. It allows users to create shopping lists using pictures and automatically categorizes products. It also provides augmented reality scene instructions to help users with ASD complete the tasks. At a supermarket, users can open the application and select one of the previously prepared shopping lists. Real-world supermarket scenes are displayed at the top, and instructions are at the bottom of the screen. Users follow instructions to take a shopping cart or basket, find products from the shopping list, wait in line, and pay. After completing one task, users move on to the next step by pressing an arrow. They can skip a product if they cannot find it in the supermarket. The application also provides simple voice instructions if a user has reading problems. Furthermore, ParaShop has an option for recognizing fruit and vegetables. When users take a picture of an item with a phone camera, the item name appears at the top of the screen. They can also use the text-to-speech option by pressing the speaker icon (Xia et al., 2021).

Virtual Action Planning Supermarket (VAP-S) is a virtual environment laptop or desktop software designed to improve shopping skills in adolescents with

ASD. VAP-S simulates a medium-sized supermarket with a full range of products and four checkouts. Users perform a procedure similar to that in a regular supermarket, i.e., they choose products according to the shopping list that appears on the screen, pay, and exit the supermarket. The software automatically records user positions to provide an overview of the route and stops made during virtual shopping (Lamash et al., 2017).

A collaborative virtual reality application based on a head-mounted display allows students and teachers to be in a virtual supermarket simultaneously and collaborate while shopping. They control their virtual avatars and use real head and hand movements. Users move through the virtual environment by moving the thumbstick on Oculus Touch controllers. They can pick up items such as shopping baskets, shopping lists, products, coins, and bills. When one user takes an item in the virtual environment, the other users can see the change of position and rotation of the item in their virtual environment. Also, users can pass interactive products to each other. Finally, students can go to a self-checkout machine to scan the items and pay using virtual coins and notes. Throughout the whole process, all participants can verbally communicate with each other (Thomsen & Adjorlu, 2021).

Goh et al. (2021) presented a serious game in which users used gestures to control their movements in a virtual supermarket with the help of Microsoft Kinect sensors. The game has three levels. At the easiest level, there are no other people, the designated route encourages players to find the section of the desired product, and they are free to buy what they want without a shopping list. The selected product is automatically moved to the virtual cart. In the end, an animation directs players to the checkout. At the next level, there are other customers at the supermarket, and players have to move items from shelves to the virtual cart themselves. In addition, there is a background noise simulating the murmur of people. The noise level varies depending on the crowd. The last level of the game introduces two more options: returning an unwanted item on a shelf and paying at the checkout.

Virtual shopping has also been used as an environment primarily aimed at teaching students with ASD to use money. Thus, Adjorlu and Serafin (2019) created an application based on a virtual reality head-mounted display. Students were placed in front of a virtual shop assistant and a table with various products. The shop assistant would state how much they needed to pay for a specific item, and the same amount appeared on the virtual cash register. Various coins and banknotes were placed on the table next to students. They could approach the table, take the desired amount using Oculus Touch controllers, and place it on the table in front of the virtual shop assistant. Taking the money and putting it in front of the virtual shop assistant were performed by physical interactions in the air while holding the touch controller. When the students chose the right amount of money, the virtual shop assistant would say thank you and perform a dance animation as a reward. If they failed to provide the correct answer, they were given verbal instructions explaining which coins and notes they should put on the table. Interestingly, the teachers who participated in the research suggested designing two additional levels to be played before the mini-game with the virtual shop assistant. Since some of their students had difficulty understanding that coins and banknotes had different values, the teachers suggested a level at which students could take a virtual coin or note and put it on a small table with appropriate images of the selected coin or note. The next level would require the student to put virtual money on virtual tables with numbers indicating the appropriate amount.

The results of evaluating the effectiveness of the applications designed to develop shopping skills are mainly positive. Significant improvements have been determined in learning the shopping procedure, focusing, and problem-solving skills (Vallefuoco et al., 2022), as well as in learning meta-cognitive strategies to increase shopping efficacy (e.g., arranging a shopping list, using signs in a supermarket, etc.) and their application in a virtual environment (Lamash et al., 2017). However, not all results are entirely positive. While testing the use of virtual reality head-mounted displays to develop shopping skills in adolescents with ASD, Adjorlu et al. (2017) found that participants located items in a real supermarket more accurately and more safely than before the intervention. However, the authors reported negative results with regard to students' self-confidence and self-satisfaction during the intervention. Furthermore, Adjorlu and Serafin (2019) found some improvements in handling money while shopping, but verbal instructions provided by the application did not prove to be adequate to help students put the correct amount of money in front of the virtual shop assistant. Apart from that, some students found the repetitiveness of the application boring. The authors believe that the results would be better if a teacher controlled the virtual shop assistant in real time, provided students with necessary feedback, and gave them new relevant tasks to help increase their motivation.

6.4.2 *Transportation*

Skills related to driving and traffic safety are among the most common goals in studies on using digital technology to teach DLS (Adjorlu, 2020). Independent transportation can improve the quality of life by increasing vocational and social opportunities and reducing dependence on caregivers (Wade et al., 2017).

6.4.2.1 Crossing the Street Safely

Many children with ASD are not independent when crossing the street. This skill is significant since it involves exposure to potentially dangerous situations and is an important step in becoming independent. Virtual reality facilitates learning in a safe environment by allowing a gradual increase in task complexity, thus resembling real-life conditions (Josman et al., 2008).

Josman et al. (2008) wanted to examine whether children with ASD were able to learn the skills necessary for crossing the street safely and generalize them in real life. They used a virtual desktop environment for crossing the street. The experimental group included six children with ASD, and the control group consisted of six typically developing children of the matching age and gender. The skills of crossing the street were tested before and after the intervention in a real training area designed for training pedestrians. The intervention was implemented on a desktop computer and included two virtual four-lane intersections—one with a pedestrian island in the middle and the other with traffic lights. The participants used avatars that had to cross the street at the beginning of each out of nine difficulty levels. A different number of virtual cars appeared on the left or right side of the avatar. The number of virtual vehicles and their speed increased with each level. The participants' task was to decide when it was safe to cross the street. They could use three keys on the keyboard to interact with the system: to look left, look right, and cross the street. A navigation card with three circles of the same colors as the stickers on the keyboard was placed near the monitor. Each circle included picture communication symbols and inscriptions matching the ones on the keys. If a student was hit by a virtual vehicle, there was a sound of brakes and an accident sign on the screen, and that level was repeated. The participants used the application at eight school sessions, once or twice a week. Each session lasted for 10–30 min. After the eighth session, all students with ASD managed to complete all training levels in the virtual environment, and half of them improved their skills for crossing the street in a real-life setting.

A natural user interface, or natural interface, is a system for human-computer interaction through intuitive activities that involve natural, everyday, human behavior. It refers to sensory inputs such as touch, speech, gestures, etc. Saiano et al. (2015) were interested in whether an integrated approach based on a virtual

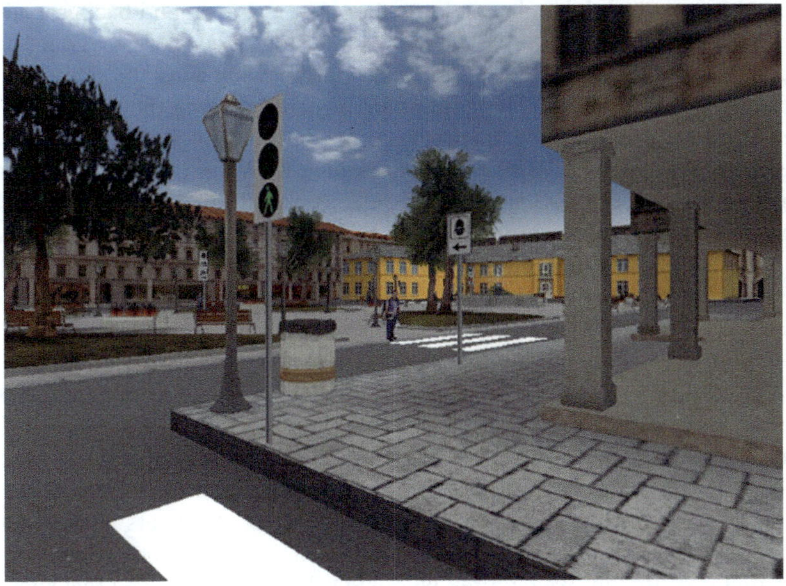

Fig. 6.2 Screenshot of the virtual environment in which walking around the town and safely crossing the street were practiced. (Reproduced from Saiano et al., 2015)

environment and natural interface was effective in teaching adults with ASD the skills needed to cross the street. Seven people with ASD explored a virtual environment representing a city (buildings, sidewalks, streets, squares), continuously displayed on a widescreen (Fig. 6.2). A markerless motion capture device recorded the participants' movements, which were translated into virtual environment control commands according to the predefined vocabulary of gestures. The treatment included ten 45-min sessions (one session a week). During the introduction phase, the participants practiced the vocabulary of gestures. In the training phase, they had to follow the signs (to a police station or pharmacy) and cross the streets with and without traffic lights. The number and type of errors were tracked while crossing and navigating the streets (walking speed, road length, and the ability to turn without stopping). Before and after the treatment, the participants had to complete a test questionnaire that evaluated their understanding of the practiced skill. Parents and caregivers of people with ASD were given another questionnaire that assessed the generalization of the learned skill to real-life situations. The participants easily learned simple body movements for interacting with a virtual environment. They improved their navigation skills during the sessions but did not significantly reduce the number of errors when crossing the streets. The test questionnaire also did not show a significant reduction in errors. Still, their parents and caregivers reported a significant improvement when crossing the streets. Their responses also indicated a significant generalization of the acquired skills to real-life situations.

Zhang et al. (2021) created a serious game for children with ASD based on virtual reality for simulating traffic scenarios at a virtual intersection. A Microsoft Kinect device and a touch screen were used for interaction. The process of learning to cross the street had three phases. First, the game character and background story were discussed with the children. A video demonstration was organized in the second phase. A teacher recorded a video tutorial showing what the children were expected to do in the game. The final phase involved playing the game. When the game character arrived at the intersection, the traffic light was red. The players needed to press the traffic light button to change it. When the traffic light turned green, the players could start crossing the intersection. They needed to lean forward to start moving in that direction. The children stated that the game phases helped them better understand the traffic rules, which were usually difficult to remember in a traditional class. The authors also reported that the children with ASD showed interest and enjoyed the game.

A mobile application combining social stories and digital storytelling was used to develop children's awareness of road traffic safety. A social story about road traffic safety was designed using digital storytelling through a 2D animation of a selected character representing a boy or a girl. The text-to-speech software was used for narration to provide clear pronunciation and a steady intonation tempo. Character customization was achieved by allowing users to select characters similar to them. The social story had three modalities—animation, text, and audio narration. The application was used in five children with ASD. The results showed that social stories and digital storytelling had the potential to foster positive attributes in children's behavior, not only in relation to road traffic safety but also in increasing their interest in learning appropriate content (Ying et al., 2016).

6.4.2.2 Walking Around the Town

My Story is a two-dimensional video game aiming to help students and young adults with intellectual disability and/or ASD improve independent living skills. The game follows the main character, who lives alone. Every day, the character performs various tasks that are part of the main goal. Each task is rewarded with a specific number of coins depending on the achievement. The coins can be used for upgrading the avatar, thus upgrading the home environment, and achieving immersion. There is no negative feedback, and the repeat function helps the player improve the result. The game assistant informs the player about the tasks and provides feedback. A tracking mechanism collects data on the players' progress and the effect of the game on learning. The game prototype includes three mini-games that focus on safely walking to a cinema/shopping mall, buying a cinema ticket, and understanding and following a map to find a clothing store (Tsikinas & Xinogalos, 2021).

Layar is a free, widely available mobile application for various platforms, including iOS and Android devices. It uses location-based augmented reality to show the selected content. There are thousands of potential content channels called "geolayars." Users choose the content by subscribing to a geolayar of a specific topic. This allows the application to function as a search engine based on the location of selected topics (e.g., employment opportunities) displayed according to the user's relative location. Visual prompts appear as icon locations when viewed through a phone camera. The icon helps inform students when making decisions while "hovering" above a specific destination. The distance to the location in miles is also displayed. The application uses Wi-Fi and other built-in cellphone tools to determine the location and orientation of users (McMahon et al., 2015).

6.4.2.3 Using Public Transport

Simões et al. (2018) wanted to develop a serious game that would provide a "safe environment" for adolescents with ASD to learn about riding a bus. The players were located in a three-dimensional town and were given various tasks, including riding a bus to specific destinations (Fig. 6.3). The game included several different buses and four predefined routes. A player could get on any of the buses, validate the ticket, take a seat, and press the STOP button to get off. Before the game started, the players could choose from seven different tasks. Four tasks were marked as simple (players took one bus to reach the destination), and three as complex (they had to change buses to reach the destination). Each task had two difficulty levels. The easy mode guided the players step by step. On the other hand, the players were only informed about the location they had to reach in the difficult mode. At the end of each task, performance was evaluated by awarding points, with regard to two

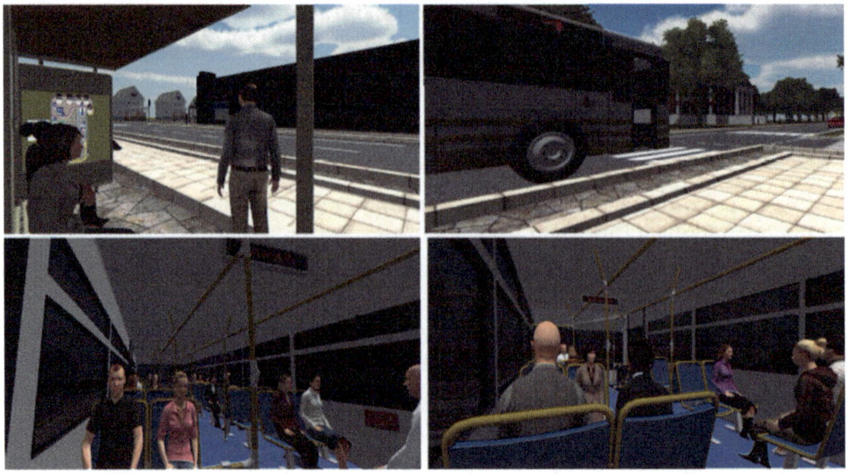

Fig. 6.3 Screenshot from the virtual environment in which adolescents with ASD learned how to ride a bus. The upper two pictures show a bus stop with a map the participants used and a bus marked with a red number. The lower two pictures show the interior of the bus. (Reproduced from Simões et al., 2018)

components: "Actions" (a player's ability to remember the norms of riding a bus and behave accordingly, e.g., validating a ticket or sitting on a non-reserved seat) and "Route" (a player's ability to plan a route to a destination, e.g., whether a player got on the right bus at the right bus stop). A laptop, head-mounted display, and gamepad were used to start and move through the game. To examine whether such an environment could be used to teach people with ASD bus riding routines and adjustment procedures, research was conducted on ten adolescents with ASD, who participated in one of three sessions, and ten of their typically developing peers who participated in one control session. The game included elements that could cause anxiety in players (people, traffic, and dogs). Thus, electrodermal activity was analyzed during the game. If a high level of anxiety was detected, chaotic stimuli were reduced. Several participants with visual impairment did not use a head-mounted display. At the end of each session, the participants were asked to describe the process of riding a bus but without receiving feedback. The answers were recorded on a checklist that included all steps of riding a bus. The results showed a significant increase in knowledge and a high degree of success in applying this knowledge while playing the game. In addition, the level of anxiety dropped, especially on a bus. The authors concluded that adolescents with ASD were most anxious while planning a trip, looking for bus stops, waiting for a bus, and anticipating the stop to get off.

Due to multiple procedures and the seemingly chaotic environment, traveling by plane can be a traumatic experience for children with ASD. Miller et al. (2020) used virtual reality-based air travel training combined with traditional functional communication training based on the air travel experience in five children with ASD and language difficulties (4–8 years of age). They used iPhone and Google Cardboard—a handheld device that launches a virtual reality experience and can be paired with almost all smartphones with appropriate applications. The researchers conducted the intervention once a week for 3 weeks. The intervention was implemented according to a narrative scenario based on social stories and was modified in accordance with each child's attention and ability to access the simulation (airport items and pictures were placed in the room in case a participant could not access virtual reality). The final session was a rehearsal at a real international airport. It included checking in, going through security, going to a gate, waiting, and walking down a jetway. It did not involve boarding the plane. To make the experience as realistic as possible, the children were encouraged to bring hand luggage or a backpack. According to the observations of researchers and parents, all children improved their air travel skills.

6.4.2.4 Driving

A driving simulator improves driving knowledge, skills, and abilities by correcting bad and risky behaviors in a safe and controlled environment (Ross et al., 2018).

Virtual reality Adaptive Driving Intervention Architecture (VADIA) consists of a virtual driving environment and a range of input and sensor peripherals. The virtual environment is a three-dimensional city model large enough to allow tasks that can last for several hours. The simulation is designed so that users can practice different aspects of driving while task parameters, such as complexity, difficulty, and duration, can be controlled. The model consists of different districts, including a city center with skyscrapers and residential and industrial zones. The roads are various, including narrow one-way streets, freeways, and sharp turns. The city contains usual features such as vehicles, pedestrians, traffic lights, and traffic signs. VADIA consists of interrelated modules, with the driving module being the central one. In addition, other modules include collecting gaze data, collecting physiological data, observer-based assessment, and electroencephalographic module. VADIA can be configured to work with different module combinations depending on the intervention goals. Also, some modules can be disabled under certain circumstances (Wade et al., 2016, 2017).

In a study that used VADIA, Wade et al. (2015) divided the adolescents with ASD according to two driving modes due to previous findings that drivers with ASD had higher vertical and right-shifted horizontal gaze direction compared to typically developing people (Reimer et al., 2013; Wade et al., 2014). In the performance-based mode, task progress depended only on driving performance, while the gaze-contingent mode required the participants to drive without error and observe key regions of interest (ROI). The performance-based mode allowed the driver three errors, while the gaze-contingent mode allowed three performance errors and three errors related to gaze direction. After any error, the drivers were given audio or text feedback explaining why the error was made and how to avoid it in the future. After the drivers successfully completed all eight attempts, they received a sound congratulation message. In the gaze-contingent mode, when the drivers failed to look at all relevant ROI for a specific situation, the attempt was repeated, and all relevant ROI were highlighted by fluorescent green light to attract the driver's attention. After the second attempt, the highlighting effect was removed when the driver looked at the ROI. The results showed that gaze direction in the gaze-contingent mode group was lower and shifted to the left compared to drivers with ASD in the performance-based mode. The authors interpreted this as a possible indication of shifting the gaze pattern toward the one in typically developing people. However, while there was a significant reduction of errors in the performance-based group, the difference compared to the period before the intervention was not statistically significant in the gaze-contingent group.

For some people with ASD, fear of driving may make it impossible to acquire and use driving privileges. One approach to alleviating such fears is gradual exposure through gaining experience in a virtual environment. Ross et al. (2018) examined the possibility of reducing fear of driving through training in virtual reality driving simulation. Data on driving attitudes were collected from parents of people with ASD and parents of neurotypical beginner drivers. According to them, drivers with ASD had fewer positive and more negative attitudes than neurotypical drivers. The training gradually progressed, from learning to respect speed limits, keeping to one lane, stopping and turning, to using direction indicators. After that, the training continued by introducing other traffic, multi-tasking, and detecting and responding to dangerous situations. All participants completed all training phases within a maximum of 12 sessions. They practiced driving with parents in their own cars on local roads to encourage generalization from virtual reality to actual driving. Parents of drivers with ASD who completed the simulator training increased the number of positive and reduced the number of negative attitudes compared to drivers with ASD who underwent regular training. However, it remained unclear whether the effects persisted when they started driving independently in the real world. Also, beginner drivers with ASD had more negative and fewer positive attitudes toward driving even after completing the virtual reality driving simulation training.

6.5 Video-Based Instruction

Different methods of VM and VP have widely been used in teaching daily living skills. Using these methods in teaching DLS increases the chances that these skills will be learned and maintained and that the overall quality of life will improve (Mellerson, 2021).

VM involves recording a video in which a person demonstrates the target skill. Trainees watch the whole video at the beginning of each training session and should then repeat the entire observed skill (Mellerson, 2021). VM was thus used to teach children with ASD, 8–14 years of age, to brush their teeth. The video, which lasted for about a minute, was sent by email every day for 3 weeks of treatment. It modeled the proper toothbrushing technique accompanied by narration and closed captioning. It started with a title screen and a sound stimulus signalizing the beginning of the video ("It's time to brush your teeth!"). Then, the video showed a 10-year-old girl applying toothpaste on a toothbrush and starting to brush her teeth. It illustrated brushing each quadrant and ended by brushing the front teeth. The results showed that dental hygiene only slightly improved, but there was a reduction of plaque, and the parents reported that the intervention was successful (Popple et al., 2016).

Unlike continuously showing the whole skill in VM, VP refers to a video display of a multi-component skill where each step is recorded separately. Students can practice each step individually and receive feedback before moving on to the next one. This pattern is repeated until the target skill is completed (Glumbić et al., 2018). One study used VP to teach three students with ASD to wash towels. The recordings, which represented the steps obtained by task analysis, lasted from 6 s to 13 s and were played on an iPhone. The instructor gave a verbal instruction ("Wash clothes"), followed by "Watch this" when the first video clip started. The procedure allowed each video to be played three times if necessary. After the video, an adult instructed the students to perform the watched activity. Correct answers were verbally praised. If the students made a mistake or failed to start the activity within 30 s, the instructor asked them to turn around and then completed the step without them looking. This was done to prepare relevant stimulus conditions for the next step (Bennett et al., 2017).

Video self-modeling is a specific form of VM that uses students as models, allowing them to watch themselves competently performing an activity. Participants watch a video of themselves performing a specific activity, but with all reinforcers and non-fluently performed parts of the activity removed from the video (Ayres et al., 2017; Mason et al., 2016). O'Handley and Allen (2017) evaluated the effect of video self-modeling on learning to fold towels, vacuum, and clean a bathroom sink and mirror in an adult man with ASD and intellectual disability. The videos, in which the model was the participant himself, were recorded with his mother's instructional prompts, whose voice was left in the background. The number of recorded attempts depended on obtaining the appropriate intervention video with no additional changes made to it. The participant was asked to watch a video before his mother asked him to perform an activity. It is interesting that large, immediate, and relatively stable effects were determined as a result of recording the videos, while small, slight, but stable improvements in task accuracy were found during the intervention when the participant watched the videos immediately before performing a task. The results showed that the learning process while recording videos may largely influence the outcomes of a video self-modeling intervention.

VM from a model's perspective is another variation called point-of-view video modeling. A skill is demonstrated from the perspective of a person performing the activity instead of someone observing the model. The video shows sequential skill performance with the accompanying explanation and hands of the person performing the task (Glumbić et al., 2018). Since people with ASD often tend to pay attention to irrelevant details, point-of-view video modeling can help students focus on key information needed to perform a skill (Gardner & Wolfe, 2013). Aldi et al. (2016) used point-of-view video modeling, with gestural prompts, in two 8-year-olds with ASD. They were taught daily living skills related to cooking, setting the table, folding clothes, and cleaning the bathroom. When a student gave an incorrect or no answer after watching a video, the researcher provided a gestural prompt. If the student again failed to answer correctly, the video was played two more times before moving on to the next step. Both participants mastered the taught skills. Although the skills did not maintain the mastery criterion level a month after the intervention, they were still better than before the intervention.

The usual course of intervention involves slowly withdrawing the prompts and triggering the activity with a discriminative stimulus (e.g., an order or a natural stimulus). However, when a person rarely performs an activity or has memory problems, providing oneself with a controlling stimulus and guiding oneself through tasks can be helpful (Ayres et al., 2017). Thus, when teaching adolescents with ASD to cook, Mechling et al. (2010) used a least-to-most prompt hierarchy controlled by the students themselves. When a personal digital assistant was activated, it showed a photograph of the prepared food (e.g., a sandwich), and the instructor told a student to begin the task. The student could then independently perform the task or, by selecting the appropriate icon, choose the desired level of prompts (picture, picture + audio, or video + audio). The results showed that students with ASD were able to adjust the level of prompts and use the device independently to complete the task.

Over the last decades, the media for displaying videos have changed from video recorders, portable DVD players, and smartboards to mobile devices, "wearables," and augmented reality. Shifting technology from optical media to smaller, mobile devices has allowed using VM in the same settings where the learned skills are used (e.g., on the street, in the kitchen) instead of a student sitting in front of a TV or computer in the classroom (Ayres et al., 2013, 2017). With regard to video-based instruction, the advantage of handheld devices, such as personal digital assistants and, recently, tablets and smartphones, is that they (a) are portable; (b) can record, store, and display pictures, audio, and video clips; (c) are becoming cheaper and more accessible; and (d) can be used by people of different ages and cognitive abilities who need different levels of support (Pérez-Fuster et al., 2019). This technology can indefinitely repeat the "perfect" pattern of behavior and allows a student to go back and review video instructions (Ayres et al., 2013).

Apart from videos, photographs and audio have also been used as prompts on mobile devices. Thus, Kellems et al. (2018) found that both VP and static pictures, when displayed on a cellphone, successfully taught children with ASD different DLS. Although some children showed greater improvement when static pictures were used, using VP generally resulted in faster skills acquisition. On the other hand, Chen and Yakubova (2019) believe that although research results have supported both audio prompting and VP, the intervention should start with VP. However, if students can acquire skills using VP, they should try and switch to audio prompting, which requires less visual attention, uses physically smaller technology, and reduces possible stigmatization.

Different VM variations in DLS have mainly been used as instructional support to master the tasks learned by chaining (Ayres et al., 2013) and have often been the element of broader instructional procedures such as various prompt-fading strategies including least to most (e.g., verbal, gesture, model, physical) and time delay (Cannella-Malone et al., 2012; Spriggs et al., 2015; Van Laarhoven & Van Laarhoven-Myers, 2006; Wu et al., 2016).

Video-based instruction has been used with the help of technology to teach a wide range of DLS: transition between daily activities (Mechling & Savidge, 2011), maintaining dental hygiene (Cihak et al., 2016; Popple et al., 2016), toileting (Drysdale et al., 2015), cooking (Aldi et al., 2016; Mechling et al., 2009, 2010; Van Laarhoven & Van Laarhoven-Myers, 2006; Van Laarhoven et al., 2010), shopping skills (Bereznak et al., 2012; Burckley et al., 2015), cleaning bathrooms and kitchens (Aldi et al., 2016; Cullen et al., 2017; O'Handley & Allen, 2017), vacuuming (O'Handley & Allen, 2017), washing clothes and dishes (Bereznak et al., 2012; Cannella-Malone et al., 2006; Pérez-Fuster et al., 2019), washing windows (Wu et al., 2016), cleaning and setting the table (Aldi et al., 2016; Cannella-Malone et al., 2012; Cullen et al., 2017; Spriggs et al., 2015; Van Laarhoven & Van Laarhoven-Myers, 2006), and folding clothes and towels (Aldi et al., 2016; O'Handley & Allen, 2017; Van Laarhoven & Van Laarhoven-Myers, 2006; Van Laarhoven et al., 2010).

Numerous studies have examined different approaches and variations within video-based instruction. Pérez-Fuster et al. (2019) compared the effects of two interventions based on prompting instructional techniques in improving dishwashing and laundry skills in four adult men with ASD. One intervention was implemented with the help of digital technology (a tablet connected to a lighting system), and the other involved traditional treatment (paper pictures and task strips). The intervention based on digital technology was more successful in terms of fewer prompts from educators and a smaller number of off-task behaviors while performing the activity.

Cannella-Malone et al. (2012) compared VP without error correction and VP with error correction in teaching cleaning and washing tables. The error correction procedure involved interrupting student errors and replaying the video. If the student repeated the mistake, a three-level least-to-most prompting hierarchy was applied for the specific skill in the task sequence. Out of three participants included in this research, only one had ASD. In his case, introducing error correction with video prompting had a minimal effect, and in vivo instructions were used to increase the number of correct answers in both skills.

One study examined three video-based instructional sequences used together with the system of least prompts for learning different DLS, such as preparing a pizza in a microwave, folding clothes, and cleaning a table. Although all three techniques were effective, the most successful combination was VM plus in vivo VP, while VM plus photo prompt sequence was more successful than isolated VM (Van Laarhoven & Van Laarhoven-Myers, 2006). Also, VP was somewhat more successful than picture prompting when learning similar skills (preparing food and folding clothes) in terms of a greater number of independently given correct answers and a smaller number of external prompts needed to complete the task, as well as the prompts provided so that the participants would use instructional materials (Van

Laarhoven et al., 2010). Furthermore, Cannella-Malone et al. (2006) found that VP was more successful than VM in learning to wash clothes and dishes.

In their review of research, Gardner and Wolfe (2013) found that VM and VP were effective in teaching people with ASD different DLS. According to them, using VM led to faster acquisition of various skills than in vivo modeling, while VP had a larger overall effect on students' achievement than picture prompting. Finally, VP was more effective than VM probably because it was easier for the limited attention span of students with ASD to cope with shorter VP segments than longer VM recordings. In a meta-analytical study, Aljehany and Bennett (2019) determined a moderate effect size of using VP in people with ASD while learning DLS. Hong et al. (2016) reported a similar effect size in their meta-analysis of using VM (including VP studies) in people with ASD and intellectual disability.

The presented studies show that digital technology can successfully be used for learning DLS in people with ASD. Its effectiveness can be compared with traditional instructional methods, even surpassing them in some segments. Over the last decades, technological advances have made virtual environments more realistic and immersive, allowing users to feel part of an authentic environment while learning. On the other hand, digital technology provides safe and predictable surroundings where mistakes do not lead to injuries and the possibility to customize difficulty levels and repeat tasks reduces the likelihood of frustration in users. However, although some results indicate that people with ASD can manage their learning process in such an environment, other studies point out that the presence of a teacher/instructor is desirable in virtual reality. Further research is needed to determine which media, methods, and approaches (or their combinations) are best for learning DLS and how some characteristics of people with ASD (e.g., the severity of symptoms, age, cognitive capacities) should influence these decisions.

References

Adjorlu, A. (2020). *Adolescent under construction: An exploration of how virtual reality can be used to teach social and daily living skills to children and adolescents diagnosed with Autism Spectrum Disorder*. Doctoral thesis, Aalborg University.

Adjorlu, A., & Serafin, S. (2019). Head-mounted display-based virtual reality as a tool to teach money skills to adolescents diagnosed with autism spectrum disorder. In A. Brooks, E. Brooks, & C. Sylla (Eds.), *Interactivity, game creation, design, learning, and innovation* (ArtsIT DLI 2018. Lecture Notes of the Institute for Computer Sciences, Social Informatics and Telecommunications Engineering) (Vol. 265). Springer. https://doi.org/10.1007/978-3-030-06134-0_48

Adjorlu, A., Høeg, E. R., Mangano, L., & Serafin, S. (2017). Daily living skills training in virtual reality to help children with autism spectrum disorder in a real shopping scenario. In *Proceedings of international symposium on mixed and augmented reality (ISMAR-Adjunct)* (pp. 294–302). https://doi.org/10.1109/ISMAR-Adjunct.2017.93

Aldi, C., Crigler, A., Kates-McElrath, K., Long, B., Smith, H., Rehak, K., & Wilkinson, L. (2016). Examining the effects of video modeling and prompts to teach activities of daily living skills. *Behavior Analysis in Practice, 9*(4), 384–388. https://doi.org/10.1007/s40617-016-0127-y

Aljehany, M. S., & Bennett, K. D. (2019). Meta-analysis of video prompting to teach daily living skills to individuals with autism spectrum disorder. *Journal of Special Education Technology, 34*(1), 17–26. https://doi.org/10.1177/0162643418780495

Alvares, G. A., Bebbington, K., Cleary, D., Evans, K., Glasson, E. J., Maybery, M. T., Pillar, S., Uljarević, M., Varcin, K., Wray, J., & Whitehouse, A. J. (2020). The misnomer of 'high functioning autism': Intelligence is an imprecise predictor of functional abilities at diagnosis. *Autism, 24*(1), 221–232. https://doi.org/10.1177/1362361319852831

Ayres, K. M., Mechling, L., & Sansosti, F. J. (2013). The use of mobile technologies to assist with life skills/independence of students with moderate/severe intellectual disability and/or autism spectrum disorders: Considerations for the future of school psychology. *Psychology in the Schools, 50*(3), 259–271. https://doi.org/10.1002/pits.21673

Ayres, K. M., Travers, J., Shepley, S. B., & Cagliani, R. (2017). Video-Based Instruction for Learners with Autism. In J. B. Leaf (Ed.), *Handbook of social skills and autism spectrum disorder* (pp. 223–239). Springer. https://doi.org/10.1007/978-3-319-62995-7_14

Aziz, M. A. B. A., Cao, Q., & Cai, Y. (2021). Design of a home bag-packing serious game for children with ASD. In Y. Cai & Q. Cao (Eds.), *When VR serious games meet special needs education: Research, development and their applications* (pp. 143–156). Springer. https://doi.org/10.1007/978-981-33-6942-9_9

Bal, V. H., Kim, S. H., Cheong, D., & Lord, C. (2015). Daily living skills in individuals with autism spectrum disorder from 2 to 21 years of age. *Autism, 19*(7), 774–784. https://doi.org/10.1177/1362361315575840

Baragash, R. S., Al-Samarraie, H., Alzahrani, A. I., & Alfarraj, O. (2020). Augmented reality in special education: A meta-analysis of single-subject design studies. *European Journal of Special Needs Education, 35*(3), 382–397. https://doi.org/10.1080/08856257.2019.1703548

Bennett, K. D., Crocco, C., Loughrey, T. O., & McDowell, L. S. (2017). Effects of video prompting without voice-over narration among students with autism spectrum disorder. *Behavioral Development Bulletin, 22*(1), 147. https://doi.org/10.1037/bdb0000058

Bereznak, S., Ayres, K. M., Mechling, L. C., & Alexander, J. L. (2012). Video self-prompting and mobile technology to increase daily living and vocational independence for students with autism spectrum disorders. *Journal of Developmental and Physical Disabilities, 24*(3), 269–285. https://doi.org/10.1007/s10882-012-9270-8

Burckley, E., Tincani, M., & Guld Fisher, A. (2015). An iPad-based picture and video activity schedule increases community shopping skills of a young adult with autism spectrum disorder and intellectual disability. *Developmental Neurorehabilitation, 18*(2), 131–136. https://doi.org/10.3109/17518423.2014.945045

Cannella-Malone, H., Sigafoos, J., O'Reilly, M., de la Cruz, B., Edrisinha, C., & Lancioni, G. E. (2006). Comparing video prompting to video modeling for teaching daily living skills to six adults with developmental disabilities. *Education and Training in Developmental Disabilities, 41*(4), 344–356.

Cannella-Malone, H., Wheaton, J. E., Wu, P., Tullis, C. A., & Park, J. H. (2012). Comparing the effects of video prompting with and without error correction on skill acquisition for students with intellectual disability. *Education and Training in Autism and Developmental Disabilities, 47*(3), 332–344.

Chang, M., Kuo, R., Lyu, C. W., & Heh, J. S. (2012). A situated game for autistic children learning activities of daily living. In *Proceedings of fourth international conference on digital game and intelligent toy enhanced learning* (pp. 217–220). https://doi.org/10.1109/DIGITEL.2012.59

Charitos, D., Karadanos, G., Sereti, E., Triantafillou, S., Koukouvinou, S., & Martakos, D. (2000). Employing virtual reality for aiding the organisation of autistic children behaviour in everyday tasks. In *Proceedings of 3rd international conference disability, virtual reality and associated technologies (ICDVRAT)* (pp. 147–152).

Chen, B. B., & Yakubova, G. (2019). Promoting independence with vocational audio and video prompting for students with ASD. *TEACHING Exceptional Children, 52*(2), 98–106. https://doi.org/10.1177/0040059919874308

Chong, S., Cao, Q., & Cai, Y. (2021). Game-assisted vocational training. In Y. Cai & Q. Cao (Eds.), *When VR serious games meet special needs education: Research, development and their applications* (pp. 129–142). Springer. https://doi.org/10.1007/978-981-33-6942-9_8

Chung, Y. P. J., Cao, Q., & Cai, Y. (2021). Design of a virtual home for special needs children to learn life skills. In Y. Cai & Q. Cao (Eds.), *When VR serious games meet special needs education: Research, development and their applications* (pp. 31–61). Springer. https://doi.org/10.1007/978-981-33-6942-9_3

Cihak, D. F., Moore, E. J., Wright, R. E., McMahon, D. D., Gibbons, M. M., & Smith, C. (2016). Evaluating augmented reality to complete a chain task for elementary students with autism. *Journal of Special Education Technology, 31*(2), 99–108. https://doi.org/10.1177/0162643416651724

Clarke, E. B., McCauley, J. B., & Lord, C. (2021). Post–high school daily living skills in autism spectrum disorder. *Journal of the American Academy of Child & Adolescent Psychiatry, 60*(8), 978–985. https://doi.org/10.1016/j.jaac.2020.11.008

Cullen, J. M., Simmons-Reed, E. A., & Weaver, L. (2017). Using 21st century video prompting technology to facilitate the independence of individuals with intellectual and developmental disabilities. *Psychology in the Schools, 54*(9), 965–978. https://doi.org/10.1002/pits.22056

De Urturi, Z. S., Zorrilla, A. M., & Zapirain, B. G. (2011). Serious Game based on first aid education for individuals with Autism Spectrum Disorder (ASD) using android mobile devices. In *Proceedings of 16th international conference on computer games (CGAMES)* (pp. 223–227). https://doi.org/10.1109/CGAMES.2011.6000343

Drysdale, B., Lee, C. Y. Q., Anderson, A., & Moore, D. W. (2015). Using video modeling incorporating animation to teach toileting to two children with autism spectrum disorder. *Journal of Developmental and Physical Disabilities, 27*(2), 149–165. https://doi.org/10.1007/s10882-014-9405-1

Duncan, A. W., & Bishop, S. L. (2015). Understanding the gap between cognitive abilities and daily living skills in adolescents with autism spectrum disorders with average intelligence. *Autism, 19*(1), 64–72. https://doi.org/10.1177/1362361313510068

Duncan, A., Ruble, L. A., Meinzen-Derr, J., Thomas, C., & Stark, L. J. (2018). Preliminary efficacy of a daily living skills intervention for adolescents with high-functioning autism spectrum disorder. *Autism, 22*(8), 983–994. https://doi.org/10.1177/1362361317716606

Duncan, A., Liddle, M., & Stark, L. J. (2021). Iterative development of a daily living skills intervention for adolescents with autism without an intellectual disability. *Clinical Child and Family Psychology Review, 24*(4), 744–764. https://doi.org/10.1007/s10567-021-00360-6

Gardner, S., & Wolfe, P. (2013). Use of video modeling and video prompting interventions for teaching daily living skills to individuals with autism spectrum disorders: A review. *Research and Practice for Persons with Severe Disabilities, 38*(2), 73–87. https://doi.org/10.2511/027494813807714555

Glumbić, N., Brojčin, B., & Đorđević, M. (2018). *Specijalna edukacija zasnovana na dokazima: bihevioralne tehnike*. Univerzitet u Beogradu-Fakultet za specijalnu edukaciju i rehabilitaciju Izdavački centar (ICF).

Goh, J. H., Cao, Q., & Cai, Y. (2021). Design of a VR supermarket serious game. In Y. Cai & Q. Cao (Eds.), *When VR serious games meet special needs education: Research, development and their applications* (pp. 177–197). Springer. https://doi.org/10.1007/978-981-33-6942-9_11

Hayes, G. R., & Hosaflook, S. W. (2013). HygieneHelper: promoting awareness and teaching life skills to youth with autism spectrum disorder. In *Proceedings of the 12th international conference on interaction design and children* (pp. 539–542). https://doi.org/10.1145/2485760.2485860

Hong, E. R., Ganz, J. B., Mason, R., Morin, K., Davis, J. L., Ninci, J., et al. (2016). The effects of video modeling in teaching functional living skills to persons with ASD: A meta-analysis of single-case studies. *Research in Developmental Disabilities, 57*, 158–169. https://doi.org/10.1016/j.ridd.2016.07.001

Josman, N., Ben-Chaim, H. M., Friedrich, S., & Weiss, P. L. (2008). Effectiveness of virtual reality for teaching street-crossing skills to children and adolescents with autism. *International*

Journal on Disability and Human Development, 7(1), 49–56. https://doi.org/10.1515/IJDHD.2008.7.1.49

Kang, Y. S., & Chang, Y. J. (2019). Using game technology to teach six elementary school children with autism to take a shower independently. *Developmental neurorehabilitation, 22*(5), 329–337. https://doi.org/10.1080/17518423.2018.1501778

Kanne, S. M., Gerber, A. J., Quirmbach, L. M., Sparrow, S. S., Cicchetti, D. V., & Saulnier, C. A. (2011). The role of adaptive behavior in autism spectrum disorders: Implications for functional outcome. *Journal of Autism and Developmental Disorders, 41*(8), 1007–1018. https://doi.org/10.1007/s10803-010-1126-4

Karami, B., Koushki, R., Arabgol, F., Rahmani, M., & Vahabie, A. H. (2021). Effectiveness of virtual/augmented reality–based therapeutic interventions on individuals with autism spectrum disorder: A comprehensive meta-analysis. *Frontiers in Psychiatry, 12*, 665326. https://doi.org/10.3389/fpsyt.2021.665326

Kellems, R. O., Frandsen, K., Cardon, T. A., Knight, K., & Andersen, M. (2018). Effectiveness of static pictures vs. video prompting for teaching functional life skills to students with autism spectrum disorders. *Preventing School Failure: Alternative Education for Children and Youth, 62*(2), 129–139. https://doi.org/10.1080/1045988X.2017.1393790

Lamash, L., Klinger, E., & Josman, N. (2017). Using a virtual supermarket to promote independent functioning among adolescents with Autism Spectrum Disorder. In *Proceedings of international conference on virtual rehabilitation (ICVR)* (pp. 1–7). https://doi.org/10.1109/ICVR.2017.8007467

Mason, R. A., Davis, H. S., Ayres, K. M., Davis, J. L., & Mason, B. A. (2016). Video self-modeling for individuals with disabilities: A best-evidence, single case meta-analysis. *Journal of Developmental and Physical Disabilities, 28*(4), 623–642. https://doi.org/10.1007/s10882-016-9484-2

McMahon, D., Cihak, D. F., & Wright, R. (2015). Augmented reality as a navigation tool to employment opportunities for postsecondary education students with intellectual disabilities and autism. *Journal of Research on Technology in Education, 47*(3), 157–172. https://doi.org/10.1080/15391523.2015.1047698

Mechling, L. C., & Savidge, E. J. (2011). Using a personal digital assistant to increase completion of novel tasks and independent transitioning by students with autism spectrum disorder. *Journal of Autism and Developmental Disorders, 41*(6), 687–704. https://doi.org/10.1007/s10803-010-1088-6

Mechling, L. C., Gast, D. L., & Seid, N. H. (2009). Using a personal digital assistant to increase independent task completion by students with autism spectrum disorder. *Journal of Autism and Developmental Disorders, 39*(10), 1420–1434. https://doi.org/10.1007/s10803-009-0761-0

Mechling, L. C., Gast, D. L., & Seid, N. H. (2010). Evaluation of a personal digital assistant as a self-prompting device for increasing multi-step task completion by students with moderate intellectual disabilities. *Education and Training in Autism and Developmental Disabilities, 45*(3), 422–439.

Mellerson, S. D. (2021). Analytical review of using video technology to teach independent and daily living skills to students with intellectual disability. *DADD Online Journal, 8*(1), 58–73.

Miller, I. T., Wiederhold, B. K., Miller, C. S., & Wiederhold, M. D. (2020). Virtual reality air travel training with children on the autism spectrum: A preliminary report. *Cyberpsychology, Behavior, and Social Networking, 23*(1), 10–15. https://doi.org/10.1089/cyber.2019.0093

O'Handley, R. D., & Allen, K. D. (2017). An evaluation of the production effects of video self-modeling. *Research in Developmental Disabilities, 71*, 35–41. https://doi.org/10.1016/j.ridd.2017.09.012

Pérez-Fuster, P., Sevilla, J., & Herrera, G. (2019). Enhancing daily living skills in four adults with autism spectrum disorder through an embodied digital technology-mediated intervention. *Research in Autism Spectrum Disorders, 58*, 54–67. https://doi.org/10.1016/j.rasd.2018.08.006

Popple, B., Wall, C., Flink, L., Powell, K., Discepolo, K., Keck, D., et al. (2016). Brief report: Remotely delivered video modeling for improving oral hygiene in children with ASD: A pilot study. *Journal of Autism and Developmental Disorders, 46*(8), 2791–2796. https://doi.org/10.1007/s10803-016-2795-4

Reimer, B., Fried, R., Mehler, B., Joshi, G., Bolfek, A., Godfrey, K. M., Zhao, N., Goldin, R., & Biederman, J. (2013). Brief report: Examining driving behavior in young adults with high functioning autism spectrum disorders: A pilot study using a driving simulation paradigm. *Journal of Autism and Developmental Disorders, 43*(9), 2211–2217. https://doi.org/10.1007/s10803-013-1764-4

Rias, R. M., & Dehkordi, S. R. (2013). Computer game approach for children with autism spectrum disorder: A pilot study. In *Proceedings of 6th WSEAS world congress: Applied computing conference* (pp. 174–179). https://doi.org/10.13140/2.1.4411.1682

Ross, V., Cox, D. J., Reeve, R., Brown, T., Moncrief, M., Schmitt, R., & Gaffney, G. (2018). Measuring the attitudes of novice drivers with autism spectrum disorder as an indication of apprehensive driving: Going beyond basic abilities. *Autism, 22*(1), 62–69. https://doi.org/10.1177/1362361317735959

Saiano, M., Pellegrino, L., Casadio, M., Summa, S., Garbarino, E., Rossi, V., Dall'Agata, D., & Sanguineti, V. (2015). Natural interfaces and virtual environments for the acquisition of street crossing and path following skills in adults with Autism Spectrum Disorders: A feasibility study. *Journal of Neuroengineering and Rehabilitation, 12*(1), 1–17. https://doi.org/10.1186/s12984-015-0010-z

Simões, M., Bernardes, M., Barros, F., & Castelo-Branco, M. (2018). Virtual travel training for autism spectrum disorder: Proof-of-concept interventional study. *JMIR Serious Games, 6*(1), e8428. https://doi.org/10.2196/games.8428

Smith, L. E., Maenner, M. J., & Seltzer, M. M. (2012). Developmental trajectories in adolescents and adults with autism: The case of daily living skills. *Journal of the American Academy of Child & Adolescent Psychiatry, 51*(6), 622–631. https://doi.org/10.1016/j.jaac.2012.03.001

Sparrow, S., Cicchetti, D., & Saulnier, C. (2016). *Vineland adaptive behavior scales* (3rd ed.). NCS Pearson.

Spriggs, A. D., Knight, V., & Sherrow, L. (2015). Talking picture schedules: Embedding video models into visual activity schedules to increase independence for students with ASD. *Journal of Autism and Developmental Disorders, 45*(12), 3846–3861. https://doi.org/10.1007/s10803-014-2315-3

Thomsen, L. A., & Adjorlu, A. (2021). A collaborative virtual reality supermarket training application to teach shopping skills to young individuals with autism spectrum disorder. In *Proceedings of IEEE conference on virtual reality and 3D user interfaces abstracts and workshops (VRW)* (pp. 50–55). https://doi.org/10.1109/VRW52623.2021.00015

Tsikinas, S., & Xinogalos, S. (2021). "This is my story": A serious game for independent living skills in special education. In *Proceedings of European conference on games based learning* (p. 880). https://doi.org/10.34190/GBL.21.154

Tsikinas, S., Xinogalos, S., & Satratzemi, M. (2017). Review on serious games for people with intellectual disabilities and autism. In *Proceedings of the 10th European conference on games based learning* (pp. 696–703).

Vallefuoco, E., Bravaccio, C., Gison, G., Pecchia, L., & Pepino, A. (2022). Personalized training via serious game to improve daily living skills in pediatric patients with autism spectrum disorder. *IEEE Journal of Biomedical and Health Informatics.* https://doi.org/10.1109/JBHI.2022.3155367

Van Laarhoven, T., & Van Laarhoven-Myers, T. (2006). Comparison of three video-based instructional procedures for teaching daily living skills to persons with developmental disabilities. *Education and Training in Developmental Disabilities, 41*(4), 365–381.

Van Laarhoven, T., Kraus, E., Karpman, K., Nizzi, R., & Valentino, J. (2010). A comparison of picture and video prompts to teach daily living skills to individuals with autism. *Focus on Autism and Other Developmental Disabilities, 25*(4), 195–208. https://doi.org/10.1177/1088357610380412

Wade, J., Bian, D., Zhang, L., Swanson, A., Sarkar, M., Warren, Z., & Sarkar, N. (2014). Design of a virtual reality driving environment to assess performance of teenagers with ASD. In

Proceedings of international conference on universal access in human-computer interaction (pp. 466–474). https://doi.org/10.1007/978-3-319-07440-5_43

Wade, J., Bian, D., Fan, J., Zhang, L., Swanson, A., Sarkar, M., Weitlauf, A., Warren, Z., & Sarkar, N. (2015). A virtual reality driving environment for training safe gaze patterns: Application in individuals with ASD. In *Proceedings of international conference on universal access in human-computer interaction* (pp. 689–697). https://doi.org/10.1007/978-3-319-20684-4_66

Wade, J., Zhang, L., Bian, D., Fan, J., Swanson, A., Weitlauf, A., Sarkar, M., Warren, Z., & Sarkar, N. (2016). A gaze-contingent adaptive virtual reality driving environment for intervention in individuals with autism spectrum disorders. *ACM Transactions on Interactive Intelligent Systems (TiiS), 6*(1), 1–23. https://doi.org/10.1145/2892636

Wade, J., Weitlauf, A., Broderick, N., Swanson, A., Zhang, L., Bian, D., Sarkar, M., Warren, Z., & Sarkar, N. (2017). A pilot study assessing performance and visual attention of teenagers with ASD in a novel adaptive driving simulator. *Journal of Autism and Developmental Disorders, 47*(11), 3405–3417. https://doi.org/10.1007/s10803-017-3261-7

Wu, P., Cannella-Malone, H. I., Wheaton, J. E., & Tullis, C. A. (2016). Using video prompting with different fading procedures to teach daily living skills: A preliminary examination. *Focus on Autism and Other Developmental Disabilities, 31*(2), 129–139. https://doi.org/10.1177/1088357614533594

Xia, M., Chen, N., Tang, Y., & Zhu, Z. (2021). ParaShop: Shopping assistance to ASD individuals with a mobile AR app. *Journal on Technology and Persons with Disabilities, 9*, 1–17. https://doi.org/10.1109/URTC51696.2020.9668867

Ying, K. T., Sah, S. B. M., & Abdullah, M. H. L. (2016). Personalised avatar on social stories and digital storytelling: Fostering positive behavioural skills for children with autism spectrum disorder. In *Proceedings of 4th international conference on user science and engineering (i-USEr)* (pp. 253–258). https://doi.org/10.1109/IUSER.2016.7857970

Zhang, Q., Cao, Q., & Cai, Y. (2021). Learning to cross roads through VR playing. In Y. Cai & Q. Cao (Eds.), *When VR serious games meet special needs education: research, development and their applications* (pp. 63–75). Springer. https://doi.org/10.1007/978-981-33-6942-9_4

Chapter 7
Employment

7.1 Challenges in Employing People with Autism

The unemployment of people with autism is three to four times higher than unemployment in the general population (Mpofu et al., 2019). Given the significant differences between the economic development of specific countries and regions, it is difficult to determine what percentage of adults with autism has found employment. The estimates mainly range from 6% to 25% (according to Mpofu et al., 2019), although in some countries, such as the USA and Australia, around 50% of young adults with autism manage to find employment (according to Hedley et al., 2017). Despite these differences in statistical indicators, all researchers agree that the unemployment rate of people with autism is higher compared to both neurotypical people and adults with different types of disabilities. Also, people with autism usually have badly paid jobs which are sometimes below their skill level and are more frequently involved in a segregated employment model such as sheltered workshops. In developed countries, appropriate legal acts stimulate competitive integrated employment of people with autism. Competitive integrated employment means that people with autism earn at least a minimum wage, work on a location within their community, and have equal advancement opportunities as their nondisabled colleagues. Despite legal changes and knowledge about the beneficial effects of community employment, many people with autism still work at sheltered workshops, daycare facilities, and other forms of segregated employment, with wages below the minimum or none at all (Bross et al., 2020).

Employing people with autism has positive economic effects, both on individuals with autism and their families and society in general; it affects social relations and encourages integration into society; it improves autonomy and independence of people with autism and consequently reduces the intensity of support needs; it improves their emotional well-being, mental health, and quality of life (García-Villamisar et al., 2002; Hedley et al., 2017; Hendricks, 2010). Therefore, it is very

N. Glumbić et al., *Digital Inclusion of Individuals with Autism Spectrum Disorder*, Autism and Child Psychopathology Series,
https://doi.org/10.1007/978-3-031-12037-4_7

important to analyze the risk factors that reduce the possibilities of getting and keeping a job in adults with autism and constantly work on improving the opportunities for their participation in the labor market.

Difficulties in verbal and nonverbal communication, lack of soft skills, stereotyped activities and interests, resistance to change and problems switching from one task to another, time management difficulties, and insufficient stress control are only some of the frequently mentioned characteristics of autism that may have adverse effects on finding and keeping employment (e.g., Tomczak, 2021). However, the unemployment phenomenon is not solely an individual's issue, and the interventions aimed only at modifying individual behaviors and developing skills will not have the desired outcomes. As we will see, contemporary vocational rehabilitation programs, job interview preparations, and workplace support still mainly focus on developing individual skills and adapting an individual with autism to potential workplace demands.

We often take it for granted that employers are aware of the diagnosis of a potential worker with autism. Disclosing the diagnosis increases the possibility of accommodating the workplace for that person. However, people with autism are reluctant to reveal their diagnosis for fear of discrimination, which leaves them without the opportunity to have working conditions adapted to their needs (Lindsay et al., 2021). Protocols designed by neurotypical people regulate work organization and complex interpersonal relationships of employees. Although an employer has no conscious intention to discriminate against people with autism, they may perceive these rules as an insurmountable system barrier that reduces the possibility of their employment and further enhances negative attitudes toward them (Lorenz et al., 2021). Employers often believe that people with autism can only do solitary and repetitive jobs, although, with appropriate support, they can also train to do activities that involve frequent social interactions (Bross et al., 2020).

Apart from explicit and implicit discrimination by employers and colleagues, problems of social inequality and different opportunities in the labor market also refer to people with autism. According to Chiang et al. (2013), annual family income is one of the significant factors that affects the employment of high school graduates with autism. People with autism from poorer families have less access to early intervention, transportation, educational, health, and social support services. They do not have access to social capital that would allow them to use social networks and relations for employment and material gain (Mpofu et al., 2019). These authors believe that, when considering the potential role of digital technologies in employing people with autism, we should bear in mind their influence on the development of skills and encouragement of independence in people with autism, and also their possible role in work relations, expanding social network, and overcoming social inequalities.

Although some countries make significant efforts to support the employment of people with autism, the achieved results are very modest. Vocational support expenses for people with autism are higher than those for people with other types of disabilities, and their support needs last longer (Scott et al., 2019). The high unemployment rate indicates that the existing support services in the transition period are not sufficiently evidence-based (Smith et al., 2020). The employment outcomes are better if support services specialize in autism (Hedley et al., 2017). These services play a significant role in recruiting, interviewing, finding and adapting a workplace, and providing permanent support (Scott et al., 2019). In order to achieve competitive integrated employment, it is necessary to provide quality programs in the transition period, before graduating from high school, and evidence-based vocational rehabilitation. It is especially important to provide intensive job services and career counseling (Schall et al., 2020). People with autism who have career counseling at high school are 5.7 times more likely to find a job than their peers with autism who do not have this service at school (Chiang et al., 2013).

Supported employment starts with establishing a job seeker profile. This phase involves making an assessment and determining personal work goals. Job development is the next phase during which a person with autism is trained how to apply for a job and attend an interview. Job training comes after getting a job. In this phase, the person learns both work skills and all other skills necessary for doing the job. The third phase lasts as long as it takes a person with autism to be independent in work activities for at least 80% of working time. Long-term support is the final fourth phase, during which employees with autism receive a work instructor's support for less than 20% of working time (Wehman et al., 2017). This support model is not universal, but its basic elements are present in most comprehensive employment support programs.

The following text will point out the possibilities of applying digital technologies in preparing people with autism for job interviews and training for specific work activities. These technologies provide greater independence, increase workplace accessibility, and reduce vocational support expenses for people with autism, which are significant limitations of existing interventions in this field (Mpofu et al., 2019).

7.2 Job Interview

Under normal circumstances, job interviews require the applicants to understand and interpret interviewers' questions, to think of possible answers and clearly state the one they consider the most appropriate. In addition to verbal elements, job applicants need to recognize, understand, and adequately produce paralinguistic communication elements, such as prosody and facial expression, which are particularly challenging for people with cognitive disorders (Đorđević et al., 2016). Many different skills and abilities become apparent at a job interview. They include emotion recognition ability, understanding mental states of others, keeping adequate distance in interpersonal communication, modulating voice according to current circumstances, ignoring irrelevant sensory stimuli, presenting one's abilities in the best possible way, elaborating a specific topic in the appropriate time, etc.

An interviewer is usually an unfamiliar person, and the interview an individual's professional future depends on is mainly conducted in an unfamiliar setting. Therefore, it is not surprising that a job interview can cause anxiety even in persons who are otherwise not prone to such reactions. Interview anxiety is a multidimensional construct with cognitive, behavioral, and physiological components. Personal factors (e.g., physical appearance, skills, previous experiences), the interviewer's behavior and characteristics, and contextual features (e.g., face-to-face or video conference, type of interview, cultural factors, etc.) all significantly influence the occurrence of interview anxiety (Constantin et al., 2021).

7.2.1 Video-Based Interventions

Video-based interventions (VBI) are various strategies that use visual and auditory signals to help a person with autism develop specific behavior patterns and skills needed for finding and keeping a job. A systematic review of the literature on the efficacy of VBI has shown that they mainly focus on the acquisition of specific working skills and very rarely on job interview skills and other skills needed for finding a job (Munandar et al., 2020b). Personal computers, tablets, or cellphones are usually sufficient for implementing an intervention that includes videos of human subjects as models of specific behavior. For video-based interventions, it is not necessary to have specialized software or a stable Internet connection in most cases. On the other hand, introducing a virtual agent in VBI implies using software solutions and special equipment still unavailable to a wider range of potential users, at least in interventions based on immersive virtual reality. Regardless of whether an intervention uses a human or a virtual agent, they are all more or less based on well-known prompting, reinforcement, and modeling techniques.

Modeling is a technique used for demonstrating desirable behavior to a learner who is expected to adopt that behavior under specific circumstances. Wong et al. (2015) point out that modeling belongs to a group of evidence-based techniques in treating people with autism. This technique has different forms and variations, and instead of being exposed to live models, it is possible to adopt desirable behavior by watching video materials. Video modeling can easily be applied in learning the skills that do not need to be broken down into smaller steps (Glumbić et al., 2018), which is why it has successfully been used in training people with autism for a job interview.

Hayes et al. (2015) developed a cellphone application in which a person with autism chooses one out of three options: observing a model, performing, or watching a practiced activity. The model in this application is a peer with similar physical characteristics as a person with autism. When an interviewer asks a question, a visual signal first appears on the screen directing the application user to the correct answer, followed by a model who answers the question. After that, the screen shows a question for the person with autism which is related to the previously modeled behavior. The application user chooses one of the given answers and receives feedback on its accuracy. The second and third options offer the possibility of video self-modeling, i.e., recording and analyzing one's behavior while answering job interview questions. Compared to the control group of participants, people with autism who used this application achieved a higher degree of coherence and clarity in answering questions, were less nervous, and paid more attention to personal appearance.

Video modeling and video self-modeling are also used in the training system developed by Munandar et al. (2020a). The training begins by filming people with autism who answer job interview questions. In the second phase of training, people with autism watch videos of their peers answering the same questions. Since the questions aim to reveal the personal experiences of interviewees, the obtained answers cannot literally be used in a future interview. Therefore, people with autism are encouraged to notice the basic components of responses and not memorize the presented answers. In the third phase, people with autism receive video feedback. They watch and analyze their recorded answers from the first phase of training. In the fourth phase, the participants are informed that they will be asked the same questions once again and that they can use graphic organizers to plan their answers. The following training phases repeat job interview filming, watching, and analyzing the recording. The results indicate an improvement in target question-answering skills in four participants with autism.

VBI that use videos with human agents do not pay much attention to the environment in which a job interview is conducted (e.g., whether the office, furniture, and other details are similar to those in an actual job interview). Environment simulation is made possible by using virtual reality (VR) technologies. Certain elements of the VR-based training program can be repeated as much as needed. Several specialized systems for developing job interview skills in adults with autism, based on non-immersive and immersive technologies, have been developed in the last decade. By using non-immersive technologies, a person with autism takes on the role of an external observer of the content shown on a computer, tablet, or cellphone. In contrast, VR interventions that use a head-mounted display provide the experience of actual presence in the virtual environment. Various training tools for job interview skills typically include numerous written or auditory instructions, conversation transcripts, specific curricula, reward systems, visual signals, schedules, etc. VR technologies can also be included in these programs.

Strickland et al. (2013) evaluated the efficacy of a web-based interviewing skills program in a small sample of adolescents with high-functioning autism. In this program, VR-based training sessions were organized in a simulated office environment with two avatars. A person with autism had the role of an interviewee, while the avatar interviewer was a clinician who remotely guided the entire interview simulation process. They provided feedback to each answer of a person with autism, pointing out that some answers were more acceptable than others from a potential employer's perspective. The clinician praised appropriate reactions of the participants but also pointed out their mistakes in response content (e.g., straying from the topic, making remarks employers would not like, etc.) and nonverbal communication (appropriate facial expressions, eye contact, greeting, etc.). It turned out that the participants included in the training program made significant progress compared to the control group, who did not practice job interview skills. However, the observed improvement was significantly greater in verbal content than in the accompanying nonverbal communication.

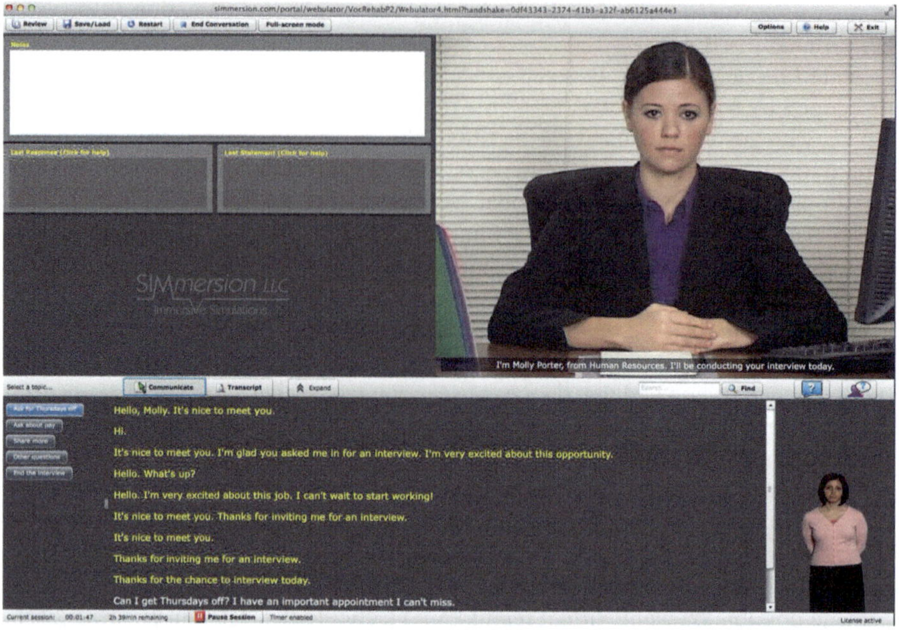

Fig. 7.1 VR-JIT-Simulated Interview Interface. (Reproduced from Smith et al., 2014)

Smith et al. (2014) obtained similar results by using the interactive simulation "Virtual Reality Job Interview Training" (VR-JIT) (Fig. 7.1). Since this intervention was originally intended for people with chronic mental illnesses, the interviewing scripts were not initially adapted for people with autism. This program uses a simulated interview interface where the interviewer is the avatar Molly. An algorithm is used to generate questions, but the interview may be changed to some extent depending on the obtained reactions. A text with multiple-choice answers appears on the screen. A person with autism chooses one answer and then reads it out loud. Speech recognition software allows Molly to "understand" what the interviewee said. A job instructor's avatar is located in the lower right corner of the screen, providing nonverbal feedback on the chosen answer by showing a thumbs-up or thumbs-down. It is also possible to get verbal feedback from the job instructor by clicking the help button. As in all similar programs, the mock interview can be repeated indefinitely. The randomized controlled study with 16 adult participants with autism included in the intervention and 10 participants with autism in the control group showed a significant improvement in job interview performance and self-confidence levels in the participants included in the training program (Smith et al., 2014). The evaluation of vocational outcomes pointed out that people with autism who completed this training program were more likely to get a competitive job than the control group 6 months after completing the training (Smith et al., 2015).

Autism specialists, community members, and program users (people with autism, their family members, teachers, potential employers) were consulted in order to adapt VR-JIT for people with autism in the transition period. The program was significantly improved and adapted for people with autism based on the feedback received. In addition to making reading and comprehension of accompanying materials easier, changes were also made to the virtual environment. Most participants in this research believed that the virtual hiring manager should not always be a Caucasian woman but that the avatar interviewers should be of different gender, race, and ethnicity and that their faces should be more expressive. Numerous adaptations were made to the number and content of multiple-choice answers, and great effort was put into making the training program fun for users with autism (Smith et al., 2020).

Similar results were obtained by using the commercial training program "Virtual Interactive Training Agents" (ViTA) in a sample of 153 participants with different types of disabilities, with most participants having autism. Virtual humans as interviewers can be of different gender, age, and ethnicity. Unlike most described training systems in which the interview is conducted in a simulated office, this program offers a possibility to choose from seven different settings. The change also applies to the behavioral disposition of the virtual interviewer, who, in addition to being kind and neutral, can sometimes also exhibit hostile behavior. During the training, which lasts for 22 weeks, individuals learn the essential skills needed for adequately presenting themselves at a job interview. The latest versions of the ViTA system are equipped with software that monitors nonverbal reactions of the participants, such as blinking frequency, keeping eye contact, head position, response latency, etc. Although progress was observed both in job interview skills and in the evaluated self-efficacy, it is still unknown whether the acquired skills have persisted over time and have actually been used to get a job (Burke et al., 2021).

Interview training systems based on non-immersive VR technology create a safe and simulated learning environment. However, the users are always aware of the distance between them as observers and the virtual environment displayed on the screen. Since there is no direct link between a user and a device, it is possible to monitor only behavioral parameters without monitoring the physiological ones that could indicate that the person is under stress. In an attempt to overcome these limitations, the InterViewR training system was developed. It uses headphones and a head-mounted display to block potential distractors, such as background noises and visual stimuli from the real environment. Good virtual environment graphics, convincing behavior of virtual humans, and adequate frame rates also contribute to a high degree of immersiveness. The level of stimulation in the virtual environment can be changed according to the users' reactions. Also, the users wear a smart shirt that provides information on heart rate, breathing, and physiological stress indicators. During each session, the users are informed in real time that some key parameters have been changed (e.g., that eye contact is lost or that a certain question has upset the participant). A usability study on a small sample of 11 people with autism showed that the platform that integrated affective feedback and immersive VR technology could help people with autism improve their job interview skills and control stress levels (Ahmed et al., 2020). Using immersive VR technologies for these purposes is still in the initial phase, and their efficacy will undoubtedly be the subject of future research.

VR technologies allow the intervention to be implemented in safe and strictly controlled conditions so that even the smallest changes in behavior can be detected and the obtained results used to improve the training program. The training does not require direct contact between people with autism and their instructors. This makes it possible to overcome the barriers that naturally arise when a potential user is not at the place where the training is conducted in direct contact or if face-to-face communication is not safe due to a pandemic or some other emergency. However, interview training based on VR technologies also has some drawbacks. Although connecting advanced technologies to cellphones would reduce costs, VR technologies at the moment, especially immersive ones, require high-performance computers, specialized equipment, and often uninterrupted Internet access. Many training programs are very expensive and therefore inaccessible to a large number of potential users. Apart from that, immersive technologies may have some adverse effects, such as asthenopia, nausea, loss of balance, increased anxiety, and sensory difficulties. Thus, gradual adaptation of people with autism during their implementation is necessary (Schmidt et al., 2021). A study conducted on a convenience sample of children with ASD is encouraging. It indicated that these children preferred immersive VR technologies to video content shown on the screen. No significant differences were observed in the level of anxiety or other adverse effects when comparing the use of a head-mounted display and a monitor-display video (Malihi et al., 2020).

Unlike VR technologies, which are based on creating artificial reality, augmented reality (AR) uses the existing, real environment in which it inserts digital information. This technique allows overlaying computer graphics with real-world objects. AR systems use cameras to detect markers, i.e., prominent objects in the environment near which a graphic image is rendered. Audio systems, infrared sensors, and biosensors are often used as additional hardware components for obtaining information about the users and their environment (Verma et al., 2021).

AR can be used as a navigation tool for finding locations where people with autism can get a job. Mobile application Layar is used for this purpose. Based on the user's location, this application shows available nearby jobs. It uses a location-based AR display for selected content. If the users select the "job opportunities" option, they get computer-generated information about the distance and the type of job at that location by looking through the camera. A young man with autism included in the postsecondary job-finding training program was much more successful in finding the desired location after a short training in using the AR application than when he used a paper or Google map (McMahon et al., 2015).

AR technologies have also been used in preparing people with autism for a job interview. Xu et al. (2015) used the Google Glass application LittleHelper to train people with autism to keep appropriate eye contact and modulate speech during a job interview. This application can detect the speech volume of a person with autism and, by using computer-generated information (up and down arrows and textual information about speech volume), direct the user to speak louder or quieter. There is also a module for interviewer detection. If the interviewer moves from the direct visual contact with the interviewee, left or right arrows are a visual reminder that head position and eye contact should be adjusted to the location of the interviewer. Hartholt et al. (2019) developed a virtual human application in AR based on the ViTA system. Unlike the desktop application, which offers various virtual environments, the AR version places a virtual human directly in the real world. The improved hardware with sensors that were not available in the desktop version makes it possible to carefully monitor six parameters during an interview: gaze direction, blinking frequency, head position, response latency, response time, and speech volume. Computer-generated information in the form of graphics and textual information provides users with autism immediate feedback on their performance. It should be pointed out that AR applications for work activities of people with autism are mainly prototypes in the alpha phase. They have been used by a small number of users mostly for the purpose of improving technical details, while their actual efficacy in finding a job or training for specific work activities is yet to be determined.

7.2.2 Robotics

Unlike VR technologies that use digitally generated visual characters to conduct interviews, robots are artificial agents placed in the real environment in which an intervention is held. Robot-based technologies are primarily used to encourage joint attention, social interactions, and communication in children with autism. Since they are among the most expensive emerging technologies, their use is mainly limited to specialized research and clinical centers (Kumm et al., 2021).

A group of Japanese authors created a tele-operating female type of android robot with human-like appearance and movements. This robot was used for job interview training in seven young people with autism. The control group included participants with autism whose training involved traditional means of reading and analyzing written instructions on adequate interview participation and answering questions. Although the 5-day training was based only on practice and exposure, with no specific, structured curriculum, the participants who practiced the interview with a robot slightly improved their self-confidence. Also, their stress level, measured by salivary cortisol concentration, was significantly lower at the end of the intervention (Kumazaki et al., 2017). By using the same android robot 2 years later, similar results were obtained regarding the self-assessed level of self-confidence and the objective assessment of stress level. Furthermore, the short job interview training was this time successfully used to develop nonverbal communication skills (Kumazaki et al., 2019a).

Bearing in mind the significance of nonverbal communication during a job interview, some researchers tried to determine the specifics of some nonverbal communication aspects in experimental settings of a mock job interview. Gaze aversion, for example, does not necessarily mean avoiding contact but can also have some important communicative functions, such as turn-taking, indicating a cognitive effort, or regulating intimacy (Acarturk et al., 2021). These authors found that the interviewers made more frequent and longer eye contact during a mock job interview than the interviewee, but the gaze aversion pattern was different. While the interviewers tended to make diagonal gaze aversions, the interviewees made sideways aversions. As suggested by the authors, these results could be used to create realistic android robots that would have the role of interviewers. However, it seems that this should also be done without exaggeration. It turned out that people with autism prefer robots to humans when practicing job interviews but only if robots have simplified facial expressions and movements. The more robots resemble humans, the greater the resistance of people with autism is (Kumazaki et al., 2019c).

One of the possible interventions in job interview training refers to observing the interview situation from the aspect of an interviewer. For that purpose, pair work role-play was organized. One person with autism had the role of an interviewee, while the other was an interviewer. The person with autism who played the interviewer operated a robot by activating questions according to a predetermined plan, repeated and practiced nonverbal communication signals, and monitored the relationship between the robot and the interviewee with autism via video. In each training session, each participant with autism had both roles of an interviewer and an interviewee. The results indicate a potential to successfully use role-play with a tele-operating android robot to improve job interview skills in people with autism (Kumazaki et al., 2019b).

7.3 The Influence of VBI on Job Performance Skills

In a systematic review of the literature on how VBI affects the work skills of people with autism, out of 19 studies that met the inclusion criteria, only 3 dealt with using VBI for finding a job, while all others examined the possibility of applying VBI in training people with autism for specific job responsibilities (Munandar et al., 2020a, b). To successfully do a job, apart from necessary knowledge and skills, a person with autism must have appropriate communication with employers, other workers, and sometimes, depending on the job, potential users or buyers. From the employers' perspective, their employees with autism must have both hard (ability to perform job duties) and soft skills (social skills, emotional regulation, planning ability, etc.) (Albright et al., 2020).

Video modeling is most frequently used in teaching soft skills to people with autism both in a simulated (Stauch & Plavnick, 2020) or real work environment (Bross et al., 2020). Five young people with autism included in the research by Bross et al. (2020) already did the jobs of box office cashiers, food deliverers for elderly people with limited mobility, amusement park ticket controllers, and other jobs for which developed soft skills are required. By using video modeling, employees with autism were taught how to greet new customers, say appropriate phrases while providing a service, and say goodbye when leaving. In addition to verbal expressions, tone of voice and body language were also modeled. The participants with autism made progress in acquiring soft skills, which persisted for 2 and 4 weeks afterward.

To successfully perform job duties, employees with autism must be able to easily manage their behavior, complete tasks on time, and switch between work activities. Executive function problems, which are quite common in people with autism, can adversely affect their ability to manage their behavior at work. Smart technologies can compensate for these limitations to some extent. Personal digital assistants (PDAs), which in their modern form represent multifunctional, easily portable, pocket-size devices, can be used for this purpose. Gentry et al. (2012) successfully used personal digital assistants for achieving different work goals in three adult participants with autism. PDA used in this research provided various types of support: task list, task reminder, videos of individual work task steps presented as video prompts, behavioral self-management adaptations, etc.

PDAs that provide video modeling and video prompting have also been successfully used to learn hard skills, i.e., to perform multicomponent tasks accurately (e.g., Burke et al., 2013). Video modeling and video prompting are the most commonly used VBI for teaching people with autism various job performance skills, such as checking out and shelving books, dye cuts, preparing food, using different devices, cleaning, photocopying, recycling, etc. (Munandar et al., 2020a, b). Based on a meta-analysis of studies dealing with the application of video modeling in teaching specific work skills to people with autism, Bross et al. (2021) conclude that it is an effective and highly recommendable technique. However, unfortunately, it is more studied in a school setting in adolescents with autism going through a transition period than in an integrated, competitive work environment.

Video self-modeling has been used very rarely. Therefore, a paper that examines the effects of video self-modeling on vocational skills (receiving orders, packaging, and delivering flowers) and social skills (engaging with customers) in participants with low-functioning autism is very significant (Parsons et al., 2020). An employee with autism participated with support in flower delivery. The videos were edited to show sequences of successfully completed activities. A gold star and recorded words of praise appeared on the video as specific individual prompting. After a series of training sessions in which special attention was paid to the gradual reduction of prompting, significant effects were achieved in both vocational and related social skills.

Researchers and practitioners are so preoccupied with developing different techniques for improving work skills of people with autism that they often forget to assess future employees' work preferences, which are crucial for their success and satisfaction at work. By using video modeling, various options of supported employment were shown to people with autism undergoing job training, and then a mobile application was used to determine their work preferences (Walsh et al., 2020). This is a classic technique of assessing preferences by exposure to pairs of stimuli from which the preferred one should be chosen; only, in this case, the application itself is set to calculate the degree of preference for specific work activities. As expected, the participants were best at jobs for which they had interest and all necessary skills. However, it turned out that even when they did not have all the required skills, people with autism could perform specific work tasks very well, provided that they highly preferred them.

The use of VR technologies in job training of people with autism is of recent date, so papers dealing with this issue are scarce. Bozgeyikli et al. (2017) developed a system based on immersive VR technology for job training of people with autism. Immersiveness was achieved by using HMD or 180° curved screens. Special modules were designed for six different transferrable skills. Work skills that can be used in many different jobs, such as cleaning, loading, shelving, etc., were deliberately chosen. The modules were structured in a way that a person with autism was gradually exposed to more and more complex tasks. At the first (tutorial) level, the trainees learned how to perform a task. At the second level, they had the opportunity to practice the task in a virtual environment without any distractions. VR distractors were introduced at the third level but only when the trainees mastered a particular activity. Since work tasks in real settings are also performed under various environmental distractors, it is necessary for potential employees with autism to get used to them. If a trainee did not complete the task at any level, verbal instructions, pictograms, or animations were used for prompting. This system was not designed to replace training with professional job instructors but as help and addition to the existing training system. Therefore, job instructors were provided with a remote control interface so that they could change and control different system parameters in each training phase.

Initial research on the application of digital technologies in employing people with autism indicates their potential advantages over traditional job training and employment programs. However, research predominantly focuses on people with high-functioning autism, especially in the studies dealing with job interview training. Research samples are typically small, and the possibility to generalize the obtained results is limited. Also, we should bear in mind that 95% of the world's population of people with autism live in low- and middle-income countries (Kumm et al., 2021), whose citizens usually have cheaper digital technologies based on the use of cellphones and personal computers. Hence, it is not surprising that the most expensive technologies based on VR and robotics are still limited to individual research and rehabilitation centers in developed world countries.

References

Acarturk, C., Indurkya, B., Nawrocki, P., Sniezynski, B., Jarosz, M., & Usal, K. A. (2021). Gaze aversion in conversational settings: An investigation based on mock job interview. *Journal of Eye Movement Research, 14*(1). https://doi.org/10.16910/jemr.14.1.1

Ahmed, S., Deneke, W., Mai, V., Veneruso, A., Stepita, M., Dawson, A., Hoefel, B., Claeys, G., Lam, N., & Sharmin, M. (2020). InterViewR: A mixed-reality based interview training simulation platform for individuals with autism. In *2020 IEEE 44th annual computers, software, and applications conference (COMPSAC)* (pp. 439–448). IEEE. https://doi.org/10.1109/COMPSAC48688.2020.0-211

Albright, J., Kulok, S., & Scarpa, A. (2020). A qualitative analysis of employer perspectives on the hiring and employment of adults with autism spectrum disorder. *Journal of Vocational Rehabilitation, 53*, 167–182. https://doi.org/10.3233/JVR-201094

Bozgeyikli, L., Bozgeyikli, E., Raij, A., Alqasemi, R., Katkoori, S., & Dubey, R. (2017). Vocational rehabilitation of individuals with autism spectrum disorder with virtual reality. *ACM Transactions on Accessible Computing (TACCESS), 10*(2), 1–25. https://doi.org/10.1145/3046786

Bross, L. A., Travers, J. C., Wills, H. P., Huffman, J. M., Watson, E. K., Morningstar, M. E., & Boyd, B. A. (2020). Effects of video modeling for young adults with autism in community employment settings. *Career Development and Transition for Exceptional Individuals, 43*(4), 209–225. https://doi.org/10.1177/2165143420941488

Bross, L. A., Travers, J. C., Huffman, J. M., Davis, J. L., & Mason, R. A. (2021). A meta-analysis of video modeling interventions to enhance job skills of autistic adolescents and adults. *Autism in Adulthood*. https://doi.org/10.1089/aut.2020.0038

Burke, R. V., Allen, K. D., Howard, M. R., Downey, D., Matz, M. G., & Bowen, S. L. (2013). Tablet-based video modeling and prompting in the workplace for individuals with autism. *Journal of Vocational Rehabilitation, 38*(1), 1–14. https://doi.org/10.3233/JVR-120616

Burke, S. L., Li, T., Grudzien, A., & Garcia, S. (2021). Brief report: Improving employment interview self-efficacy among adults with autism and other developmental disabilities using virtual interactive training agents (ViTA). *Journal of Autism and Developmental Disorders, 51*(2), 741–748. https://doi.org/10.1007/s10803-020-04571-8

Chiang, H. M., Cheung, Y. K., Li, H., & Tsai, L. Y. (2013). Factors associated with participation in employment for high school leavers with autism. *Journal of Autism and Developmental Disorders, 43*(8), 1832–1842. https://doi.org/10.1007/s10803-012-1734-2

Constantin, K. L., Powell, D. M., & McCarthy, J. M. (2021). Expanding conceptual understanding of interview anxiety and performance: Integrating cognitive, behavioral, and physiological features. *International Journal of Selection and Assessment, 29*(2), 234–252. https://doi.org/10.1111/ijsa.12326

Đorđević, M., Glumbić, N., & Brojčin, B. (2016). Paralinguistic abilities of adults with intellectual disability. *Research in Developmental Disabilities, 48*, 211–219. https://doi.org/10.1016/j.ridd.2015.11.001

García-Villamisar, D., Wehman, P., & Navarro, M. D. (2002). Changes in the quality of autistic people's life that work in supported and sheltered employment. A 5-year follow-up study. *Journal of Vocational Rehabilitation, 17*(4), 309–312.

Gentry, T., Lau, S., Molinelli, A., Fallen, A., & Kriner, R. (2012). The Apple iPod Touch as a vocational support aid for adults with autism: Three case studies. *Journal of Vocational Rehabilitation, 37*(2), 75–85. https://doi.org/10.3233/JVR-2012-0601

Glumbić, N., Brojčin, B., & Đorđević, M. (2018). *Specijalna edukacija zasnovana na dokazima: Bihevioralne tehnike*. Univerzitet u Beogradu – Fakultet za specijalnu edukaciju i rehabilitaciju.

Hartholt, A., Mozgai, S., Fast, E., Liewer, M., Reilly, A., Whitcup, W., & Rizzo, A. S. (2019). Virtual humans in augmented reality: A first step towards real-world embedded virtual roleplayers. In *Proceedings of the 7th international conference on human-agent interaction* (pp. 205–207). https://doi.org/10.1145/3349537.3352766

Hayes, G. R., Custodio, V. E., Haimson, O. L., Nguyen, K., Ringland, K. E., Ulgado, R. R., Waterhouse, A., & Weiner, R. (2015). Mobile video modeling for employment interviews for individuals with autism. *Journal of Vocational Rehabilitation, 43*(3), 275–287. https://doi.org/10.3233/JVR-150775

Hedley, D., Uljarević, M., Cameron, L., Halder, S., Richdale, A., & Dissanayake, C. (2017). Employment programmes and interventions targeting adults with autism spectrum disorder: A systematic review of the literature. *Autism, 21*(8), 929–941. https://doi.org/10.1177/1362361316661855

Hendricks, D. (2010). Employment and adults with autism spectrum disorders: Challenges and strategies for success. *Journal of Vocational Rehabilitation, 32*(2), 125–134.

Kumazaki, H., Warren, Z., Corbett, B. A., Yoshikawa, Y., Matsumoto, Y., Higashida, H., Yuhi, T., Ikeda, T., Ishiguro, H., & Kikuchi, M. (2017). Android robot-mediated mock job interview sessions for young adults with autism spectrum disorder: A pilot study. *Frontiers in Psychiatry, 8*, 169. https://doi.org/10.3389/fpsyt.2017.00169

Kumazaki, H., Muramatsu, T., Yoshikawa, Y., Corbett, B. A., Matsumoto, Y., Higashida, H., Yuhi, T., Ishiguro, H., Mimura, M., & Kikuchi, M. (2019a). Job interview training targeting nonverbal communication using an android robot for individuals with autism spectrum disorder. *Autism, 23*(6), 1586–1595. https://doi.org/10.1177/1362361319827134

Kumazaki, H., Muramatsu, T., Yoshikawa, Y., Matsumoto, Y., Ishiguro, H., Mimura, M., & Kikuchi, M. (2019b). Role-play-based guidance for job interviews using an android robot for individuals with autism spectrum disorders. *Frontiers in Psychiatry, 10*, 239. https://doi.org/10.3389/fpsyt.2019.00239

Kumazaki, H., Muramatsu, T., Yoshikawa, Y., Matsumoto, Y., Miyao, M., Ishiguro, H., Mimura, M., Minabe, Y., & Kikuchi, M. (2019c). How the realism of robot is needed for individuals with autism spectrum disorders in an interview setting. *Frontiers in Psychiatry, 10*, 486. https://doi.org/10.3389/fpsyt.2019.00486

Kumm, A. J., Viljoen, M., & de Vries, P. J. (2021). The digital divide in technologies for autism: Feasibility considerations for low-and middle-income countries. *Journal of Autism and Developmental Disorders*, 1–14. https://doi.org/10.1007/s10803-021-05084-8

Lindsay, S., Osten, V., Rezai, M., & Bui, S. (2021). Disclosure and workplace accommodations for people with autism: A systematic review. *Disability and Rehabilitation, 43*(5), 597–610. https://doi.org/10.1080/09638288.2019.1635658

Lorenz, T., Brüning, C. R., Waltz, M., & Fabri, M. (2021). Not a stranger to the dark: Discrimination against autistic students and employees. *Advances in Autism, 7*(1), 60–72. https://doi.org/10.1108/AIA-10-2019-0036

Malihi, M., Nguyen, J., Cardy, R. E., Eldon, S., Petta, C., & Kushki, A. (2020). Short report: Evaluating the safety and usability of head-mounted virtual reality compared to monitor-displayed video for children with autism spectrum disorder. *Autism, 24*, 1924–1929. https://doi.org/10.1177/1362361320934214

McMahon, D., Cihak, D. F., & Wright, R. (2015). Augmented reality as a navigation tool to employment opportunities for postsecondary education students with intellectual disabilities and autism. *Journal of Research on Technology in Education, 47*(3), 157–172. https://doi.org/10.1080/15391523.2015.1047698

Mpofu, E., Tansey, T., Mpofu, N., Tu, W. M., & Li, Q. (2019). Employment practices with people with autism spectrum disorder in the digital age. In *Theory, research and dynamics of career wellbeing* (pp. 309–326). Springer.

Munandar, V. D., Bross, L. A., Zimmerman, K. N., & Morningstar, M. E. (2020a). Video-based intervention to improve storytelling ability in job interviews for college students with autism. *Career Development and Transition for Exceptional Individuals*, 2165143420961853. https://doi.org/10.1177/2165143420961853

Munandar, V. D., Morningstar, M. E., & Carlson, S. R. (2020b). A systematic literature review of video-based interventions to improve integrated competitive employment skills among youth and adults with autism spectrum disorder. *Journal of Vocational Rehabilitation, 53*(1), 29–41. https://doi.org/10.3233/jvr-201083

Parsons, N., D'Aprano, F., Hughes, M., Parish, A., & Outsikas, N. (2020). *Using video self-modelling to teach combined vocational and social skills to an adult with autism spectrum disorder*. https://doi.org/10.31234/osf.io/ra879

Schall, C., Wehman, P., Avellone, L., & Taylor, J. P. (2020). Competitive integrated employment for youth and adults with autism: Findings from a scoping review. *Child and Adolescent Psychiatric Clinics of North America, 29*(2), 373–397. https://www.sciencedirect.com/science/article/pii/S1056499319301208

Schmidt, M., Newbutt, N., Schmidt, C., & Glaser, N. (2021). A process-model for minimizing adverse effects when using head mounted display-based virtual reality for individuals with autism. *Frontiers in Virtual Reality, 2*, 13. https://doi.org/10.3389/frvir.2021.611740

Scott, M., Milbourn, B., Falkmer, M., Black, M., Bolte, S., Halladay, A., Lerner, M., Taylor, J. L., & Girdler, S. (2019). Factors impacting employment for people with autism spectrum disorder: A scoping review. *Autism, 23*(4), 869–901. https://doi.org/10.1177/1362361318787789

Smith, M. J., Ginger, E. J., Wright, K., Wright, M. A., Taylor, J. L., Humm, L. B., Olsen, D., Bell, M., & Fleming, M. F. (2014). Virtual reality job interview training in adults with autism spectrum disorder. *Journal of Autism and Developmental Disorders, 44*(10), 2450–2463. https://doi.org/10.1007/s10803-014-2113-y

Smith, M. J., Fleming, M. F., Wright, M. A., Losh, M., Humm, L. B., Olsen, D., & Bell, M. D. (2015). Brief report: Vocational outcomes for young adults with autism spectrum disorders at six months after virtual reality job interview training. *Journal of Autism and Developmental Disorders, 45*(10), 3364–3369. https://doi.org/10.1007/s10803-015-2470-1

Smith, M. J., Pinto, R. M., Dawalt, L., Smith, J. D., Sherwood, K., Miles, R., Taylor, L., Hume, K., Dawkins, T., Baker-Ericzén, M., Frazier, T., Humm, L., & Steacy, C. (2020). Using community-engaged methods to adapt virtual reality job-interview training for transition-age youth on the autism spectrum. *Research in Autism Spectrum Disorders, 71*, 101498. https://doi.org/10.1016/j.rasd.2019.101498

Stauch, T. A., & Plavnick, J. B. (2020). Teaching vocational and social skills to adolescents with autism using video modeling. *Education and Treatment of Children, 43*, 137–151. https://doi.org/10.1007/s43494-020-00020-4

Strickland, D. C., Coles, C. D., & Southern, L. B. (2013). JobTIPS: A transition to employment program for individuals with autism spectrum disorders. *Journal of Autism and Developmental Disorders, 43*(10), 2472–2483. https://doi.org/10.1007/s10803-013-1800-4

Tomczak, M. T. (2021). Employees with autism spectrum disorders in the digitized work environment: Perspectives for the future. *Journal of Disability Policy Studies, 31*(4), 195–205. https://doi.org/10.1177/1044207320919945

Verma, V., Sharma, A., Jain, K. K., & Adlakha, S. (2021). Digital assistant with augmented reality. In *ICT systems and sustainability* (pp. 395–404). Springer. https://doi.org/10.1007/978-981-15-8289-9_38

Walsh, E., Lydon, H., & Holloway, J. (2020). An evaluation of assistive technology in determining job-specific preference for adults with autism and intellectual disabilities. *Behavior Analysis in Practice, 13*(2), 434–444. https://doi.org/10.1007/s40617-019-00380-3

Wehman, P., Schall, C. M., McDonough, J., Graham, C., Brooke, V., Riehle, J. E., Brooke, A., Ham, W., Lau, S., Allen, J., & Avellone, L. (2017). Effects of an employer-based intervention on employment outcomes for youth with significant support needs due to autism. *Autism, 21*(3), 276–290. https://doi.org/10.1177/1362361316635826

Wong, C., Odom, S. L., Hume, K. A., Cox, A. W., Fettig, A., Kucharczyk, S., Brock, M. E., Plavnick, J. B., Fleury, V. P., & Schultz, T. R. (2015). Evidence-based practices for children, youth, and young adults with autism spectrum disorder: A comprehensive review. *Journal of Autism and Developmental Disorders, 45*(7), 1951–1966. https://doi.org/10.1007/s10803-014-2351-z

Xu, Q., Cheung, S. C. S., & Soares, N. (2015). LittleHelper: An augmented reality glass application to assist individuals with autism in job interview. In *2015 Asia-Pacific signal and information processing association annual summit and conference (APSIPA)* (pp. 1276–1279). IEEE. https://doi.org/10.1109/APSIPA.2015.7415480

Chapter 8
Technology-Aided Instruction and Intervention

8.1 Technology-Aided Instruction and Intervention: Definition and Scientific Basis

Autism in combination with technology first appeared in WoS papers in 1992. According to Carmona-Serrano et al. (2020), the research period can be divided into two parts—from 1992 to 2009 and from 2009 to the present. The first interval is characterized by fewer research studies and topics focusing on children. In the second period, the number of publications has significantly increased, and the topics are more frequently related to interventions. The focus of interventions has changed over the years. First, they aimed to improve communication, then support everyday activities, and finally, improve social skills. Although there are certain differences between these two intervals, coincidences have also been noted in 35% of cases. Carmona-Serrano et al. (2020) explain this by the fact that, along with establishing new research goals, the scientific community still maintains the existing ones, i.e., traditional approaches that are the basis for further research. With regard to this time division, it is not surprising that the US National Autism Center recognized a special category of interventions in 2009, called "technology-based treatment," considering them the interventions in which technology had a central place and was used to support different skills (NAC, 2009). In a report published in 2015, the National Autism Center referred to these interventions by a slightly different name—"technology-based intervention"—and classified them in the group of interventions with the emerging level of evidence, i.e., interventions that may lead to favorable outcomes but require further research to prove that (NAC, 2015). Steinbrenner et al. (2020) used the phrase "technology-aided instruction and intervention" to denote these interventions in the report for the National Clearinghouse on Autism Evidence and Practice (NCAEP). Technology-aided instruction and intervention involve using any electronic devices, equipment, applications, or networks to improve or

N. Glumbić et al., *Digital Inclusion of Individuals with Autism Spectrum Disorder*, Autism and Child Psychopathology Series,
https://doi.org/10.1007/978-3-031-12037-4_8

maintain skills related to an individual's quality of life (Odom et al., 2015). In the mentioned report, Steinbrenner et al. (2020) indicate that these interventions belong to the category of focused approaches, i.e., they are aimed at specific outcomes and skills, and their application is usually shorter compared to comprehensive interventions. Furthermore, Steinbrenner et al. (2020) point out that conditions have been met for these interventions to join the group of evidence-based practices.

According to the National Professional Development Center on Autism Spectrum Disorder (2017), technology-aided instruction and intervention are a science-based approach for ages 0–22 years in the following areas: pre-academic and academic skills, adaptive and self-help skills, cognitive skills, communication, joint attention, school readiness, and social skills. Evidence of their scientific basis in challenging behavior, mental health, motor skills, and play has so far been confirmed for ages 0–14 years. Areas for which, by the time of publishing this report, no science-based effects have been determined include vocational and self-determination skills (National Professional Development Center on Autism Spectrum Disorder, 2017).

Apart from inconsistencies in attitudes regarding the scientific basis and terminology of these interventions, there is also a discrepancy in relation to their content. Thus, for example, Whitehouse et al. (2021) include augmentative and alternative communication interventions (interventions involving various procedures and technologies that enhance or replace speech) in this group of treatments. On the other hand, Steinbrenner et al. (2020) point out that augmentative and alternative communication interventions are a special group and that speech-generating devices belong to them and not the group of technology-based treatments. Barton et al. (2017) divided these interventions into three subcategories—augmentative and alternative communication, computer-assisted instruction (interventions that use computers to improve academic, language, and cognitive skills, usually with the help of modeling and computer tutors), and virtual reality. In terms of the used devices, these authors mention mobile devices, personal computers, speech-generating devices, virtual reality, the Internet, and shared active surface. Discussing what constitutes a technology-based intervention, Goldsmith and LeBlanc (2004) distinguish five categories within which they combine interventions with the used devices—tactile and auditory prompting devices, video-based instruction and feedback, computer-aided instruction, virtual reality, and robotics.

8.2 Advantages and Limitations of Technology-Based Interventions

In their report for Autism CRC, Whitehouse et al. (2021) state that technology-based interventions can be helpful in working with children and adults with autism spectrum disorder (ASD) because they show an affinity for using technology very often and because these interventions reduce social interactions and social demands to a minimum. A study that confirmed these claims used two types of robots (a

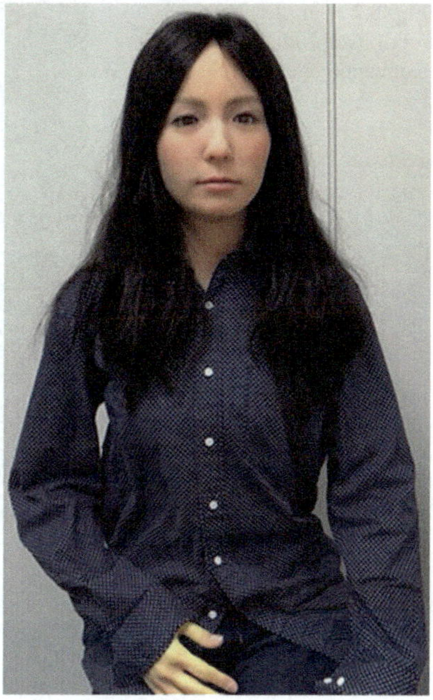

Fig. 8.1 Android robot. (Reproduced from Kumazaki et al., 2019)

human-like android robot and a humanoid robot with a simple face) and a digital, screen-based avatar to determine how children with ASD at a younger preschool age reacted to their instructions. The results showed that children with ASD responded better and more often to the humanoid robot and avatar than to the android robot (Kumazaki et al., 2019) (Figs. 8.1, 8.2, and 8.3). Bekele et al. (2014) confirm that, when faced with a real person and an android robot, children with ASD focus on the robot. All this indicates that technologies stimulate greater motivation in people with ASD.

Another advantage of using technology in interventions in people with autism, compared to other approaches, is consistent and timely application, as well as a wide range of extrinsic rewards (which can be personalized or enhanced by adding different functions) (Constantin et al., 2017). Frequently mentioned advantages also include the availability of these interventions at any time (e.g., any time during 24 h) and space (e.g., rural areas) and the possibility to adapt them to the users' language (Baggett et al., 2010). In favor of technology-based interventions, Hansen and Winn (2019) state that the devices and equipment are often portable; that they can provide clear visual information, necessary predictability, and clarity; and that they can be a motivator for acquiring new knowledge and skills in people with ASD.

Furthermore, the value of technology-based interventions is reflected in their flexibility, i.e., the ability to incorporate the bases of other science-based approaches and treatments. Thus, it is not surprising that applications based on applied behavior analysis (e.g., Autistic Behavior and Computer-based Didactic Software, ABA Find It!, Jacob's Lessons, AB Pathfinder, TOBY) have been developed in recent years.

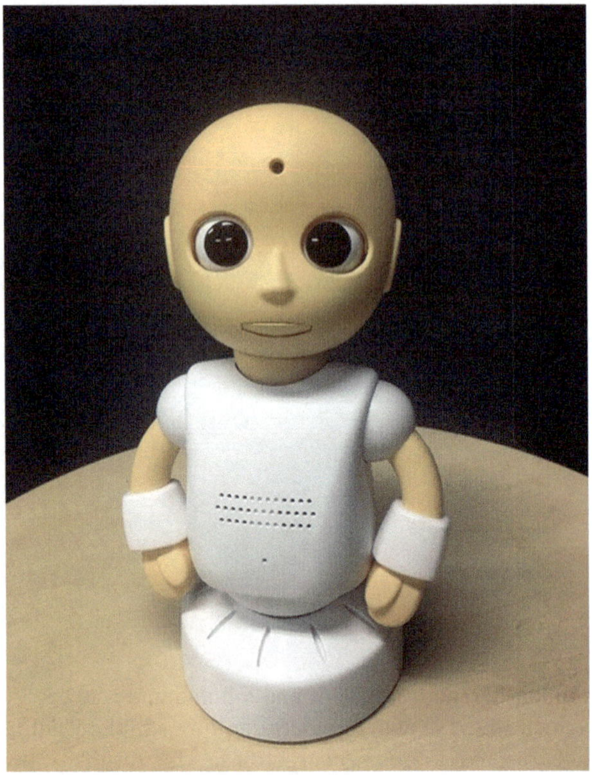

Fig. 8.2 Simple humanoid robot. (Reproduced from Kumazaki et al., 2019)

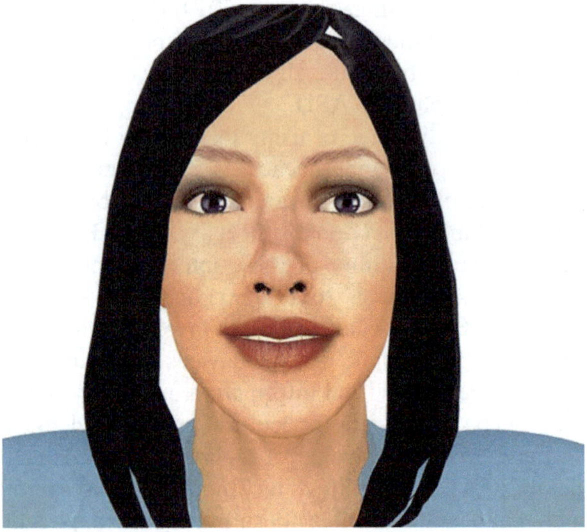

Fig. 8.3 Digital avatar. (Reproduced from Kumazaki et al., 2019)

These applications save practitioners' time, are adapted to users' specific characteristics, and allow accurate and fast assessment of the achieved outcomes (Artoni et al., 2018; Granich et al., 2016). Technologies are also combined with parent-implemented interventions (Hampshire & Allred, 2018; Meadan et al., 2016), peer-mediated instruction and intervention (Baldwin, 2013; Trottier et al., 2011; Wu et al., 2020), visual supports (Shane et al., 2012; Schlosser et al., 2017), social skills training (Rice et al., 2015; Yun et al., 2017), etc. In addition, technology can be used in the dissemination of other science-based interventions, i.e., in training adults (parents, caregivers, and professionals) to use the recommended interventions (Baggett et al., 2010).

Although the advantages of using technology in working with people with autism are mentioned most frequently, researchers also point out some concerns and limitations. One of the limitations of using technology in interventions is the fact that applications or technological devices are usually aimed at a specific skill. In other words, using a digital program or tool in working with people with autism most often does not facilitate their comprehensive learning (Artoni et al., 2018).

Furthermore, since technology-based interventions are appealing and easy to use and do not require the engagement of many different professionals, it sometimes happens that these technological solutions change or suppress the existing evidence-based approaches instead of supplementing them (Pellecchia et al., 2020a). Heng et al. (2020) indicate that the skills acquired with the help of technology-based interventions should be generalized and additionally practiced with people from a real-life environment.

Sharmin et al. (2018) point out that the devices used in interventions may also have certain shortcomings. For example, portable devices can be quite conspicuous or have a battery life problem. On the other hand, some applications (especially those that are free) can be rigid, cannot be customized, or cannot provide the necessary feedback. The main objections to the use of robots include a high price that prevents wide availability and the requirement for the process to be supervised by a trained technician (Sharmin et al., 2018).

Discussing augmentative and alternative communication, Light et al. (2019) point out that the main obstacles to its application include (1) marginalization of people with severe disabilities (e.g., this type of technology is often unavailable or insufficiently adapted to them; they may find it nonfunctional, expensive, unattainable, or inapplicable to all living spaces); (2) lack of research to determine the actual needs of users, how useful the available tools are to them, and what cognitive, linguistic, and social demands are imposed on technology users; (3) an insufficient number of programmers and researchers in this field; and (4) the gap between science and practice (e.g., not applying scientifically confirmed approaches and insufficient training of practitioners).

8.3 Areas in Which Technology-Based Interventions Have Most Commonly Been Used with Regard to the Age of People with ASD

8.3.1 Early Childhood

From the literature review, Heng et al. (2020) conclude that technology-based interventions are most commonly used to improve communication, social interaction, and play skills at an early age in children with ASD, by using video modeling and reinforcement with the help of mobile devices and computers. On the other hand, Pham et al. (2019) point out that social-communication skills can most often be developed by using speech-generating devices, computer-assisted instruction, video-based instruction, virtual reality, and robot-mediated interventions. Reed et al. (2011) indicate that not all topics within the area of social communication are equally represented in technology-based interventions in early childhood, i.e., that these interventions have more often been applied in teaching children to initiate a conversation, master play skills, and adequately respond to other people, while nonverbal social behavior and problem-solving have been less present in research goals when applying technology-based interventions.

Speech-generating devices are computerized devices of different complexity levels, with recorded or synthesized voice messages, which enable people with ASD to communicate (Pham et al., 2019). Analyzing 20 studies on the effects of speech-generating devices in children with ASD 3–8 years of age, Muharib and Alzrayer (2017) determined that these devices could be used in different environments (family homes, schools, clinics, childcare institutions, etc.), that they were most often used in working directly with a child (one on one at a table), but that there were also cases in which a speech-generating device was incorporated into a child's daily routine and could be used on different devices (usually an iPad, iPod, iPad mini) with the help of different applications (e.g., *Proloquo2Go*, *GoTalk*, *SoundingBoard*, *My Choice Board*, *Lexigrams*, *Pick-A-Word*, and *Scene & Heard*). According to the results of this meta-analysis, speech-generating devices were most commonly used to improve manding, tacting, and intraverbal skills in children with ASD at an early age. In 13 studies, a large effect was found in teaching verbal behavior, more specifically, for teaching single-step manding, multistep manding, multistep tacting, and multistep intraverbal, while the effect was medium in four studies (in single-step tacting) and insufficient in one study (in vocal production). Muharib and Alzrayer (2017) concluded that speech-generating devices were portable, available, applicable, and effective in minimally verbal children with ASD. Lorah et al. (2021) compared the effects of speech-generating devices and other alternative forms of communication in nine studies in which the average age of children with ASD was 7 years. The results showed that children with ASD generally had little success in using different communication techniques without additional instructions, support, and teaching. In addition, behavioral approaches proved to be compatible with teaching children with ASD to communicate. Thus, all the interventions used some of the recommended techniques, such as reinforcement, prompting, time delay, discrete trial training, and task analysis. Since this meta-analysis compared speech-generating devices with no-tech manual sign and low-tech picture exchange, the results indicated that after the applied intervention with speech-generating devices, children with ASD showed an average intervention performance level of 63.8%, while their performance level was 53.1% after using low-tech picture exchange, and 22.9% after no-tech manual sign. With regard to the effect size estimations, the use of speech-generating devices usually achieved medium and large effects compared to no-tech manual sign and low-tech picture exchange. Aydin and Diken (2020) analyzed 21 studies in which different augmentative and alternative communication applications were used in children with ASD. The results showed that these applications were most often used in preschool and school children, while they were minimally applied in adolescence and adulthood, although communication difficulties persisted. The requesting skills were the most common of the skills practiced through augmentative and alternative communication applications. Communication improvement applications were often combined with techniques such as error correction, reinforcement, discrete trial teaching, and time delay procedure. Some of the analyzed studies compared the effects of different applications, most commonly PECS, speech-generating devices, and manual sign applications. The results showed that children with ASD preferred applications with speech-generating devices. Manual sign applications were the least effective. Possible reasons could be inadequate motor skills in children with ASD and the complexity of these movements. However, Aydin and Diken (2020) indicate that despite such general findings, there are studies in which manual sign applications are more effective than others because some children with ASD prefer them.

Moon et al. (2019) performed a meta-analysis in which they included seven studies aiming to improve different skills in small children with the help of applications. The studies were mostly conducted in the USA, Great Britain, Australia, and Ireland, with samples of different sizes (from 25 to 75 participants), 3–10 years of age. The results showed that applications could successfully be used to improve fine motor skills and visual information processing at a young age. Applications have also often been developed to improve social-communication skills in children with ASD. Fletcher-Watson et al. (2016) presented the FindMe application that aims to develop joint attention, i.e., paying attention to others and following social signals. Within this application, a child has to mark people who appear on the screen or objects and phenomena the people point at, followed by a reward the child gets by collecting a specific number of correct answers. Although Fletcher-Watson et al. (2016) found that joint attention skills improved in the application, they reported that there were no expected generalizations. Pérez-Fuster et al. (2022) examined the effects of augmented reality technology called *Pictogram Room* on the development of joint attention in children with ASD 3–8 years of age. The participants took part in six 30-min sessions within which they played in the *Pictogram Room* (the *Gaze following* game) and practiced the ability to understand and recognize the gaze direction of a doll they had previously met in the presence of a therapist who gave instructions. While playing, the participants could see their own and the therapist's bodies (the player was marked in yellow, and the therapist in gray) (Fig. 8.4). The results showed that all players improved their joint attention skills, which persisted a month after the intervention. However, practicing joint attention on a screen also has its drawbacks. Although interacting with players, virtual characters remain fixed on a screen. Thus, robots are offered as a potential solution (Chevalier et al., 2020). In practicing joint attention, robots can be seen as social mediators (Robins et al., 2004). Furthermore, it is believed that their gradual involvement can achieve similar effects as when the intervention is implemented by people (David et al., 2018) or even better (Kumazaki et al., 2018).

Robots are also often used in early childhood to improve other aspects of social engagement in children with ASD. In a study by Goodrich et al. (2012), children participated in a toy game with a mobile robot (*Troy*) that could perform basic pro-social activities (e.g., push toys, press buttons, show toys, wave and greet, show basic emotions). The participants showed great interest and motivation to participate in the activities involving the robot. After the game, their social engagement skills improved even when the robot was not present (e.g., in contact with therapists). Tapus et al. (2012) monitored the extent to which the *NAO* robot influenced the improvement of social engagement and initiative in children with ASD. While interacting with the robot (that responded to children's questions, gave answers, and changed the color of its eyes), the children showed interest, which gradually decreased with the duration of the session. Different children had different reactions to the robot, so the variability of the achieved effects was great. Although the authors expected that the interaction with the *NAO* robot would lead to a greater initiative in children compared to interactions with therapists, that was not confirmed in all participants. Since the results were mixed, Tapus et al. (2012) assumed that robots could successfully be used only in a specific group of children with ASD, which should be further examined in the future. Costa et al. (2015) used a humanoid robot called *KASPAR* (Fig. 8.5) to teach children with ASD which touches in communication were gentle and which were inappropriate and rough. They used different

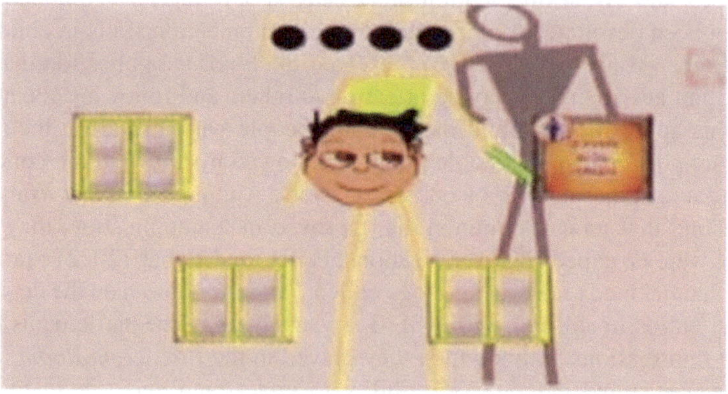

Fig. 8.4 A segment from the joint attention game in the *Pictogram Room*. (Reproduced from Pérez-Fuster et al., 2022)

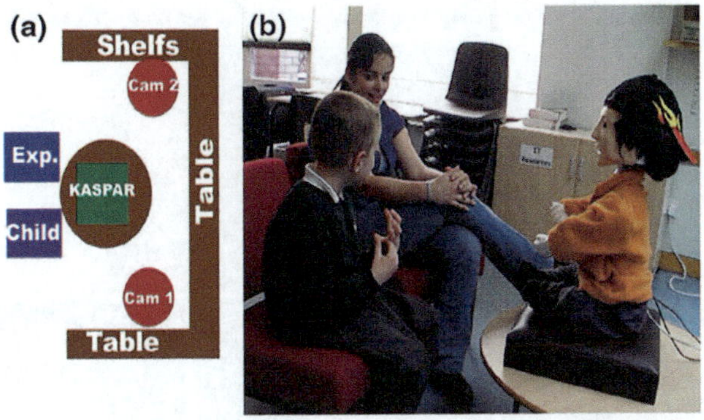

Fig. 8.5 Organization of the room in which the KASPAR robot was used and the child's position. (**a**) Room setup schematic, (**b**) positioning of the participants in the room (Reproduced from Costa et al., 2015)

interactions in the robot-therapist-child triad, practicing gaze direction, demonstration, and imitation. The obtained results showed that the children's interest in the robot was great and constant throughout the sessions and that their interest in interacting with the therapist increased. The *KASPAR* robot also contributed to improving joint attention and learning about tactile communication in general. Using the humanoid *NAO* robot, Warren et al. (2015) found that, apart from showing great and continuous interest in the robot, children were also successful in carrying out its orders and showed improvement in joint attention activities. These authors indicate that the potential of using robots is great but that we should not have unrealistic expectations that robot technology is sufficient and applicable in all areas of needed support in children with ASD.

Since the ability to recognize, interpret, and make facial expressions is related to the general development of social skills, some authors have patented various technological solutions in this area. Golan et al. (2010) developed *The Transporters* consisting of animations and quizzes (Fig. 8.6) in which vehicles have human-like facial expressions and show contextually meaningful emotions. One episode lasts for 5 min and covers 1 out of 15 emotions. The authors assumed that children with high-functioning autism would unconsciously improve their skills of naming and recognizing emotions by watching these videos. The results showed that the children's skills of recognizing and understanding emotions improved in a relatively short time (4 weeks) and that they were very motivated and interested in watching these videos. Golan et al. (2010) did not examine to what extent these acquired skills generalized to a real-life context. *Qunatiandi is an Android or iOS application developed for the Chinese market, relying on teacher-mediated instruction, visual support, behavioral principle of reinforcement, and embedded adaptive training. It includes seven domains, one of which aims to improve emotion recognition and*

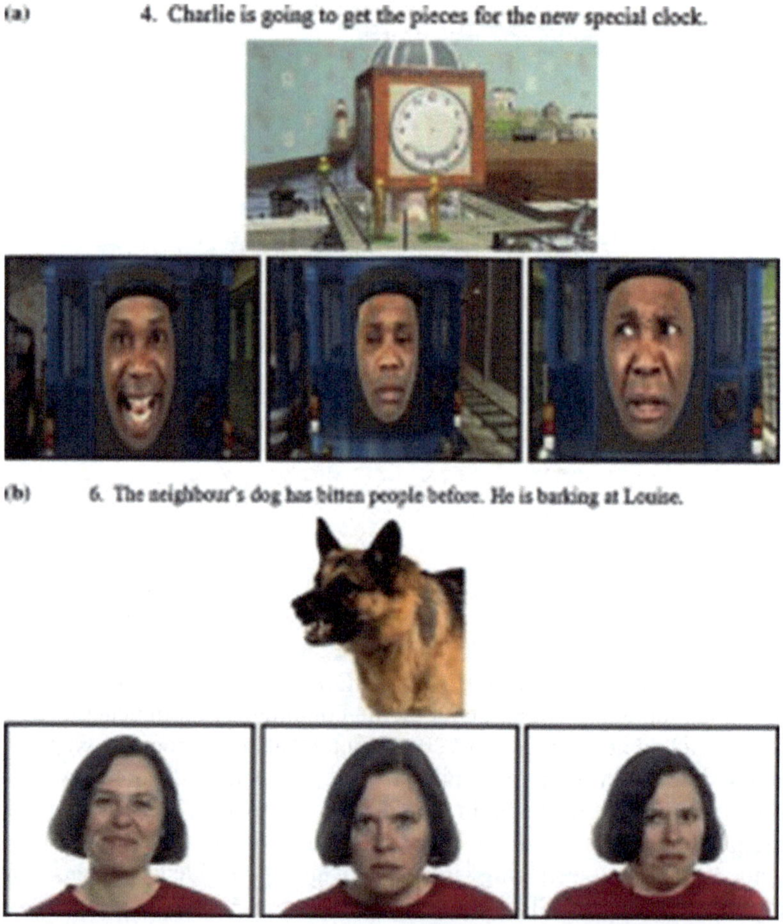

Fig. 8.6 Examples of questions from the quiz that accompanies videos in *The Transporters*. (**a**) Level 1 Task: match familiar scenes from the series with familiar faces. (**b**) Level 3 Task: match novel scenes and faces using real human faces (Reproduced from Golan et al., 2010)

management with the help of animations, video clips, clear and automatic instructions, and the freedom to choose an animated reward. It was tested in preschool children and proved to be effective (Zhang et al., 2019).

Since strengthening social-communication and language skills does not automatically imply better interaction with peers and adults, many authors test the effects of technology-based interventions, including developing relationships with people from the environment. Visual scene display technology allows children to perform activities in the natural surroundings with the help of photographs and recordings from their real life, for which they are highly motivated and which they should imitate (Laubscher et al., 2020). Chapin et al. (2021) state that, to enrich vocabulary, it is important to start with the concepts children with ASD are interested in. With regard to that, they point out that interventions based on visual scene display technology can be very useful. These interventions involve showing recordings of the objects for which the child is highly motivated. The videos are automatically interrupted every 30 s in unexpected places. The screen then shows the picture of the object, and by pressing a part of the screen (i.e., the shown object), the child can hear the name of that object part, after which the video continues. (For example, the video shows a construction site and a digging excavator. After pausing the video, the screen shows the picture of the excavator with focal points on its parts. By pressing the point on the crane, the word "crane" is heard, and the video continues.) Every time before the video was continued, the therapist practiced establishing interaction with the child, asking a question about what was shown on the screen. It was monitored to what extent the child managed to interact with the therapist, face them, look at them, give comments, etc. The results confirmed that video sequences combined well with other technological approaches and with treatment goals in children with ASD. The advantages of visual scene display technology include its easy use, minimal motor requirements, limited cognitive requirements, and contextually adapted vocabulary. Therrien and Light (2018) used an iPad with the *GoTalk NOW* application combined with visual scene display technology as a shared device between peer pairs for practicing turn-taking in leafing through a book. The application included previously recorded messages that appeared when a child pressed specific points on the screen (e.g., laughter, sighs like oh, ah, etc.). It was determined that sharing a device during a meaningful activity, accompanied by fun vocabulary, reduced barriers to social interactions and improved waiting and turn-taking skills.

Video modeling is often used to improve play skills in children with ASD. Within this intervention, a child watches a video showing how specific activities are performed and then imitates that. Petursdottir and Gudmundsdottir (2021) used videos on the iPod touch®, after which children with ASD could apply and practice play skills with carefully selected peers, prepared for this type of interaction. The results showed that the use of video modeling in children with ASD contributed to the increase in the duration of playing, a higher level of initiative, communication improvement, and generalization of acquired skills to other peers. In addition to developing play and improving social interactions (Ezzeddine et al., 2019; Karabekir & Akmanoğlu, 2018; Kouo, 2019; Lee et al., 2021), video modeling can also be used to encourage communication (Rodrigues & Almeida, 2020; Qi et al., 2017). Joint video modeling is another intervention that has been applied in children with ASD by involving peers to encourage joint play activities. Dueñas et al. (2019) monitored the effects that joint watching and imitating play videos had on pretend play in children with ASD with a low verbalization level. The results showed an improvement in scripted and unscripted verbalization and play skills in all children. Dueñas et al. (2019) believed that the involvement of typically developing peers significantly contributed to the improvement of unscripted verbalization, i.e., that the differences in dyad pairs and their reactions led to different outcomes in the behavior of children with ASD.

In addition to using technology in social-communication aspects, Mazumdar et al. (2021) indicate that applications from the category of computer-assisted interventions are applicable and effective in early childhood. Their aim is to prepare children for school, i.e., improve pre-academic skills (pre-math, pre-reading, prewriting), self-care (by using videos), and social skills (by using computerized social stories). *TeachTown* is an example of such a program that includes cognitive and language activities. It involves working on a computer, with lessons based on applied behavior analysis and animated rewards that appear at unequal intervals. This application was more effective than the commonly used approaches at a younger age (3–6 years) (Whalen et al., 2010), while that was not the case at an older age (5–9 years) (Pellecchia et al., 2020b).

8.3.2 School Age and Adolescence

Social communication is a treatment priority in school-age children and adolescents (Domínguez-Lucio et al., 2022; Zeng et al., 2021). Immersive technologies, avatars, visual scene display technology, games (serious, collaborative, somatic), etc., have often been used to improve social-communication skills. Immersive technologies include augmented reality (combines technology and real-world elements by overlaying digital content on real-world elements), virtual reality (allows digital simulation of the environment), mixed reality (combines augmented reality and virtual reality), and extended reality (collects various individual data to make the virtual experience as real as possible). Mosher et al. (2021) analyzed 41 studies (experimental, quasi-experimental, and single case studies) that used immersive technologies and mainly included children 8–13 years of age. It is interesting that over 70% of the analyzed studies used immersive technology interventions to treat multiple social skills, while the remaining 30% focused on individual skills. The skills related to developing relationships with others were treated most often. Approximately half of the studies reported that the acquired social skills were generalized and 30% that they were maintained. Mosher et al. (2021) indicated that the students' age was not related to the success of immersive technology interventions, i.e., that students with ASD, at both elementary and high school age, equally acquired social skills with the help of this technology. On the other hand, it was found that the severity of ASD symptoms correlated with accepting and applying immersive technology, i.e., that students with lower intelligence levels did not fully accept these technologies, were less successful in using them, and needed more time to perform certain activities. The analysis of intervention types and effects determined that most success was achieved by using augmented reality, followed by immersive virtual reality.

Almurashi et al. (2022) analyzed augmented reality-based interventions and found that these interventions were usually implemented through computers, cellphones, and tablets but that there were some that used smart glasses. Target skills most often included social communication and emotion recognition, followed by academic skills, and very rarely daily living skills. Berenguer et al. (2020) reviewed 20 research studies examining the effects of augmented reality in children and adolescents with ASD. They indicated that the samples most often included participants with high-functioning autism and that most studies aimed to improve social interactions, social communication, and pragmatics. Some studies focused on improving the ability to understand emotions and facial expressions, while only a few studies aimed to improve selective attention and motor skills. Berenguer et al. (2020) pointed out that most interventions in the reviewed studies had positive effects, were meaningful and pleasant, offered an interesting experience, and increased motivation in children with ASD. Vahabzadeh et al. (2018a) showed that *Empowered Brain* (Fig. 8.7), which is a representative of augmented reality and a computerized smart glasses intervention (an intervention that uses smart glasses that provide the person wearing them with prosocial guidance through visual and auditory reinforcement and feedback), was applicable in a school context in students with ASD. This assistive technology reduced irritability, hyperactivity, and social withdrawal in students with ASD. In addition, Vahabzadeh et al. (2018a) indicated that teachers positively

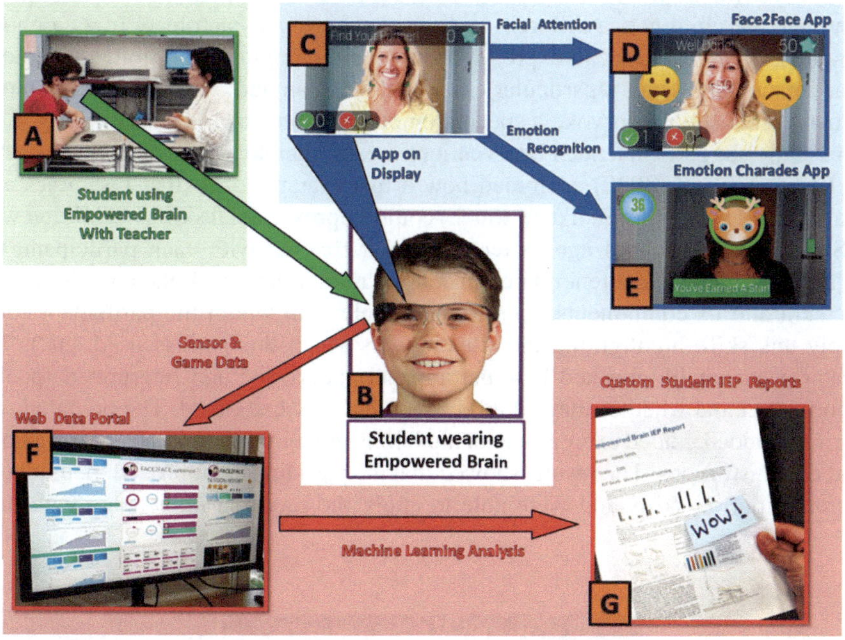

Fig. 8.7 The use of smart glasses in interacting with a therapist (**a**); in a classroom (**b**); information on the screen of the applied *Empowered Brain* program (**c**); a screenshot on the optical display of the glasses (**d**); an example of screen stimuli designed to improve the ability to focus on a face and make eye contact (**e**); an example of metrics offered by the applied *Empowered Brain* program (**f**), generating custom reports (**g**). (Reproduced from Vahabzadeh et al., 2018a)

evaluated this technology, pointing out that it was superior to other technology-based approaches in interventions. Keshav et al. (2019) showed that, apart from improving social-communication aspects, using *Empowered Brain* technology in digital games in children with ASD could contribute to better detection of hyperactivity symptoms in these children. Furthermore, Vahabzadeh et al. (2018b) indicated that *Empowered Brain* was successfully used in elementary and high school students with ASD to treat the symptoms of hyperactivity.

With regard to virtual reality, Mesa-Gresa et al. (2018) analyzed 31 studies and concluded that, in about 50% of them, virtual reality intervention aimed to improve social skills, while other topics, such as emotions (e.g., recognizing basic emotions, regulation, and reciprocity), daily living skills (e.g., driving, shopping), cognition (e.g., attention, executive functions, cognitive flexibility), and communication (e.g., social-communication strategies, nonverbal communication), were less common. Virtual reality-based interventions most frequently involved avatars, games, and virtual reality scenarios.

White et al. (2018) developed *Facial Emotion Expression Training* (FEET) for practicing emotional expression. It is based on a Kinect sensor that enables a three-dimensional representation of a child's facial expression. The child goes through four levels for each emotion. Along with verbal instruction to show the required emotion, the child gets a different additional stimulus at each level (e.g., a photograph of an animated facial expression showing the required emotion, a video of a real person expressing a particular emotional state, an audiovisual description of a situation that should provoke a specific emotion, or an avatar's activity) (Fig. 8.8). This study suggests that such interventions are acceptable and have lasting effects.

Charlton et al. (2020) examined how a fish avatar *Marla* (that resembles animated characters children like to watch) could improve social skills in children with ASD at younger school age. After the initial greeting with each participant, the avatar presented the content related to conversation initiation skills (e.g., describing the skill and its components, identifying people with whom the participant could apply this skill, highlighting the situations in which this skill is used, etc.). The avatar occasionally checked how participants understood and interpreted specific information and whether they could repeat what they had heard. The prepared scenarios included guided exercises with modeling and reinforcement, guessing games, and demonstrations. The results showed that the participants improved their conversation initiation skills and were able to apply the acquired knowledge with their

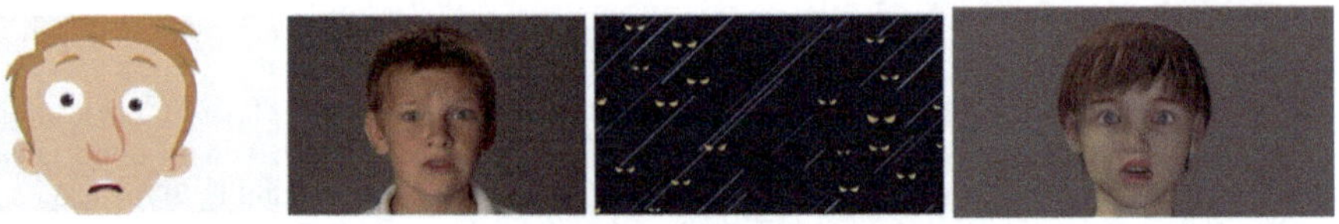

Fig. 8.8 Different stimuli in the task of expressing fear. (Reproduced from White et al., 2018)

peers. Furthermore, the parents stated that they noticed slight improvements in their children.

Also, visual scene display technology was used on an iPad to improve peer communication, more precisely, communicative turns taken while playing different games with real toys (e.g., a veterinary set, a set of ocean animals, etc.). A video with specific game scenarios was created for each toy, and each video contained focal points that included different language messages (words, short phrases, and exclamations) (Laubscher et al., 2019).

Another type of technology-based intervention is the use of digital games. Researching gamified interventions, Valencia et al. (2019) point out that digital intervention games usually use points, different levels, feedback, and rewards to be more appealing. Serious games have an educational purpose, are not designed just for fun, and are usually based on augmented reality. They are suitable for learning some skills that are demanding and insufficiently motivating for people with ASD, which the person can use in a real-life environment (Whyte et al., 2015). Hassan et al. (2021) analyzed 40 serious games designed to develop social skills, concluding they were applicable to people with ASD and intellectual disability. These games mainly aimed to improve emotion recognition and expression abilities. However, out of 40 games, only 7 met the quality criteria. Thus, the authors pointed out that many design issues related to narrative, game dynamics, genre, user profile, etc. should be considered in the future. In addition to improving emotional competencies, serious games have also been used for improving functional uses of eye gaze cues (Griffin et al., 2021), practicing team play (Terlouw et al., 2021), improving health through nutrition games (Santini et al., 2022), reducing stress and anxiety (Carlier et al., 2020; Wijnhoven et al., 2015), and improving motor skills (Vukićević et al., 2019). Somatic games are special types of games that insist on players' body movements and physical engagement in dynamic exercises, usually by using the following three types of motion detection sensors—Nintendo Wii, Microsoft Kinect, and Sony PlayStation (Xianmei, 2017). These games mostly involve ball activities, participating in sports games, or dancing. Their duration is limited, usually to a few minutes, and the tasks are simple. Somatic games mainly aim to improve balance, visual-motor coordination, imitation, attention, etc. Xianmei (2017) points out that their careless use can cause physical injury in children with ASD. As it is not practical to create different games to satisfy various interests of each child with ASD, somatic games should be flexible and adaptable to individual players (e.g., in terms of the game category, levels, pairing or grouping options, etc.). Collaborative games on large tablets are another approach used to improve social interactions and group work skills in adolescents with ASD. Some examples include *SIDES: Shared Interfaces to Develop Effective Social Skills*, where players jointly help a frog find its way from point A to point B (Piper et al., 2006), and *Collaborative Puzzle Game*, in which participants use a finger to jointly drag pieces of puzzles on the screen and get audiovisual feedback (Battocchi et al., 2010; Ben-Sasson et al., 2013).

In addition to treating social communication and motor skills, technology-based interventions have also been used in school-age children and adolescents to encourage independence. Odom et al. (2015) point out that these interventions can be used to achieve independence, raise the level of expertise and competencies in some activities, or achieve specific academic goals (Odom et al., 2015). Kang and Chang (2018) examined the effect of the gamification of training intervention (playing video games through engaging in the target behavior and then applying that behavior in real-life activities) with the help of Kinect sensors to teach children with ASD to shower. In addition to playing the game, Kang and Chang (2018) used video modeling and the principle of breaking down activities into 25 individual steps. The research included six school-age participants who all improved their independent showering skills in a real-life context. The parents also stated that they were very satisfied with this type of intervention.

Although it can be noticed that there are many similarities between the interventions applied in early childhood and adolescence, augmentative and alternative communication interventions are much less frequently applied after starting school. In their review of 16 studies involving only 19 adolescents and adults with ASD, Holyfield et al. (2017) showed that these interventions were effective, most often used to encourage expressing desires and needs, and focused on individual work with a researcher. They also indicate that augmentative and alternative communication interventions should be applied and examined to a greater extent in slightly older people with ASD.

You can read about technology-based interventions in adulthood in the following chapters: Employment, Daily Living, Community Living, and Leisure Activities.

References

Almurashi, H., Bouaziz, R., Alharthi, W., Al-Sarem, M., Hadwan, M., & Kammoun, S. (2022). Augmented reality, serious games and picture exchange communication system for people with ASD: Systematic literature review and future directions. *Sensors, 22*(3), 1250–1297. https://doi.org/10.3390/s22031250

Artoni, S., Bastiani, L., Buzzi, M. C., Buzzi, M., Curzio, O., Pelagatti, S., & Senette, C. (2018). Technology-enhanced ABA intervention in children with autism: A pilot study. *Universal Access in the Information Society, 17*(1), 191–210. https://doi.org/10.1007/s10209-017-0536-x

Aydin, O., & Diken, I. H. (2020). Studies comparing augmentative and alternative communication systems (AAC) applications for individuals with autism spectrum disorder: A systematic review and meta-analysis. *Education and Training in Autism and Developmental Disabilities, 55*(2), 119–141.

Baggett, K. M., Davis, B., Feil, E. G., Sheeber, L. L., Landry, S. H., Carta, J. J., & Leve, C. (2010). Technologies for expanding the reach of evidence-based interventions: Preliminary results for promoting social-emotional development in early childhood. *Topics in Early Childhood Special Education, 29*(4), 226–238. https://doi.org/10.1177/0271121409354782

Baldwin, B. (2013). *Peer-mediated intervention and technology: Mobile device application use in implementation of peer buddy training* [Doctoral dissertation, The Florida State University]. https://www.proquest.com/openview/49091227123028abde347aaf23b87ce0/1?pq-origsite=gscholar&cbl=18750

Barton, E. E., Pustejovsky, J. E., Maggin, D. M., & Reichow, B. (2017). Technology-aided instruction and intervention for students with ASD: A meta-analysis using novel methods of estimating effect sizes for single-case research. *Remedial and Special Education, 38*(6), 371–386. https://doi.org/10.1177/0741932517729508

Battocchi, A., Ben-Sasson, A., Esposito, G., Gal, E., Pianesi, F., Tomasini, D., Venuti, P., & Zancanaro, M. (2010). Collaborative puzzle game: A tabletop interface for fostering collaborative skills in children with autism spectrum disorders. *Journal of Assistive Technology, 4*(1), 4–13. https://doi.org/10.5042/jat.2010.0040

Bekele, E., Crittendon, J. A., Swanson, A., Sarkar, N., & Warren, Z. E. (2014). Pilot clinical application of an adaptive robotic system for young children with autism. *Autism, 18*(5), 598–608. https://doi.org/10.1177/1362361313479454

Ben-Sasson, A., Lamash, L., & Gal, E. (2013). To enforce or not to enforce? The use of collaborative interfaces to promote social skills in children with high functioning autism spectrum disorder. *Autism, 17*(5), 608–622. https://doi.org/10.1177/1362361312451526

Berenguer, C., Baixauli, I., Gómez, S., Andrés, M. D. E. P., & De Stasio, S. (2020). Exploring the impact of augmented reality in children and adolescents with autism spectrum disorder: A systematic review. *International Journal of Environmental Research and Public Health, 17*(17), 6143–6158. https://doi.org/10.3390/ijerph17176143

Carlier, S., Van der Paelt, S., Ongenae, F., De Backere, F., & De Turck, F. (2020). Empowering children with ASD and their parents: Design of a serious game for anxiety and stress reduction. *Sensors, 20*(4), 966–1007. https://doi.org/10.3390/s20040966

Carmona-Serrano, N., López-Belmonte, J., Cuesta-Gómez, J. L., & Moreno-Guerrero, A. J. (2020). Documentary analysis of the scientific literature on autism and technology in web of science. *Brain Sciences, 10*(12), 985–1002. https://doi.org/10.3390/brainsci10120985

Chapin, S. E., McNaughton, D., Light, J., McCoy, A., Caron, J., & Lee, D. L. (2021). The effects of AAC video visual scene display technology on the communicative turns of preschoolers with autism spectrum disorder. *Assistive Technology, 33*, 1–11. https://doi.org/10.1080/10400435.2021.1893

Charlton, C. T., Kellems, R. O., Black, B., Bussey, H. C., Ferguson, R., Goncalves, B., Jensen, M., & Vallejo, S. (2020). Effectiveness of avatar-delivered instruction on social initiations by children with autism spectrum disorder. *Research in Autism Spectrum Disorders, 71*, 101494. https://doi.org/10.1016/j.rasd.2019.101494

Chevalier, P., Kompatsiari, K., Ciardo, F., & Wykowska, A. (2020). Examining joint attention with the use of humanoid robots – A new approach to study fundamental mechanisms of social cognition. *Psychonomic Bulletin & Review, 27*(2), 217–236. https://doi.org/10.3758/s13423-019-01689-4

Constantin, A., Johnson, H., Smith, E., Lengyel, D., & Brosnan, M. (2017). Designing computer-based rewards with and for children with autism spectrum disorder and/or intellectual disability. *Computers in Human Behavior, 75*, 404–414. https://doi.org/10.1016/j.chb.2017.05.030

Costa, S., Lehmann, H., Dautenhahn, K., Robins, B., & Soares, F. (2015). Using a humanoid robot to elicit body awareness and appropriate physical interaction in children with autism. *International Journal of Social Robotics, 7*(2), 265–278. https://doi.org/10.1007/s12369-014-0250-2

David, D. O., Costescu, C. A., Matu, S., Szentagotai, A., & Dobrean, A. (2018). Developing joint attention for children with autism in robot-enhanced therapy. *International Journal of Social Robotics, 10*(5), 595–605. https://doi.org/10.1007/s12369-017-0457-0

Domínguez-Lucio, S., Compañ-Gabucio, L. M., Torres-Collado, L., & de la Hera, M. G. (2022). Occupational therapy interventions using new technologies in children and adolescents with autism spectrum disorder: A scoping review. *Journal of Autism and Developmental Disorders, 52*, 1–27. https://doi.org/10.1007/s10803-022-05431-3

Dueñas, A. D., Plavnick, J. B., & Bak, M. Y. (2019). Effects of joint video modeling on unscripted play behavior of children with autism spectrum disorder. *Journal of Autism and Developmental Disorders, 49*(1), 236–247. https://doi.org/10.1007/s10803-018-3719-2

Ezzeddine, E. W., DeBar, R. M., Reeve, S. A., & Townsend, D. B. (2019). Using video modeling to teach play comments to dyads with ASD. *Journal of Applied Behavior Analysis, 53*(2), 767–781. https://doi.org/10.1002/jaba.621

Fletcher-Watson, S., Petrou, A., Scott-Barrett, J., Dicks, P., Graham, C., O'Hare, A., Helen, P., & McConachie, H. (2016). A trial of an iPad™ intervention targeting social communication skills in children with autism. *Autism, 20*(7), 771–782. https://doi.org/10.1177/1362361315605624

Golan, O., Ashwin, E., Granader, Y., McClintock, S., Day, K., Leggett, V., & Baron-Cohen, S. (2010). Enhancing emotion recognition in children with autism spectrum conditions: An intervention using animated vehicles with real emotional faces. *Journal of Autism and Developmental Disorders, 40*(3), 269–279. https://doi.org/10.1007/s10803-009-0862-9

Goldsmith, T. R., & LeBlanc, L. A. (2004). Use of technology in interventions for children with autism. *Journal of Early and Intensive Behavior Intervention, 1*(2), 166–178. https://doi.org/10.1037/h0100287

Goodrich, M. A., Colton, M., Brinton, B., Fujiki, M., Atherton, J. A., Robinson, L., Ricks, D., Maxfield, M. H., & Acerson, A. (2012). Incorporating a robot into an autism therapy team. *IEEE Intelligent Systems, 27*, 52–59.

Granich, J., Dass, A., Busacca, M., Moore, D., Anderson, A., Venkatesh, S., Duong, T., Vellanki, P., Richdale, A., Trembath, D., Cairns, D., Wendy, M., Rodwell, T., Rayner, M., & Whitehouse, A. J. (2016). Randomised controlled trial of an iPad based early intervention for autism: TOBY playpad study protocol. *BMC Pediatrics, 16*(1), 1–12. https://doi.org/10.1186/s12887-016-0704-9

Griffin, J. W., Geier, C. F., Smyth, J. M., & Scherf, K. S. (2021). Improving sensitivity to eye gaze cues in adolescents on the autism spectrum using serious game technology: A randomized controlled trial. *JCPP Advances, 1*(3), e12041. https://doi.org/10.1002/jcv2.12041

Hampshire, P. K., & Allred, K. W. (2018). A parent-implemented, technology-mediated approach to increasing self-management homework skills in middle school students with autism. *Exceptionality, 26*(2), 119–136. https://doi.org/10.1080/09362835.2016.1216848

Hansen, J. M., & Winn, L. M. (2019). *Developmental toxicology: Methods and protocols*. Humana Press. https://doi.org/10.1007/978-3-030-15374-8_8

Hassan, A., Pinkwart, N., & Shafi, M. (2021). Serious games to improve social and emotional intelligence in children with autism. *Entertainment Computing, 38*, 100417. https://doi.org/10.1016/j.entcom.2021.1004

Heng, E., Lanovaz, M., & Beauregard, A. (2020). Research on technological interventions for young children with autism spectrum disorders: A scoping review. *Review Journal of Autism and Developmental Disorders, 8*(2), 253–263. https://doi.org/10.1007/s40489-020-00215-w

Holyfield, C., Drager, K. D., Kremkow, J., & Light, J. (2017). Systematic review of AAC intervention research for adolescents and adults with autism spectrum disorder. *Augmentative and Alternative Communication, 33*(4), 201–212. https://doi.org/10.1080/07434618.2017.1370495

Kang, Y.-S., & Chang, Y.-J. (2018). Using game technology to teach six elementary school children with autism to take a shower independently. *Developmental Neurorehabilitation, 22*(5), 329–337. https://doi.org/10.1080/17518423.2018.1501778

Karabekir, E. P., & Akmanoğlu, N. (2018). Effectiveness of video modeling presented via smartboard for teaching social response behavior to children with autism. *Education and Training in Autism and Developmental Disabilities, 53*(4), 363–377.

Keshav, N. U., Vogt-Lowell, K., Vahabzadeh, A., & Sahin, N. T. (2019). Digital attention-related augmented-reality game: Significant correlation between student game performance and validated clinical measures of attention-deficit/hyperactivity disorder (ADHD). *Children, 6*(6), 72–85. https://doi.org/10.3390/children6060072

Kouo, J. L. (2019). The effectiveness of a packaged intervention including point-of-view video modeling in teaching social initiation skills to children with autism spectrum disorders. *Focus on Autism and Other Developmental Disabilities, 34*(3), 141–152. https://doi.org/10.1177/1088357618815887

Kumazaki, H., Yoshikawa, Y., Yoshimura, Y., Ikeda, T., Hasegawa, C., Saito, D. N., Tomiyama, S., An, K., Shimaya, J., Ishiguro, H., Matsumoto, Y., Minabe, Y., & Kikuchi, M. (2018). The impact of robotic intervention on joint attention in children with autism spectrum disorders. *Molecular Autism, 9*(1), 1–10. https://doi.org/10.1186/s13229-018-0230-8

Kumazaki, H., Warren, Z., Swanson, A., Yoshikawa, Y., Matsumoto, Y., Yoshimura, Y., Shimaya, J., Ishiguro, H., Sarkar, N., Wade, J., Mimura, M., Minabe, Y., & Kikuchi, M. (2019). Brief report: Evaluating the utility of varied technological agents to elicit social attention from children with autism spectrum disorders. *Journal of Autism and Developmental Disorders, 49*(4), 1700–1708. https://doi.org/10.1007/s10803-018-3841-1

Laubscher, E., Light, J., & McNaughton, D. (2019). Effect of an application with video visual scene displays on communication during play: Pilot study of a child with autism spectrum disorder and a peer. *Augmentative and Alternative Communication, 35*(4), 299–308. https://doi.org/10.1080/07434618.2019.1699160

Laubscher, E., Raulston, T. J., & Ousley, C. (2020). Supporting peer interactions in the inclusive preschool classroom using visual scene displays. *Journal of Special Education Technology*, 016264342098156. https://doi.org/10.1177/0162643420981561

Lee, G. T., Hu, X., Liu, Y., & Ren, Y. (2021). Effects of video modeling on the acquisition, maintenance, and generalization of playing with imaginary objects in children with autism spectrum disorder. *Behavior Modification, 45*(6), 1041–1069. https://doi.org/10.1177/0145445520939856

Light, J., McNaughton, D., Beukelman, D., Fager, S. K., Fried-Oken, M., Jakobs, T., & Jakobs, E. (2019). Challenges and opportunities in augmentative and alternative communication: Research and technology development to enhance communication and participation for individuals with complex communication needs. *Augmentative and Alternative Communication, 35*(1), 1–12. https://doi.org/10.1080/07434618.2018.1556732

Lorah, E. R., Holyfield, C., Miller, J., Griffen, B., & Lindbloom, C. (2021). A systematic review of research comparing mobile technology speech-generating devices to other AAC modes with individuals with autism spectrum disorder. *Journal of Developmental and Physical Disabilities, 34*, 187–210. https://doi.org/10.1007/s10882-021-09803-y

Mazumdar, A., Banerjee, M., Chatterjee, B., Saha, S., & Gupta, G. S. (2021). Mobile application based early educational intervention for children with autism – A pilot trial. *Disability and Rehabilitation: Assistive Technology, 16*, 1–8. https://doi.org/10.1080/17483107.2021.1927

Meadan, H., Snodgrass, M. R., Meyer, L. E., Fisher, K. W., Chung, M. Y., & Halle, J. W. (2016). Internet-based parent-implemented intervention for young children with autism: A pilot study. *Journal of Early Intervention, 38*(1), 3–23. https://doi.org/10.1177/1053815116630327

Mesa-Gresa, P., Gil-Gómez, H., Lozano-Quilis, J. A., & Gil-Gómez, J. A. (2018). Effectiveness of virtual reality for children and adolescents with autism spectrum disorder: An evidence-based systematic review. *Sensors, 18*(8), 2486–2501. https://doi.org/10.3390/s18082486

Moon, S. J., Hwang, J., Hill, H. S., Kervin, R., Birtwell, K. B., Torous, J., McDougle, C. J., & Kim, J. W. (2019). Mobile device applications and treatment of autism spectrum disorder: A systematic review and meta-analysis of effectiveness. *Archives of Disease in Childhood, 105*(5), 458–462. https://doi.org/10.1136/archdischild-2019-318258

Mosher, M. A., Carreon, A. C., Craig, S. L., & Ruhter, L. C. (2021). Immersive technology to teach social skills to students with autism spectrum disorder: A literature review. *Review Journal of Autism and Developmental Disorders, 8*, 1–17. https://doi.org/10.1007/s40489-021-00259-6

Muharib, R., & Alzrayer, N. M. (2017). The use of high-tech speech-generating devices as an evidence-based practice for children with autism spectrum disorders: A meta-analysis. *Review Journal of Autism and Developmental Disorders, 5*(1), 43–57. https://doi.org/10.1007/s40489-017-0122-4

National Autism Center. (2009). *National standards report*. National Autism Center.

National Autism Center. (2015). *Findings and conclusions: National standards project, phase 2*. Author.

National Professional Development Center on Autism Spectrum Disorder. (2017). *Matrix of evidence-based practices by outcome and age*. The University of North Carolina, Frank Porter Graham Child Development Institute.

Odom, S. L., Thompson, J. L., Hedges, S., Boyd, B. A., Dykstra, J. R., Duda, M. A., Szidon, K. L., Smith, L. E., & Bord, A. (2015). Technology-aided interventions and instruction for adolescents with autism spectrum disorder. *Journal of Autism and Developmental Disorders, 45*(12), 3805–3819. https://doi.org/10.1007/s10803-014-2320-6

Pellecchia, M., Beidas, R. S., Lawson, G., Williams, N. J., Seidman, M., Kimberly, J. R., Cannuscio, C., & Mandell, D. S. (2020a). Does implementing a new intervention disrupt use of existing evidence-based autism interventions? *Autism, 24*(7), 1713–1725. https://doi.org/10.1177/1362361320919248

Pellecchia, M., Marcus, S. C., Spaulding, C., Seidman, M., Xie, M., Rump, K., Reisinger, E. M., & Mandell, D. S. (2020b). Randomized trial of a computer-assisted intervention for children with autism in schools. *Journal of the American Academy of Child & Adolescent Psychiatry, 59*(3), 373–380. https://doi.org/10.1016/j.jaac.2019.03.029

Pérez-Fuster, P., Herrera, G., Kossyvaki, L., & Ferrer, A. (2022). Enhancing joint attention skills in children on the autism spectrum through an augmented reality technology-mediated intervention. *Children, 9*(2), 258–283. https://doi.org/10.3390/children9020258

Petursdottir, A.-L., & Gudmundsdottir, T. (2021). Supporting social play skill acquisition and generalization of children with autism through video modeling. *Journal of Autism and Developmental Disorders, 51*, 1–12. https://doi.org/10.1007/s10803-021-05204-4

Pham, A. V., Bennett, K. D., & Zetina, H. (2019). Technology-aided interventions for individuals with autism: Implications for policy and practice. *Policy Insights From the Behavioral and Brain Sciences, 6*(2), 202–209. https://doi.org/10.1177/2372732219857750

Piper, A. M., O'Brien, E., Morris, M. R., & Winograd, T. (2006). SIDES: A cooperative tabletop computer game for social skills development. In P. Hinds (Ed.), *Proceedings of the 2006 20th conference on Computer Supported Cooperative Work (CSCW'06)* (pp. 1–10). Association for Computing Machinery.

Qi, C. H., Barton, E. E., Collier, M., & Lin, Y.-L. (2017). A systematic review of single-case research studies on using video modeling interventions to improve social communication skills for individuals with autism spectrum disorder. *Focus on Autism and Other Developmental Disabilities, 33*(4), 249–257. https://doi.org/10.1177/1088357617741282

Reed, F. D. D., Hyman, S. R., & Hirst, J. M. (2011). Applications of technology to teach social skills to children with autism. *Research in Autism Spectrum Disorders, 5*(3), 1003–1010. https://doi.org/10.1016/j.rasd.2011.01.022

Rice, L. M., Wall, C. A., Fogel, A., & Shic, F. (2015). Computer-assisted face processing instruction improves emotion recognition, mentalizing, and social skills in students with ASD. *Journal of Autism and Developmental Disorders, 45*, 2176–2186. https://doi.org/10.1007/s10803-015-2380-2

Robins, B., Dickerson, P., Stribling, P., & Dautenhahn, K. (2004). Robot-mediated joint attention in children with autism: A case study in robot-human interaction. *Interaction Studies, 5*(2), 161–198. https://doi.org/10.1075/is.5.2.02rob

Rodrigues, V., & Almeida, M. A. (2020). Implementation of PECS associated with point-of-view video modeling in early childhood education for children with autism. *Revista Brasileira de Educação Especial, 26*, 403–420. https://doi.org/10.1590/1980-54702020v26e0092

Santini, F., Tauro, G., Mazzali, M., Grazioli, S., Mauri, M., Rosi, E., Pozzi, M., Tarabelloni, A., Tizzoni, F., Villa, F. M., Molteni, M., Nobile, M., Sacco, M., Arlati, S., & Colombo, V. (2022). A serious game for nutritional education of children and adolescents with neurodevelopmental disorders. In H. Lewy, R. Barkan, & R. (Eds.), *International conference on pervasive computing technologies for healthcare* (pp. 240–250). Springer. https://doi.org/10.1007/978-3-030-99194-4_16

Schlosser, R. W., O'Brien, A., Yu, C., Abramson, J., Allen, A. A., Flynn, S., & Shane, H. C. (2017). Repurposing everyday technologies to provide just-in-time visual supports to children with intellectual disability and autism: A pilot feasibility study with the Apple Watch®. *International Journal of Developmental Disabilities, 63*(4), 221–227. https://doi.org/10.1080/20473869.2017.1305138

Shane, H. C., Laubscher, E. H., Schlosser, R. W., Flynn, S., Sorce, J. F., & Abramson, J. (2012). Applying technology to visually support language and communication in individuals with autism spectrum disorders. *Journal of Autism and Developmental Disorders, 42*(6), 1228–1235. https://doi.org/10.1007/s10803-011-1304-z

Sharmin, M., Hossain, M. M., Saha, A., Das, M., Maxwell, M., & Ahmed, S. (2018, April). From research to practice: Informing the design of autism support smart technology. In R. Mandryk (Ed.), *Proceedings of the 2018 CHI conference on human factors in computing systems* (pp. 1–16). https://doi.org/10.1145/3173574.3173676

Steinbrenner, J. R., Hume, K., Odom, S. L., Morin, K. L., Nowell, S. W., Tomaszewski, B., Szendrey, S., McIntyre, N. S., Yücesoy-Özkan, S., & Savage, M. N. (2020). *Evidence-based practices for children, youth, and young adults with autism*. The University of North Carolina at Chapel Hill, Frank Porter Graham Child Development Institute, National Clearinghouse on Autism Evidence and Practice Review Team.

Tapus, A., Peca, A., Aly, A., Pop, C., Jisa, L., Pintea, S., Rusu, A., & David, D. O. (2012). Children with autism social engagement in interaction with Nao, an imitative robot: A series of single case experiments. *Interaction Studies, 13*(3), 315–347. https://doi.org/10.1075/is.13.3.01tap

Terlouw, G., Kuipers, D., van't Veer, J., Prins, J. T., & Pierie, J. P. E. (2021). The development of an escape room – Based serious game to trigger social interaction and communication between high-functioning children with autism and their peers: Iterative design approach. *JMIR Serious Games, 9*(1), e19765. https://doi.org/10.2196/19765

Therrien, M. C., & Light, J. C. (2018). Promoting peer interaction for preschool children with complex communication needs and autism spectrum disorder. *American Journal of Speech-Language Pathology, 27*(1), 207–221. https://doi.org/10.1044/2017_AJSLP-17-0104

Trottier, N., Kamp, L., & Mirenda, P. (2011). Effects of peer-mediated instruction to teach use of speech-generating devices to students with autism in social game routines. *Augmentative and Alternative Communication, 27*(1), 26–39. https://doi.org/10.3109/07434618.2010.546810

Vahabzadeh, A., Keshav, N. U., Abdus-Sabur, R., Huey, K., Liu, R., & Sahin, N. T. (2018a). Improved socio-emotional and behavioral functioning in students with autism following school-based smartglasses intervention: Multi-stage feasibility and controlled efficacy study. *Behavioral Sciences, 8*(10), 85–102. https://doi.org/10.3390/bs8100085

Vahabzadeh, A., Keshav, N. U., Salisbury, J. P., & Sahin, N. T. (2018b). Improvement of attention-deficit/hyperactivity disorder symptoms in school-aged children, adolescents, and young adults with autism via a digital smartglasses-based socioemotional coaching aid: Short-term, uncontrolled pilot study. *JMIR Mental Health, 5*(2), e9631. https://doi.org/10.2196/mental.9631

Valencia, K., Rusu, C., Quiñones, D., & Jamet, E. (2019). The impact of technology on people with autism spectrum disorder: A systematic literature review. *Sensors, 19*(20), 4485–4507. https://doi.org/10.3390/s19204485

Vukićević, S., Đorđević, M., Glumbić, N., Bogdanović, Z., & Đurić Jovičić, M. (2019). A demonstration project for the utility of kinect-based educational games to benefit motor skills of children with ASD. *Perceptual and Motor Skills, 126*(6), 1117–1144. https://doi.org/10.1177/0031512519867521

Warren, Z. E., Zheng, Z., Swanson, A. R., Bekele, E., Zhang, L., Crittendon, J. A., Weitlauf, A., & Sarkar, N. (2015). Can robotic interaction improve joint attention skills? *Journal of Autism and Developmental Disorders, 45*(11), 3726–3734. https://doi.org/10.1007/s10803-013-1918-4

Whalen, C., Moss, D., Ilan, A. B., Vaupel, M., Fielding, P., Macdonald, K., Cernich, S., & Symon, J. (2010). Efficacy of TeachTown: Basics computer-assisted intervention for the intensive comprehensive autism program in Los Angeles unified school district. *Autism, 14*(3), 179–197. https://doi.org/10.1177/1362361310363282

White, S. W., Abbott, L., Wieckowski, A. T., Capriola-Hall, N. N., Aly, S., & Youssef, A. (2018). Feasibility of automated training for facial emotion expression and recognition in autism. *Behavior Therapy, 49*(6), 881–888. https://doi.org/10.1016/j.beth.2017.12.010

Whitehouse, A., Varcin, K., Waddington, H., Sulek, R., Bent, C., Ashburner, J., Eapen, V., Goodall, E., Hudry, K., Roberts, J., Silove, N., & Trembath, D. (2021). *Interventions for children on the autism spectrum: A synthesis of research evidence*. Autism CRC.

Whyte, E. M., Smyth, J. M., & Scherf, K. S. (2015). Designing serious game interventions for individuals with autism. *Journal of Autism and Developmental Disorders, 45*(12), 3820–3831. https://doi.org/10.1007/s10803-014-2333-1

Wijnhoven, L. A., Creemers, D. H., Engels, R. C., & Granic, I. (2015). The effect of the video game Mindlight on anxiety symptoms in children with an autism spectrum disorder. *BMC Psychiatry, 15*(1), 1–9. https://doi.org/10.1186/s12888-015-0522-x

Wu, Y. P., Chen, M. C., Lo, Y. Y., & Chiang, C. H. (2020). Effects of peer-mediated instruction with AAC on science learning and communitive responses of students with significant cognitive disabilities in Taiwan. *Research and Practice for Persons with Severe Disabilities, 45*(3), 178–195. https://doi.org/10.1177/1540796919900955

Xianmei, L. (2017). A review of somatic games intervention for children with autism spectrum disorders. *Journal of Exceptional People, 2*(11), 83–92.

Yun, S. S., Choi, J., Park, S. K., Bong, G. Y., & Yoo, H. (2017). Social skills training for children with autism spectrum disorder using a robotic behavioral intervention system. *Autism Research, 10*(7), 1306–1323. https://doi.org/10.1002/aur.1778

Zeng, S., Zhao, H., Hu, X., Pereira, B. A., Pan, Q., Meng, C., Reyes, A., & Stone-MacDonald, A. (2021). Systematic review of single case design meta-analyses for school-age students with autism spectrum disorders: Current trend and future direction. *Psychology in the Schools, 59*(5), 980–1000. https://doi.org/10.1002/pits.22599

Zhang, S., Xia, X., Li, S., Shen, L., Liu, J., Zhao, L., & Chen, C. (2019). Using technology-based learning tool to train facial expression recognition and emotion understanding skills of Chinese pre-schoolers with autism spectrum disorder. *International Journal of Developmental Disabilities, 65*(5), 378–386. https://doi.org/10.1080/20473869.2019.1656384

Chapter 9
Health

9.1 Challenges in Conducting Medical Interventions

Autism spectrum disorder (ASD) is often accompanied by additional health problems. Numerous medical conditions such as immune dysregulation, gastrointestinal diseases, neurological conditions, obesity, dyslipidemia, hypertension, diabetes, and major psychiatric disorders (depression, anxiety, bipolar disorder, obsessive-compulsive disorder, schizophrenia) are significantly more frequent in people with autism than their neurotypical peers (Buro et al., 2022; Croen et al., 2015; Weiss et al., 2018).

Although health systems are not adequately adapted to the specific needs of people with autism, the greatest attention is still on the characteristics of individuals with ASD that can hinder and sometimes completely prevent access to quality health care. This primarily refers to communication difficulties, attention disorders and hyperactivity, repetitive movements, lower tolerance to unfamiliar and aversive stimuli, etc. (Walsh et al., 2021). Medical phobias cause strong emotional reactions and avoidant behavior, so even routine heart and lungs checkups and measuring blood pressure, body weight, and height can be challenging (Cavalari et al., 2013; Cuvo et al., 2010; Gillis et al., 2009). Some interventions that involve blood sampling, biopsy, or catheterization are much more invasive. As a rule, the more intense and unfamiliar sensory experience related to medical interventions is, the more resistance a person with ASD will put up (Allen & Kupzyk, 2016).

Rare interventions can be particularly challenging for people with autism. Some techniques, such as electroencephalography (EEG) (Slifer et al., 2008), require tolerance of medical devices, unfamiliar environment, and keeping still, while thyroid scintigraphy using a gamma camera requires a specific head position as well (Glumbić et al., 2022a) (Fig. 9.1).

In addition, some procedures such as neuroimaging scans (magnetic resonance imaging (MRI) and positron emission tomography (PET)) create unbearable noise.

N. Glumbić et al., *Digital Inclusion of Individuals with Autism Spectrum Disorder*, Autism and Child Psychopathology Series,
https://doi.org/10.1007/978-3-031-12037-4_9

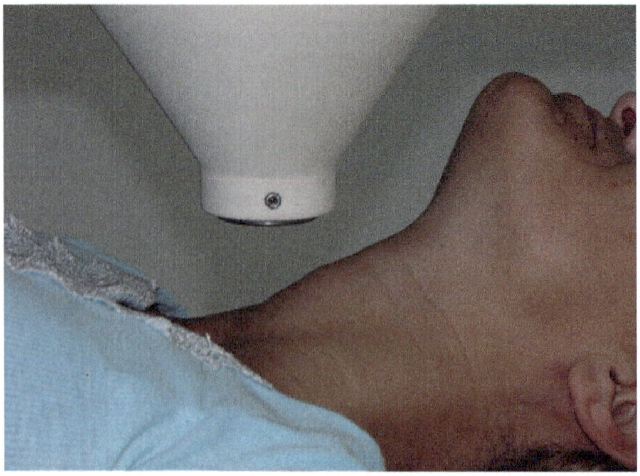

Fig. 9.1 Recommended head position during thyroid scintigraphy (personal archive)

The sound pressure level can reach 118 dB, which is equivalent to the sound of a plane takeoff. Thus, various means are used to reduce the sound pressure level to the acceptable 60 dB, which is equivalent to restaurant noise (Hendrix & Thomason, 2022). However, noise reduction is not an acceptable solution for hypersensitive people with ASD. The additional problem is that there is no specific scheme for sound emission, and it can be changed with no warning. Furthermore, scanners often have narrow bores, which increases the possibility of claustrophobia and panic attacks. The table on which a patient lies occasionally vibrates and may move abruptly. The imaging room is relatively cold to avoid overheating (Stogiannos et al., 2021). Therefore, the medical examination environment may be very unpleasant for people with autism.

If the examination is necessary and the autistic patient does not cooperate, restraint, either physical or pharmacological, is one of the options. Physical restraint can cause injury and psychological trauma, and it involves numerous ethical and legal concerns (Zaami et al., 2020). Apart from that, interns and full-time physicians typically do not have adequate knowledge about restraining people with ASD and are not familiar with protocols or possible alternatives (Salvatore et al., 2021). Unlike mechanical restraint, which is considered in blood sampling or other short interventions, various imaging procedures that require tolerating noise, controlling movements, and a high degree of cooperation can be performed with sedation or anesthesia. However, these procedures also have their downsides. General anesthesia and sedation do not allow patients to acquire the skills that would help them undergo future examinations; although considered safe for people with autism, they can still have some side effects (adverse respiratory and cardiovascular events); using sedation and anesthesia can change the obtained data, and the patient must be awake during functional MRI; the examination cost is three times higher with sedation, and ten times more with anesthesia than when the patient is awake (Cox et al., 2017; Grider et al., 2012; Kuschner et al., 2021; Nordahl et al., 2016; Tziraki et al., 2021). Thus, Stogiannos et al. (2021) recommend that sedation or anesthesia be given only to those patients with autism who are not cooperative, provided that the perceived benefits outweigh the possible risks.

9.2 Training Individuals with ASD to Be Compliant with Medical Procedures

In a systematic review of interventions used for improving healthcare experiences of people with autism, Walsh et al. (2021) have found that more than half of these interventions focus on patients with autism, while a significantly smaller number of programs focus on organizational issues and systematic solutions. Patient-focused interventions are a set of different interventions aimed at people with autism who receive support in tolerating and anticipating medical procedures or healthcare settings (Walsh et al., 2021).

Such most common highly efficient interventions are based on various behavioral techniques (task analysis, graduate exposure, escape extinction, reinforcement, modeling, etc.), visual support, relaxation techniques, and cooperation with parents (e.g., Cox et al., 2017; Meindl et al., 2019; Pineda & Mullett, 2018; Walsh et al., 2021). Digital technologies are often used as a medium for realizing specific techniques (e.g., video modeling, distraction), and their significance is crucial in the gradual habituation of people with autism to specific clinical settings and procedures.

Compliance of patients with autism is crucial for the successful performance of many medical interventions and treatment outcomes. The role of modern technologies in patient compliance is observed from a broader perspective in the general population. Technological applications and tools can be used to familiarize patients with a particular procedure, to remind them to take a medication or make an appointment. However, a lot of contradictory information in the online environment may be confusing and frustrating for patients and raise their doubts about the health system (Planel-Ratna & Juwaheer, 2021). Studies on the compliance of people with ASD are generally aimed only at reaching the optimal level of tolerance to perform a medical examination.

9.2.1 *Videos*

Videos are easy to make, do not require specific or expensive equipment, and can easily be changed and adapted to the individual needs of users. They are most commonly used for modeling, reinforcement, or distraction in the context of health.

Cuvo et al. (2010) have recorded a 9-min DVD of typically developing children who go through physical examination without any difficulty and resistance, in order to develop compliance in children with autism. The children in the video undergo regular heart and lungs stethoscope checkups, abdomen palpation, and ear, nose, and throat examination. During each examination step, the narrator is a dinosaur toy that rewards the children's appropriate behavior. Occasionally, there are close-ups of the used medical equipment for the purpose of video priming. Video modeling has also been used in more complex procedures such as acquiring MRI data in children with ASD and comorbid intellectual disability. Nordahl et al. (2016) created a fun Spider-Man video for their research, showing all scanning phases in a simulated environment. Parents could show video models of the MRI procedure at home unlimited times. A training protocol for preparing adults with ASD for simultaneous PET and MRI scans was developed in a similar way (Smith et al., 2019). It includes an introductory 4-min video for home training, describing the entire procedure from entering the hospital to scanning, and five videos with nonverbal instructions showing specific PET/MRI imaging components.

Gradual exposure is a commonly used technique in training children with autism to tolerate medical interventions. This technique involves slowly reducing spatial distance from an aversive stimulus (e.g., a needle), prolonging exposure to an unwanted stimulus, or achieving the appropriate level of tolerance to a larger number of aversive stimuli. Tolerance is usually increased by reinforcing any behavior that is one step closer to a desired goal (e.g., a child who had a violent reaction to seeing a needle is reinforced if they tolerate being near one without getting very upset or trying to escape). The reinforcers are highly individualized, and for some children, videos can be ideal reinforcers. Slifer et al. (2008) used a similar technique to achieve tolerance to electroencephalography (EEG) equipment. Being aware that their patients with autism would put up strong resistance to EEG leads and probably try to take them off, they designed an intervention based on modeling, escape extinction, and other behavioral techniques, including differential reinforcement of other behaviors. While the children cooperated in placing EEG leads, their favorite video was played. The video was turned off briefly when the children tried to take the leads off.

In the clinical and technical magnetoencephalography (MEG) protocol of nonverbal and minimally verbal children with autism, favorite videos have also been used to reinforce compliant behavior and as distractors during the examination. Due to excellent temporal and spatial information, MEG provides a better image of brain activity than EEG. Also, compared to MRI, it is much more comfortable for the patient who can sit or lie down and is not exposed to loud noise. Only a few sensors are placed on the head, and the child should keep still during the examination (Kuschner et al., 2021). Kuschner et al. (2021) monitored the brain response of children with low-functioning autism to simple auditory stimuli. The children were not required to consciously direct their attention to sound, while the videos and films were used as distractors. A favorite video was also used to hold the attention of a young man with autism who received a medication administered through a hypodermic needle due to advanced psoriasis (Grider et al., 2012). According to the designed protocol, the video was played 30 s before the needle was placed, during the procedure itself, and immediately after it.

Functional MRI examinations, where a patient has to be awake and still, are especially challenging for clinicians since the images are subject to artifacts due to possible head movements. Thus, Vanderwal et al. (2015) created a moving paradigm Inscapes consisting of films without narration, stage cuts, and explicit social references. The film shows only abstract shapes (Fig. 9.2).

In the mentioned research, head movements were significantly reduced in typical participants of different ages, which resulted in quality images. This was the motive

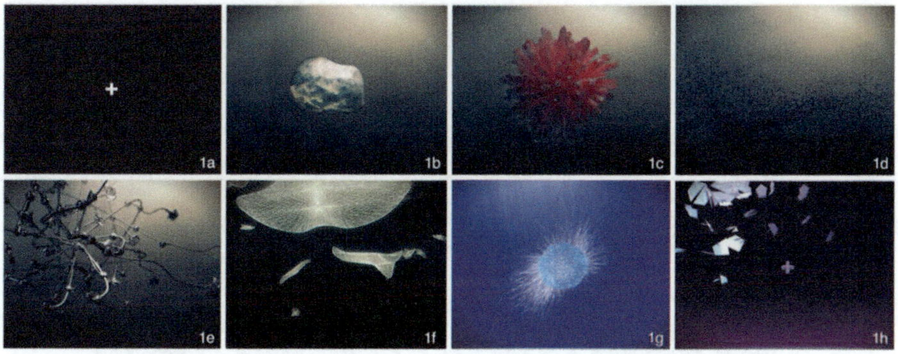

Fig. 9.2 Inscapes abstract shapes. (Reproduced from Vanderwal et al., 2015)

to use the Inscapes paradigm in participants with ASD. Gabrielsen et al. (2018) examined brain connectivity in people with autism and their typically developing peers. Since the research aim was to determine possible differences between high-functioning and low-functioning participants with ASD, it was necessary to ensure a high level of compliance and minimize mobility. This research used various videos. In the preparation phase, a video was used to model desirable behavior during individual steps in the MRI procedure. The participants were shown their favorite YouTube video during the structural scan to achieve greater comfort and reduce head movements, while the Inscapes videos were played during the functional MRI. Although, as expected, the mobility of low-functioning participants with ASD was greater than that of participants with high-functioning autism and typically developing ones, the recordings of all participants were good enough for analysis. Similar effects were achieved in a recent study during MEG in typically developing children, children with ASD, and those with ADHD (Vandewouw et al., 2021).

9.2.2 *Mock Equipment*

As shown, various behavioral techniques and videos have successfully been used to increase the compliance of people with ASD with medical procedures. No special technical devices are needed in preparing for interventions such as general physical examination, venipuncture, and other simple and short procedures. However, certain diagnostic procedures require the use of sophisticated technology, which can cause anxiety both because of an unfamiliar setting and the need to tolerate high-intensity sounds and limited space, which is all especially pronounced in neuroimaging technologies. Thus, some authors have used commercial mock scanners or toy scanners to prepare participants with ASD for scanning. Nordahl et al. (2016) used a mock scanner consisting of a conical bore, movable bed, head coil, head stabilization system, and auditory and visual presentations (Fig. 9.3).

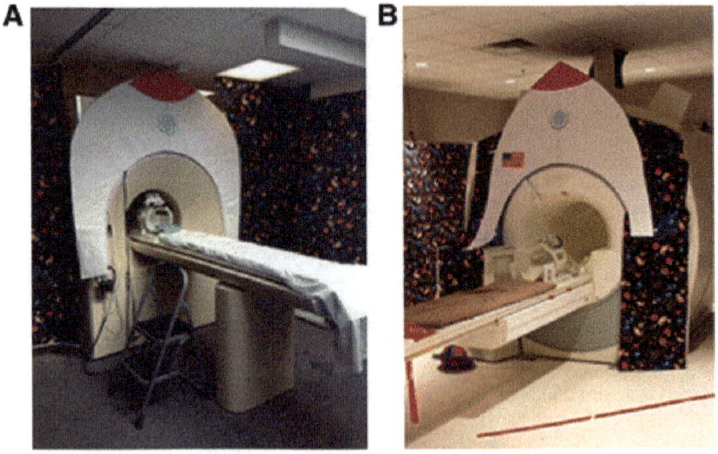

Fig. 9.3 A pediatric-friendly space theme environment for (**a**) mock MRI scanner and (**b**) 3 T MRI scanner. (Reproduced from Nordahl et al., 2016)

Similarly, Cox et al. (2017) used a mock scanner to prepare patients with ASD for scanning by using numerous behavioral techniques to get the patients to approach the "scanner," take the appropriate position, and keep still. Only after the adequate level of compliance was reached did they start using the real MRI. Both studies paid particular attention to getting used to noise and measuring head movements.

Some authors have certain reservations about the use of mock devices because they are often unavailable; their use is not time-saving; after getting used to a mock scanner, participants have to go through the additional procedure of getting used to real devices; the size of real and mock scanners is sometimes significantly different; there is usually no special room for "injecting" radiotracers, and the question of generalizing the acquired skills to a real clinical environment remains (Gabrielsen et al., 2018; Kuschner et al., 2021; Smith et al., 2019).

Sometimes a combination of real and mock equipment is used to get accustomed to cheap and technically less demanding procedures from the clinicians' perspective, which can be very challenging for patients with ASD due to their duration and numerous instruments used. Paasch et al. (2016) used real and mock polysomnography components that are irreplaceable in diagnosing obstructive sleep apnea. For a successful procedure, the child must be asleep. Polysomnography involves using specific devices to monitor heart rate and arm and leg movements; a belt is placed around the abdomen and chest to measure respiratory effort; a nasal cannula is necessary for airflow, while a pulse oximeter is necessary for oxygen saturation.

Although many studies use videos or devices to get children and adults with ASD to comply with medical interventions, it is difficult to determine their effectiveness since they are never used in isolation but as an integral part of behavioral packages and other interventions.

9.2.3 Virtual Reality Technologies

Virtual reality (VR) technologies enable the simulation of a real environment where people with ASD can safely and gradually get used to medical interventions. Although the application of VR technologies in people with ASD of different ages and functioning levels has been researched for almost three decades, studies dealing with the use of these technologies for medical purposes are scarce. Cognitive behavioral therapy with gradual exposure to threat stimuli in a virtual environment has reduced specific phobias in young people with autism (Maskey et al., 2014). In this study, participants with autism were exposed to virtual stimuli in the so-called blue room. No additional devices are needed for moving around the blue room, but the whole room provides an immersive and interactive experience. The drawback of this technology is that it requires a special setting, and its potential application would be very expensive. Headset technology is a much more affordable alternative. Preliminary studies show that, regardless of the level of intellectual functioning, most participants with autism enjoy head-mounted displays, giving high scores to subjective immersive experience (Newbutt et al., 2016). By using 360-degree headset technology, a specific virtual environment was created to get a young man with autism to tolerate a blood sampling procedure (Meindl et al., 2019). The young man's father went through the procedure, filming it with a VR camera held at chest height. The camera was equipped with lenses that simultaneously recorded two 180-degree video images. The impression of three-dimensionality is achieved when these images are simultaneously observed. The autistic user, watching a 360-degree video with a VR headset, could look in any direction and see the whole room where a nurse was taking his father's blood sample. A therapist watched the same video on a screen, trying to expose the autistic participant to the same sensations (e.g., applying a tourniquet) simultaneously with the blood sampling phases shown in the video. Gradual exposure to the virtual environment with reinforcement proved to be very effective as the compliant behavior generalized to different settings and persisted over time.

9.2.4 Robots

The development of robotics and artificial intelligence has provided numerous opportunities for using robots in the healthcare system. Thus, nowadays, there are care robots, hospital robots, rehabilitation robots, and walking assisting robots (Kyrarini, 2021). Using robots to get children with autism to comply with medical procedures is still in the initial phase. One of the scarce studies used two robots in a sample of five children with autism: a humanoid NAO robot that could talk, dance, sing, and give instructions and another zoomorphic MiRo robot behaving like a dog that runs and barks (Di Nuovo et al., 2020). At the beginning of the treatment, NAO introduced itself and then entertained the children by telling them stories, playing music, and asking them to imitate it. Then, a simulated clinical procedure was introduced, in which a nurse had to put a cast on a child's arm. In order to understand the procedure better, children with autism were asked to put a cast on the robot's arm. After that, NAO told the children to follow MiRo to a sink to wash their hands, after which they were allowed to play with robots (Fig. 9.4). The autistic children followed the orders of the humanoid robot better, while the "dog" was interesting only during free play.

Many robotics platforms are still in the research phase, while commercially available robots are very expensive and thus rarely used in healthcare institutions. In addition, the use of robots in educational, social, and healthcare facilities for people with ASD raises numerous ethical issues that will become increasingly relevant in the years to come.

9.3 Dental Care

People with ASD have poorer dental and oral health than their typically developing peers, and dental care is at the very top of the infamous list of unmet healthcare needs (e.g., Isong et al., 2014; Narzisi et al., 2020; Suresh & George, 2019). The literature lists various factors that influence the increased prevalence of oral and dental diseases in individuals with ASD. They can be categorized as follows: poor oral hygiene; habits, diseases, and behaviors that increase the risk of dental problems; the characteristics of autism that make it difficult to comply with dental procedures; and underdeveloped dental care services.

Poor oral hygiene is one of the most significant risk factors for caries and other dental diseases. Inadequate manual skills and uncooperativeness of children with autism, difficulties they have in following the procedure of brushing their teeth, and consequent overinvolvement of parents in maintaining hygiene are considered the

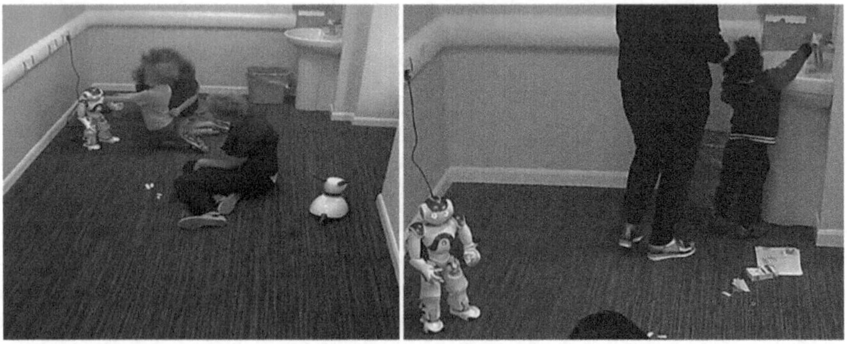

Fig. 9.4 Using robots in getting children with autism to comply with medical procedures. (Reproduced from Di Nuovo et al., 2020)

main reasons why dental hygiene is poor, which increases the need for various dental interventions (Barry, 2012; Bondioli et al., 2018).

Some eating habits (selective food intake, preference of soft and sweetened food they keep in their mouth for a long time), bruxism, and self-harm cause frequent dental trauma and disease. Gastroesophageal reflux accompanied by regurgitation of gastric contents can lead to tooth erosion. We should also mention the frequent use of anticonvulsants and psychotropic drugs that can cause gingival hyperplasia, delayed teeth eruption, caries, and xerostomia (dry mouth) (Barry, 2012; Lefer et al., 2019; Logrieco et al., 2021).

Some of the main symptoms of autism, such as social communication disorder, resistance to change, and sensory hypersensitivity, make dental procedures challenging. Dental procedures often involve unusual and unpleasant suction sounds, or sounds of ultrasonic scalers, dental micromotors, and drills; specific flavors of pastes and other dental materials used for prophylaxis or fissure sealing; bright lights above the dental chair; etc. (Bondioli et al., 2018; Narzici et al., 2020). In addition, the patient must cooperate. Examination with a dental mirror is short, but during fissure and pit sealing, the patient's mouth has to be open the whole time. Some procedures are even more challenging. Dental burrs can cause oral tissue injury if a person with autism makes a sudden movement, while restoration with adhesive material requires a dry oral environment, which means salivation control (Narzici et al., 2020).

Based on a questionnaire completed by 142 mothers of children with ASD, Alshihri et al. (2021) found that the behavior of children with autism was an obstacle to dental services in 45% of the cases, while three-quarters of the participants stated that financial inability to cover the intervention costs and unavailability of a qualified dentist were the main problems. Other studies also state that dentists and dental surgeons are not adequately trained to work with people with ASD, which is why they openly refuse patients with autism or do not know how to adapt the intervention to their needs (e.g., Curri et al., 2022; Duker et al., 2017; Lefer et al., 2018).

Anesthesia and sedation can have adverse effects, while standard techniques for preparing patients for dental interventions, such as tell-show-do, voice control, positive reinforcement, systematic desensitization, and other behavioral techniques, have limited efficacy when applied in people with ASD (Curri et al., 2022; Isong et al., 2014; Suresh et al., 2019). Since people with autism have a propensity for visual content, information and communication technologies (ICTs) are increasingly used to improve their oral hygiene, familiarize them with dental procedures and the environment, reduce anxiety, and increase cooperation.

9.3.1 Non-personalized Tools and Content

Within her Ph.D. research in pediatric dentistry, Barry (2012) evaluated the effectiveness of various techniques for preparing children with ASD for dental examinations. To familiarize the children with the examination procedure, she used photographs of the dental clinic and staff, social stories, a comic with customized pictures and content, and a dental application for tablets and smartphones. The application enabled the patients to make a virtual tour through the dental clinic from home and familiarize themselves with the staff, environment, devices, and usual sounds. All mentioned interventions were more effective in children with ASD than in the control group of their typically developing peers.

For similar purposes, experts from São Paulo have developed a free mobile application—Autistic Child Going to the Dentist. The home screen shows easy-to-use icons, so the choice of content can be customized. The content includes a text explaining each procedure step-by-step, appropriate images, and audio comments. The user can select one out of three languages (English, Portuguese, and Spanish), the narrator's gender, and background music. Children with autism who used this application complied with preventive dental examinations much faster than the group of autistic children who used only the Picture Exchange Communication System to prepare for dental interventions (Zink et al., 2018).

Isong et al. (2014) had more complex aims and methodological solutions. Their study examined the possible role of two electronic media in reducing dental fear and increasing the cooperation of children with autism. In this randomized controlled study, 80 children with autism, aged 7–17, were classified into 1 of the 4 groups after the first visit to a dentist when their anxiety and cooperativeness were evaluated. The first control group included children with autism who received usual dental care. In the second group, a video-modeling technique was applied by recording a special DVD showing various activities such as entering the dental clinic, checking in, the examination, cleaning and polishing teeth, fluoride varnish, dental radiography, etc. The models in the DVD were the participants' peers. The DVD was distributed to the families of children with autism to play at home. In addition, this DVD was played to all children in this group in the waiting room, 15 min before the examination. The third group used video goggles to watch favorite films during the examination, and the fourth group used the DVD for peer modeling and video goggles for distraction. The children from the third and fourth group made significant improvements between the first and the control examination, which reflected in their increased cooperativeness and reduced anxiety. No significant changes were determined in the first two groups.

What all mentioned studies have in common are digital technologies based on visual content used to achieve compliance of people with ASD during dental examinations and the fact that the participants were mostly passive users of the presented digital content. Understanding the drawbacks of this approach, some authors search for technical solutions that would be more personalized.

9.3.2 *Personalized Tools and Content*

One of the few studies that used a personalized program for improving compliance, based on TEACCH (Treatment and Education of Autistic and related Communication-handicapped CHildren), in children and adults with ASD, was conducted in Spain (Orellana et al., 2014). The research included 72 participants and had 3 phases: a basic oral assessment, 5 training sessions, and a final assessment. The whole oral assessment process was divided into ten steps, from entering the dental office to assessing dental occlusion. Each step was explained in simple terms. The activities were demonstrated on a toy model, after which the participants had the opportunity to apply a specific procedure to the model. Furthermore, photographs and pictograms were shown on a laptop so that a participant could anticipate the examination phases. Much attention was given to modeling in this research. Modeling was first conducted in person. During the examination, a model stood directly in front of a person with autism showing them what to do. The same model was recorded participating in different examination phases, which was later used in video modeling. Elements of program personalization were most prominent in self-modeling. For this purpose, photographs of the participants with autism were used. These photographs were made during dental examinations and later edited and modified to remove undesirable behaviors from them. The authors indicated a statistically significant improvement in the number of mastered steps and compliance with a dental examination after the program.

French authors (Lefer et al., 2018, 2019) designed the çATED application as a digital diary showing different examination phases. Pictograms, photographs, and visual schedules were personalized in a way that children with autism and their parents participated in their choice. During the 8-month training program, an iPad with the application was the mediator between a child with autism and a dentist. The intervention that combined behavioral techniques and visual pedagogy with ICTs proved to be effective in reducing dental fear and increasing the compliance of participants with autism.

A significant improvement has been made in personalizing multimedia content used to prepare children with autism for dental interventions in the last few years. The first visit to a dentist is usually used to determine how much a child cooperates and collect data about dental hygiene, sensory hypersensitivity, habits in using ICTs, etc. Bondioli et al. (2018) created a team consisting of researchers, dentists, psychologists, developers, dental technology experts, and parents of children with autism to design a personalized multimedia kit, based on the principles of participatory design, to be used at home between two visits to a dentist. The photographs and videos show a patient's activities from entering the clinic to sitting on a dental chair, certain examination phases, and dental equipment and setting. The children were allowed to make their own photographs and videos at each examination, which were later added to the multimedia material. In addition, various cognitive games and interactive PDFs with sound effects were designed to give patients with autism the most realistic insight into the procedures that await them.

Similar multimedia content has also been successfully used in the My Dentist application (Narzisi et al., 2020). Apart from the content designed for home use, this application allows patients with ASD to observe themselves during the examination (mirror mode), relax by watching a favorite video (distractor mode), or have fun after the examination (reinforcement mode).

Watching films, listening to favorite music, counting, and even casual chatting with the staff are frequently applied distraction techniques in dental care. However, using VR technologies as distractors during dental interventions is still in the initial phase. The first results of the study conducted by Suresh and George (2019) are encouraging. They achieved significant anxiety reduction during dental examinations by providing patients with autism with a fully immersive experience, blocking all potentially aversive stimuli from the dental office environment.

9.4 Telehealth

The Health Resources and Services Administration of the US Department of Health and Human Services defines telehealth as "the use of electronic information and telecommunication technologies to support long-distance clinical health care, patient and professional health-related education, health administration, and public health" (HRSA, 2021). Telehealth services can be transmitted in synchronous and asynchronous modes. Synchronous telehealth means that a trained expert or a team of experts provide remote services using different technologies in real time. Asynchronous telehealth services are based on a store-and-forward method when, for example, parents upload videos of their children's behavior to a certain web portal, which are then analyzed by a team of experts (Alfuraydan et al., 2020; Glumbić & Đorđević, 2020; Lamash et al., 2022). Depending on the purpose of telehealth services, availability of ICTs, digital literacy of potential users, and available time, these services can be provided in a variety of ways—phone calls, videoconferencing, emails, instant messengers, forums, online platforms, mobile and web applications, national platforms for Internet-delivered treatments, and sometimes specially designed software for interventions in people with autism (Dahiya et al., 2020; Ellison et al., 2021; Lamash et al., 2022; Панцырь & Шведовский, 2020).

Telehealth services can be a convenient way to overcome the obstacles in using support services that many families of people with autism face. It is known that autism is diagnosed later, and support services are less available in rural communities, which are geographically distant from large urban areas, and in individuals living below the poverty line compared to wealthier users from urban areas (Antezana et al., 2017).

The COVID-19 pandemic created additional difficulties in providing direct support to people with autism and their families. However, it was at the same time a great impetus for the development of telehealth services. Telehealth services soon replaced interventions that were until then performed in direct contact. The main advantages of telepractice are the following: availability to a wider range of users, cost-effectiveness, possibility to perform the intervention in a natural environment, and satisfaction of the parents of people with ASD (Alfuraydan et al., 2020; Dahiya et al., 2020; Ellison et al., 2021). However, the introduction of telehealth interventions did not go smoothly. At the beginning of the pandemic, almost 40% of the surveyed parents refused to use telehealth services. As it soon became clear that the pandemic would last much longer than the seasonal flu, an increasing number of families started using telehealth services. By comparing the families of children with autism who accepted with the ones who refused telehealth support, it was found that neither sociodemographic variables (gender, age, socioeconomic status, ethnicity, language) nor adaptive and speech-language abilities of people with autism significantly affected their decision. It turned out that parents who provided their autistic children with more intensive behavioral interventions and more speech and occupational therapy before the pandemic were more inclined to use telehealth technology to continue with the interventions (Aranki, 2022).

Adapting to telehealth support services involves both internal and external contexts. Motivating users to accept remote interventions, reorganizing working methods, rules, management, and redistribution of resources refer to the internal context. The most important external contextual factor is the technology itself. The existing digital divide is further deepened in crises such as a pandemic if attention is not paid to the pragmatic adaptation of telehealth services. In South Africa, such adaptation involved providing remote support in the asynchronous mode because many families did not have a stable and fast Internet connection (Franz et al., 2022).

Telehealth is used for assessment, intervention, and counseling in people with autism. Two review studies, published in a relatively short period (Ellison et al., 2021; Sutherland et al., 2018), found that assessment-related research was significantly rarer than research dealing with different interventions.

Telehealth is used for autism screening and diagnosis, functional assessment, preference assessment, speech and language assessment, etc. Remote screening is an important current issue since access to many services has been limited due to the epidemiological situation. Videoconferencing is usually used for remote screening, allowing a team of experts to evaluate a child in the natural environment. Another approach is based on mobile and web applications. By using these applications, parents can share important information about their children's developmental history, complete a screening instrument, or upload videos of their children in different situations. Some applications provide ecological momentary assessment, i.e., dynamic assessment of symptoms that may vary at different times of day (Dahiya et al., 2020).

Interventions are mostly aimed at training parents and, to a much lesser extent, at training experts or working directly with people with autism. Telehealth is mainly used for early intervention, using behavioral techniques, functional communication training, social skills training, language interventions, consultations, etc. (Ellison et al., 2021; Sutherland et al., 2018). Behavioral interventions usually include technology-based training and coaching. Technology-based training is provided so that people who conduct the intervention become familiar with the theoretical foundations of a technique or program to be used by using technological devices. On the other hand, coaching is individual training in performing an intervention followed by feedback (Ferguson et al., 2019). Video coaching can also be organized for a group of parents. Garnett et al. (2022) provided training for the parents of 11 participants with autism in implementing the Hanen More Than Words program aimed at encouraging social communication. The parents pointed out positive changes in their children and listed interactive learning opportunities, group participation, video coaching, and service individualization as advantages of the program.

The accuracy of autism diagnosis made by the telehealth method ranges from 80% to 91% compared to traditional in-person diagnosis (Stavropoulos et al., 2022). Telehealth interventions have been effective in at least one of the outcome variables related to children with ASD, with positive effects on parents' self-confidence and high social validity ratings. Usually, there is no significant difference in the quality of interventions performed using the traditional or the telehealth method (Drew et al., 2022; Ellison et al., 2021; Ferguson et al., 2019; Garnett et al., 2022; Glumbić et al., 2022b). Studies dealing with the reduction of autistic symptoms and improvement of mental health in adolescents with autism through telehealth services are scarce and do not yet provide sufficient empirical evidence for their efficacy (Lamash et al., 2022).

Despite the encouraging results of published studies on using the telehealth approach in assessing and treating people with ASD, there are still some limitations in their application. Some barriers are related to the disparity in the accessibility of ICTs and the disability digital divide also present in people with autism, especially those living in poorer and rural areas. Most research studies on the effects of telehealth interventions in people with autism included white people belonging to the upper-middle class from Europe and America (Franz et al., 2022). Even when potential problems related to the availability of telehealth technologies are solved, we face difficulties related to gestural or positional prompting and accurate interpretation of facial expressions in the synchronous mode of telehealth services. Although existing research shows positive effects of telehealth interventions, they are based on a small number of participants, and their quality ratings are, as a rule, low (Ferguson et al., 2019).

References

Alfuraydan, M., Croxall, J., Hurt, L., Kerr, M., & Brophy, S. (2020). Use of telehealth for facilitating the diagnostic assessment of Autism Spectrum Disorder (ASD): A scoping review. *PLoS One, 15*(7), e0236415. https://doi.org/10.1371/journal.pone.0236415

Allen, K. D., & Kupzyk, S. (2016). Compliance with medical routines. In J. K. Luiselli (Ed.), *Behavioral health promotion and intervention in intellectual and developmental disabilities* (pp. 21–42). Evidence-Based Practices in Behavioral Health. https://doi.org/10.1007/978-3-319-27297-9_2

Alshihri, A. A., Al-Askar, M. H., & Aldossary, M. S. (2021). Barriers to professional dental care among children with autism spectrum disorder. *Journal of Autism and Developmental Disorders, 51*(8), 2988–2994. https://doi.org/10.1007/s10803-020-04759-y

Antezana, L., Scarpa, A., Valdespino, A., Albright, J., & Richey, J. A. (2017). Rural trends in diagnosis and services for autism spectrum disorder. *Frontiers in Psychology, 8*, 590. https://doi.org/10.3389/fpsyg.2017.00590

Aranki, J., Wright, P., Pompa-Craven, P., & Lotfizadeh, A. D. (2022). Lotfizadeh Acceptance of telehealth therapy to replace in-person therapy for autism treatment during covid-19 pandemic: An assessment of patient variables. *Telemedicine and e-Health*. https://doi.org/10.1089/tmj.2021.0397

Barry, S. M. (2012). *Improving access and reducing barriers to dental care for children with autism spectrum disorder*. University of Leeds.

Bondioli, M., Buzzi, M. C., Buzzi, M., Pelagatti, S., & Senette, C. (2018, July). ICT to support dental care of children with autism: An exploratory study. In *International conference on universal access in human-computer interaction* (pp. 475–492). Springer. https://doi.org/10.1007/978-3-319-92049-8_34

Buro, A. W., Salinas-Miranda, A., Marshall, J., Gray, H. L., & Kirby, R. S. (2022). Obesity and co-occurring conditions among adolescents with autism spectrum disorder: The National Survey of Children's Health 2017–2018. *Research in Autism Spectrum Disorders, 92*, 101927. https://doi.org/10.1016/j.rasd.2022.101927

Cavalari, R. N. S., DuBard, M., Luiselli, J. K., & Birtwell, K. (2013). Teaching an adolescent with autism and intellectual disability to tolerate routine medical examination: Effects of a behavioral compliance training package. *Clinical Practice in Pediatric Psychology, 1*(2), 121–128. https://doi.org/10.1037/cpp0000013

Cox, A. D., Virues-Ortega, J., Julio, F., & Martin, T. L. (2017). Establishing motion control in children with autism and intellectual disability: Applications for anatomical and functional MRI. *Journal of Applied Behavior Analysis, 50*(1), 8–26. https://doi.org/10.1002/jaba.351

Croen, L. A., Zerbo, O., Qian, Y., Massolo, M. L., Rich, S., Sidney, S., & Kripke, C. (2015). The health status of adults on the autism spectrum. *Autism, 19*(7), 814–823. https://doi.org/10.1177/1362361315577517

Curi, D. S. C., Miranda, V. E. V. L., da Silva, Z. B., de Lucena Bem, M. C., de Pinho, M. D., & Zink, A. G. (2022). Strategies used for the outpatient dental care of people with autism spectrum disorder: An integrative review. *Research in Autism Spectrum Disorders, 91*, 101903. https://doi.org/10.1016/j.rasd.2021.101903

Cuvo, A. J., Reagan, A. L., Ackerlund, J., Huckfeldt, R., & Kelly, C. (2010). Training children with autism spectrum disorders to be compliant with a physical exam. *Research in Autism Spectrum Disorders, 4*(2), 168–185. https://doi.org/10.1016/j.rasd.2009.09.001

Dahiya, A. V., McDonnell, C., DeLucia, E., & Scarpa, A. (2020). A systematic review of remote telehealth assessments for early signs of autism spectrum disorder: Video and mobile applications. *Practice Innovations, 5*(2), 150–164. https://doi.org/10.1037/pri0000121

Di Nuovo, A., Bamforth, J., Conti, D., Sage, K., Ibbotson, R., Clegg, J., Westaway, A., & Arnold, K. (2020). An explorative study on robotics for supporting children with autism spectrum disorder during clinical procedures. In *Companion of the 2020 ACM/IEEE International Conference on Human-Robot Interaction* (pp. 189–191). https://doi.org/10.1145/3371382.3378277

Drew, C. M., Machalicek, W., Crowe, B., Glugatch, L., Wei, Q., & Erturk, B. (2022). Parent-implemented behavior interventions via telehealth for older children and adolescents. *Journal of Behavioral Education, 1-20*. https://doi.org/10.1007/s10864-021-09464-z

Duker, L., Henwood, B. F., Bluthenthal, R. N., Juhlin, E., Polido, J. C., & Cermak, S. A. (2017). Parents' perceptions of dental care challenges in male children with Autism Spectrum Disorder: An initial qualitative exploration. *Research in Autism Spectrum Disorders, 39*, 63–72. https://doi.org/10.1016/j.rasd

Ellison, K. S., Guidry, J., Picou, P., Adenuga, P., & Davis, T. E. (2021). Telehealth and autism prior to and in the age of COVID-19: A systematic and critical review of the last decade. *Clinical Child and Family Psychology Review, 24*(3), 599–630. https://doi.org/10.1007/s10567-021-00358-0

Ferguson, J., Craig, E. A., & Dounavi, K. (2019). Telehealth as a model for providing behaviour analytic interventions to individuals with autism spectrum disorder: A systematic review. *Journal of Autism and Developmental Disorders, 49*(2), 582–616. https://doi.org/10.1007/s10803-018-3724-5

Franz, L., Howard, J., Viljoen, M., Sikich, L., Chandrasekhar, T., Kollins, S. H., Lee, L., Ndlovu, M., Sabatos-De Vito, M., Seris, N., Shabalala, N., Spanos, M., de Vries, P. J., & Dawson, G. (2022). Pragmatic adaptations of telehealth-delivered caregiver coaching for children with autism in the context of COVID-19: Perspectives from the United States and South Africa. *Autism, 26*(1), 270–275. https://doi.org/10.1177/13623613211022585

Gabrielsen, T. P., Anderson, J. S., Stephenson, K. G., Beck, J., King, J. B., Kellems, R., Top, D. N., Russell, N. C. C., Anderberg, E., Lundwall, R. A., Hansen, B., & South, M. (2018). Functional MRI connectivity of children with autism and low verbal and cognitive performance. *Molecular Autism, 9*(1), 1–14. https://doi.org/10.1186/s13229-018-0248-y

Garnett, R., Davidson, B., & Eadie, P. (2022). Parent perceptions of a group telepractice communication intervention for Autism. *Autism & Developmental Language Impairments.* https://doi.org/10.1177/23969415211070127

Gillis, J. M., Hammond Natof, T., Lockshin, S. B., & Romanczyk, R. G. (2009). Fear of routine physical exams in children with autism spectrum disorders: Prevalence and intervention effectiveness. *Focus on Autism and Other Developmental Disabilities, 24*, 156–168. https://doi.org/10.1177/1088357609338477

Glumbić, N., & Đorđević, M. (2020). On-line podrška osobama s autizmom, njihovim porodicama i terapeutima tokom vanrednog stanja. *Specijalna edukacija i rehabilitacija, 19*(1), 59–70. https://doi.org/10.5937/specedreh19-26342

Glumbić, N., Đorđević, M., Brojčin, B., & Matović, M. (2022a). Priprema osoba sa autizmom za scintigrafiju štitnjače. *Specijalna edukacija i rehabilitacija.*

Glumbić, N., Grujičić, R., Stupar, S., Petrović, S., & Pejović-Milovančević, M. (2022b). Positive effects of the caregiver skills training programme on children with developmental disabilities: Experiences from Serbia. *Frontiers in Psychiatry*, 1181.

Grider, B., Luiselli, J. K., Turcotte-Shamski, W. (2012). Graduated exposure positive reinforcement and stimulus distraction in a compliance-with-blood-draw intervention for an adult with Autism. *Clinical Case Studies, 11*(3), 253–260. https://doi.org/10.1177/1534650112448921

Hendrix, C. L., & Thomason, M. E. (2022). A survey of protocols from 54 infant and toddler neuroimaging research labs. *Developmental Cognitive Neuroscience*, 101060. https://doi.org/10.1016/j.dcn.2022.101060

HRSA. (2021). What is telehealth? Available at https://www.hrsa.gov/rural-health/telehealth/what-is-telehealth

Isong, I. A., Rao, S. R., Holifiedl, C., Iannuzzi, D., Hanson, E., Ware, J., & Nelson, L. P. (2014). Addressing dental fear in children with autism spectrum disorders: A randomized controlled pilot using electronic screen media. *Clinical Pediatrics, 53*, 230–237. https://doi.org/10.1177/0009922813517169

Kuschner, E. S., Kim, M., Bloy, L., Dipiero, M., Edgar, J. C., & Roberts, T. P. (2021). MEG-PLAN: A clinical and technical protocol for obtaining magnetoencephalography data in minimally verbal or nonverbal children who have autism spectrum disorder. *Journal of Neurodevelopmental Disorders, 13*(1), 1–17. https://doi.org/10.1186/s11689-020-09350-1

Kyrarini, M., Lygerakis, F., Rajavenkatanarayanan, A., Sevastopoulos, C., Nambiappan, H. R., Chaitanya, K. K., Babu, A. R., Mathew, J., & Makedon, F. (2021). A survey of robots in healthcare. *Technologies, 9*(1), 8. https://doi.org/10.3390/technologies9010008

Lamash, L., Little, L., & Hen-Herbst, L. (2022). Telehealth interventions to promote health and behavior-related outcomes in adolescents with autism spectrum disorder. *Journal of Autism and Developmental Disorders, 1-19*. https://doi.org/10.1007/s10803-022-05440-2

Lefer, G., Bourdon, P., Mercier, C., & Lopez-Cazaux, S. (2018). Apprentissage du brossage dentaire chez des enfants présentant un trouble du spectre autistique: Effets de l'utilisation de tablettes tactiles. *Santé Publique, 30*, 297–306. https://doi.org/10.3917/spub.183.0297

Lefer, G., Rouches, A., Bourdon, P., & Cazaux, S. L. (2019). Training children with autism spectrum disorder to undergo oral assessment using a digital iPad® application. *European Archives of Paediatric Dentistry, 20*(2), 113–121. https://doi.org/10.1007/s40368-018-0398-9

Logrieco, M. G. M., Ciuffreda, G. N., Sinjari, B., Spinelli, M., Rossi, R., D'Addazio, G., Lionett, F., Caputi, S., & Fasolo, M. (2021). What happens at a dental surgery when the patient is a child with autism spectrum disorder? An Italian study. *Journal of Autism and Developmental Disorders, 51*(6), 1939–1952. https://doi.org/10.1007/s10803-020-04684-0

Maskey, M., Lowry, J., Rodgers, J., McConachie, H., & Parr, J. R. (2014). Reducing specific phobia/fear in young people with autism spectrum disorders (ASDs) through a virtual reality environment intervention. *PLoS One, 9*(7), e100374. https://doi.org/10.1371/journal.pone.0100374

Meindl, J. N., Saba, S., Gray, M., Stuebing, L., & Jarvis, A. (2019). Reducing blood draw phobia in an adult with autism spectrum disorder using low-cost virtual reality exposure therapy. *Journal of Applied Research in Intellectual Disabilities, 32*(6), 1446–1452. https://doi.org/10.1111/jar.12637

Narzisi, A., Bondioli, M., Pardossi, F., Billeci, L., Buzzi, M. C., Buzzi, M., Pinzino, M., Senette, C., Semucci, V., Tonacci, A., Uscidda, F., Vagelli, B., Giuca, M. R., & Pelagatti, S. (2020). "Mom Let's Go to the Dentist!" preliminary feasibility of a tailored dental intervention for children with autism spectrum disorder in the Italian public health service. *Brain Sciences, 10*(7), 444. https://doi.org/10.3390/brainsci10070444

Newbutt, N., Sung, C., Kuo, H. J., Leahy, M. J., Lin, C. C., & Tong, B. (2016). Brief report: A pilot study of the use of a virtual reality headset in autism populations. *Journal of Autism and Developmental Disorders, 46*(9), 3166–3176. https://doi.org/10.1007/s10803-016-2830-5

Nordahl, C. W., Mello, M., Shen A. M., Shen M. D., Vismara L. A., Li, D., Harrington, K., Tanase, C., Goodlin-Jones, B., Rogers, S., Abbeduto, L., & Amaral, D. G. (2016). Methods for acquiring MRI data in children with autism spectrum disorder and intellectual impairment without the use of sedation. *Journal of Neurodevelopmental Disorders, 8*(1), 20. https://doi.org/10.1186/s11689-016-9154-9

Orellana, L. M., Martinez-Sanchis, S., & Silvestre, F. J. (2014). Training adults and children with an autism spectrum disorder to be compliant with a clinical dental assessment using a TEACCH-based approach. *Journal of Autism and Developmental Disorders, 44*, 776–785. https://doi.org/10.1007/s10803-013-1930-8

Paasch, V., Leibowitz, L., Accardo, J., & Slifer, K. (2016). Preparing children with autism spectrum disorders for overnight sleep studies: A case series. *Clinical Practice in Pediatric Psychology, 4*(2), 153–163. https://doi.org/10.1037/cpp0000139

Pineda, J., & Mullett, J. (2018). Medical procedures: Challenges and strategies. In E. Hazen & C. McDougle (Eds.), *The Massachusetts General Hospital Guide to Medical Care in Patients with Autism Spectrum Disorder* (pp. 43–57). Humana Press. https://doi.org/10.1007/978-3-319-94458-6_4

Planel-Ratna, C., & Juwaheer, T. D. (2021). Assessing the impact of digitalization and technology on patient compliance in healthcare services. *HighTech and Innovation Journal, 2*(3), 216–223. https://doi.org/10.28991/HIJ-2021-02-03-06

Salvatore, G. L., Simmons, C. A., & Tremoulet, P. D. (2021). Physician perspectives on severe behavior and restraint use in a hospital setting for patients with autism spectrum disorder. *Journal of Autism and Developmental Disorders, 1-14*. https://doi.org/10.1007/s10803-021-05327-8

Slifer, K. J., Avis, K. T., & Frutchey, R. A. (2008). Behavioral intervention to increase compliance with electroencephalographic procedures in children with developmental disabilities. *Epilepsy & Behavior, 13*(1), 189–195. S1525505008000140. https://doi.org/10.1016/j.yebeh.2008.01.013

Smith, C. J., Bhanot, A., Norman, E., Mullett, J. E., Bilbo, S. D., McDougle, C. J., Zürcher, N. R., & Hooker, J. M. (2019). A protocol for sedation free MRI and PET imaging in adults with autism spectrum disorder. *Journal of Autism and Developmental Disorders, 49*(7), 3036–3044. https://doi.org/10.1007/s10803-019-04010-3

Stavropoulos, K. K. M., Bolourian, Y., & Blacher, J. (2022). A scoping review of telehealth diagnosis of autism spectrum disorder. *PLoS One, 17*(2), e0263062. https://doi.org/10.1371/journal.pone.0263062

Stogiannos, N., Carlier, S., Harvey-Lloyd, J. M., Brammer, A., Nugent, B., Cleaver, K., McNulty, J. P., Dos Reis, C. S., & Malamateniou, C. (2021). A systematic review of person-centred adjustments to facilitate magnetic resonance imaging for autistic patients without the use of sedation or anaesthesia. *Autism*, 13623613211065542. https://doi.org/10.1177/13623613211065542

Suresh, L. R., & George, C. (2019). Virtual reality distraction on dental anxiety and behavior in children with autism spectrum disorder. *Journal of International Dental and Medical Research, 12*(3), 1004–1010.

Sutherland, R., Trembath, D., & Roberts, J. (2018). Telehealth and autism: A systematic search and review of the literature. *International Journal of Speech-Language Pathology, 20*(3), 324–336. https://doi.org/10.1080/17549507.2018.1465123

Tziraki, M., Garg, S., Harrison, E., Wright, N. B., Hawkes, R., Akhtar, K., Green, J., & Stivaros, S. (2021). A neuroimaging preparation protocol tailored for autism. *Autism Research, 14*(1), 65–74. https://doi.org/10.1002/aur.2427

Vanderwal, T., Kelly, C., Eilbott, J., Mayes, L. C., & Castellanos, F. X. (2015). Inscapes: A movie paradigm to improve compliance in functional magnetic resonance imaging. *NeuroImage, 122*, 222–232. https://doi.org/10.1016/j.neuroimage.2015.07.069

Vandewouw, M. M., Dunkley, B. T., Lerch, J. P., Anagnostou, E., & Taylor, M. J. (2021). Characterizing inscapes and resting-state in MEG: Effects in typical and atypical development. *NeuroImage, 225*, 117524. https://doi.org/10.1016/j.neuroimage.2020.117524

Walsh, C., O'Connor, P., Walsh, E., & Lydon, S. (2021). A systematic review of interventions to improve healthcare experiences and access in autism. *Review Journal of Autism and Developmental Disorders, 1-18*. https://doi.org/10.1007/s40489-021-00279-2

Weiss, J. A., Isaacs, B., Diepstra, H., Wilton, A. S., Brown, H. K., McGarry, C., & Lunsky, Y. (2018). Health concerns and health service utilization in a population cohort of young adults with autism spectrum disorder. *Journal of Autism and Developmental Disorders, 48*(1), 36–44. https://doi.org/10.1007/s10803-017-3292-0

Zaami, S., Rinaldi, R., Bersani, G., & Marinelli, E. (2020). Restraints and seclusion in psychiatry: Striking a balance between protection and coercion. Critical overview of international regulations and rulings. *Rivista di Psichiatria, 55*(1), 16–23. https://doi.org/10.1708/3301.32714

Zink, A. G., Molina, E. C., Diniz, M. B., Santos, M. T. B. R., & Guaré, R. O. (2018). Communication application for use during the first dental visit for children and adolescents with autism spectrum disorders. *Pediatric Dentistry, 40*(1), 18–22.

Панцырь, С. Н., & Шведовский, Е. Ф. (2020). Возможности и условия дистанционного консультирования семей, воспитывающих детей с расстройствами аутистического спектра. In *Вызовы пандемии COVID-19: психическое здоровье, дистанционное образование, интернет-безопасность* (pp. 444–457).

Chapter 10
Risks Related to Digital Technology Use

10.1 Problematic Internet Use

In the late 1990s, the first case studies were published, describing the negative consequences of excessive Internet use on daily functioning, social relations, and work achievement (Young, 1996). Papers from that period often used the term Internet addiction as an umbrella term that included various forms of addictive behavior in the online space, regardless of whether it referred to social media activities or addiction to games, gambling, pornography, shopping, etc. The concept of Internet addiction has been widely criticized. Some authors point out that the Internet is just a medium for conducting certain activities. Thus, using the term Internet addiction to denote a specific addictive behavior in the online space would make as much sense as saying that a person addicted to a psychoactive substance is actually addicted to the bottle containing the substance (e.g., Kuss & Griffiths, 2017). The term addiction can also be questionable since various forms of excessive Internet use are often transient, while substance abuse is usually chronic. In addition, there is a justified fear that the uncritical use of the term addiction could underestimate the severity of "real" addictions on the one hand and pathologize common forms of behavior on the other (Király & Demetrovics, 2021). Therefore, we will mainly use the term problematic Internet use (PIU) in this chapter.

Since the concept of normal Internet use has been changing due to technological advances, generalized PIU is difficult to define. However, most authors agree that the main symptoms include preoccupation with the Internet, not being able to control the time spent online with the increasing need for more, mood swings that become especially intensified when the Internet is denied, and negative consequences of excessive Internet use (Murray et al., 2021). Some research shows that the core symptoms of PIU (i.e., those highly related to other symptoms) change with age. The core symptoms of PIU include increasing time for satisfaction and

N. Glumbić et al., *Digital Inclusion of Individuals with Autism Spectrum Disorder*, Autism and Child Psychopathology Series,
https://doi.org/10.1007/978-3-031-12037-4_10

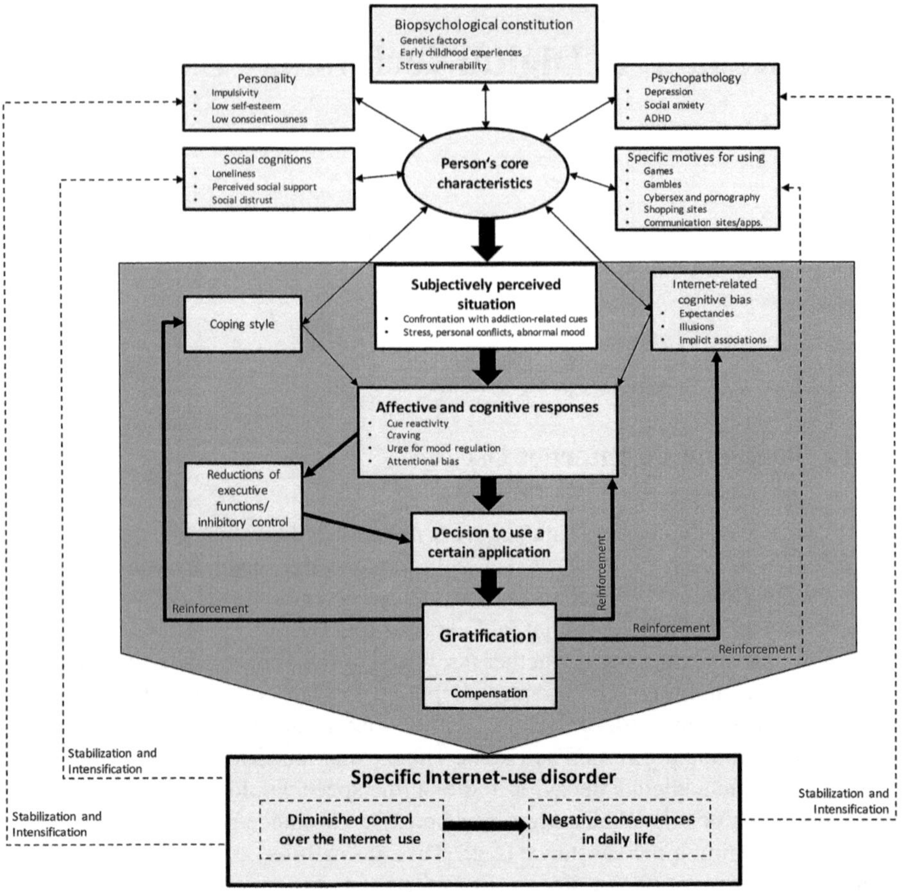

Fig. 10.1 The model on the development and maintenance of a specific Internet use disorder. Bold arrows represent the main pathways of the addiction process. (Reproduced from Brand et al., 2016)

empty life in early adolescence, the lack of sleep, failure to stop, and depression in middle adolescence, and just depression in late adolescence (Liu et al., 2022).

Brand et al. (2016) developed a theoretical framework for understanding the processes leading to PIU—Interaction of Person-Affect-Cognition-Execution (I-PACE) (Fig. 10.1). According to this model, PIU results from the interaction between predisposing factors (e.g., genetic factors, traumatic childhood experiences, and comorbid conditions such as depression, anxiety, and ADHD) and affective and cognitive reactions to internal and external stimuli (e.g., dysfunctional stress-coping patterns, belief that the Internet could help to escape problems, achieve satisfaction, and regulate mood). Insufficiently developed executive functions have a significant role in PIU development, as well as gratification, which is achieved at least in the initial phases of PIU development, additionally increasing the need for Internet use.

Although I-PACE needs further empirical assessment, it is important to consider the interaction of complex factors that result in PIU in the specific population of people with ASD.

10.1.1 Problematic Internet Use in People with Autism

People with ASD are considered particularly vulnerable to PIU, primarily due to the main characteristics of the disorder, such as difficulties in social interaction, limited interests, repetitive activities, their propensity to use digital technologies, and preference for visual stimuli (Normand et al., 2021). In addition, it is known that PIU is associated with anxiety, depression, and ADHD (Moreno et al., 2022) and that these psychiatric disorders are common comorbidities in people with ASD (Leader et al., 2022).

Research generally shows that PIU is much more common in people with autism compared to their typically developing (TD) peers. These studies have usually used a cross-sectional study design, while self-report measures have been used to assess PIU. Convenience samples have usually included children and adolescents with a clinical ASD diagnosis.

One of the scarce studies in which the assessment was based on parental reports found that the participants with ASD had significantly higher scores on a scale assessing excessive Internet use than their TD peers and that the negative consequences of using electronic media were much more frequent in the subsample of children with autism (MacMullin et al., 2016).

Three self-report Japanese studies used Young's Internet Addiction Test (YIAT, Young, 1998) to assess PIU. The total score on this questionnaire ranges from 20 to 100 points. Some authors consider 70 points the addiction cutoff score, noting that participants with 40–69 points may be addicted to the Internet (So et al., 2017, 2019). Kawabe et al. (2019) believe that participants with 50 and more points on YIAT show signs of addiction. In relation to the set criteria, So et al. (2017) found that the prevalence of addictive Internet use in adolescents with ASD was 10.8% and 12.5% in participants with ADHD. Every fifth participant with autism and comorbid ADHD exceeded the cutoff score on YIAT. Two-thirds of the sample from this research were included in the follow-up study 2 years later. A high correlation was determined between the YIAT scores on the first and repeated testing. The scores were above the cutoff values in 8.9% of children with ASD and 22.2% of children with ASD and ADHD. Significant individual variations were noted. Remission occurred in 60% of participants with autism, but new cases of addictive behavior were also found (So et al., 2019). Since the cutoff score was lower compared to previously mentioned studies (So et al., 2017, 2019), Kawabe et al. (2019) quite expectedly concluded that the PIU prevalence in adolescents with ASD was much higher (45.5%). These authors found that the participants with autism who showed signs of PIU differed from their peers with ASD with no PIU symptoms in pronounced ADHD traits.

In a clinical sample of 60 participants with ASD in Turkey, Coskun et al. (2020) found that 23 (38.3%) had PIU. The participants with PIU spent on average 4.54 h a day online, while "normal" Internet users spent just under 2 h a day in online activities.

One of the scarce studies of this type included adult participants 20–75 years of age (Umeda et al., 2021). In this research, the prevalence of PIU in adults with autism was 26.4%. Adults with ASD were 2.6 times more likely to have Internet addiction than the TD participants in the control group.

Shane-Simpson et al. (2016) brought rare dissonance in the already formed concept of the high PIU prevalence in people with autism. They found no statistically significant differences in compulsive Internet use between students with ASD and their neurotypical peers. These authors found a relationship between compulsive Internet use and nonsocial autism symptoms. They concluded that the main reason for excessive online activities was the abundance of possibilities the Internet provided to meet their specific interests. The results of a network analysis of PIU symptoms were in accordance with the mentioned claims, showing that the relation between "Life is boring and empty without the Internet" and preoccupation with the Internet was much stronger in people with ASD than in TD participants (Hirota et al., 2021).

In a systematic review of PIU in people with autism, Normand et al. (2021) list the most common PIU correlates: time spent online, age at which an individual started using the Internet, depression, inattention, hyperactivity, impulsivity, defiance, and escapism.

10.2 Gaming Disorder

Although Internet addiction and PIU are recognized as important research topics, there is a growing belief that these generalized concepts should be replaced by specific online activities that are considered problematic (Király & Demetrovics, 2021). Gaming disorder (GD) is a specific form of PIU, and all global issues about the relationship between excessive and addictive Internet use are also relevant for GD. However, unlike Internet addiction, which is (still) not recognized as a separate clinical entity, GD has been included in the ICD-11 classification developed by WHO (2022) as a diagnostic category. GD is characterized by "persistent or recurrent gaming behavior ('digital gaming' or 'video-gaming') which may be online (i.e., over the Internet) or offline" and manifested by:

- Loss of control over gaming.
- Giving priority to gaming to the extent that all other life activities become less important.
- Continuation of gaming despite the negative consequences of such behavior.

For making the diagnosis, the observed symptoms should last for at least a year and significantly affect personal, family, and social life, education, work, and other areas of functioning (WHO, 2022).

The American Psychiatric Association (APA, 2013) is much more cautious about the nosological status of the Internet gaming disorder (IGD), classifying it as a "condition for further study." In order to make a diagnosis, at least five out of nine diagnostic criteria should be present for 1 year:

- An individual is preoccupied with gaming; they constantly think about previous games and the ones yet to be played.
- Irritability, anxiety, sadness, and other withdrawal symptoms that occur when an individual is prevented from gaming.
- Tolerance manifested in the gradual increase in the need to spend more and more time gaming.
- Unsuccessful attempts to control online gaming.
- Loss of interest in hobbies and other fun activities that have been "suppressed" by gaming.
- Continuation of gaming despite psychosocial problems.
- Concealing information about the time spent online from parents, therapists, and other people.
- Using gaming as a means to avoid negative feelings.
- Negative consequences of gaming in social relations and educational and work activities.

Although there are numerous studies on GD, there is still no reliable data on the prevalence of this disorder. In a meta-analysis of 61 studies conducted in 29 countries, Kim et al. (2022) found that the overall pooled prevalence of GD was 3.3% and that by selecting representative sample studies, the prevalence decreased to 2.4%. High heterogeneity in evaluating the prevalence of GD can be attributed to various factors such as the way of forming the sample, assessment instruments, participants' age, the region, cultural factors, quality of research, etc. (Kim et al., 2022).

10.2.1 Gaming Disorder in People with Autism

People with ASD are considered vulnerable to PIU in general, which is also true for specific activities such as gaming. Studies on children and adolescents have found a positive relationship between autism and GD (MacMullin et al., 2016; Mazurek & Wenstrup, 2013; Mazurek & Engelhardt, 2013a; Paulus et al., 2020) with medium or large effect sizes. It has also been determined that adults with ASD spend more time daily playing computer games, spend most of their free time in these activities, and show more symptoms of pathological gaming than the TD population (Engelhardt et al., 2017). Comparing adults with autism and neurotypical people

Murray et al. (2022) found similar results. GD criteria were met by 9.1% of participants with autism and 2.9% of neurotypical participants in their study.

Although research studies conducted in different countries, on different samples, and using numerous assessment instruments have noticeably similar results, the obtained findings should be considered with caution since most studies regard gaming as a continuous variable and do not use a specific cutoff score to distinguish excessive and addictive gaming (Craig et al., 2021). In addition, the issue of distinguishing between addictive and repetitive behavior has not yet been fully resolved (Paulus et al., 2020). The narrow and limited interests of people with autism can be directed at gaming. Unlike TD individuals who often change their interests in adolescence, people with autism can focus on one area for a longer time (Coutelle et al., 2021). However, the time spent on gaming cannot be the only GD criterion. Although the function of gaming is mainly fun, some people do these activities professionally. Esports are becoming increasingly recognized as sports activities, and the "athletes" who invest great time and energy in preparing for competitions should be distinguished from ordinary gamers (Kaye et al., 2021). Gaming function should also always be considered in people with ASD since it could have significant implications for the treatment. Another limitation of the existing research is related to participants' sociodemographic characteristics. The samples usually included male children and adolescents, and almost three-quarters of the participants had average intellectual abilities (Coutelle et al., 2021), which brings the possibility of generalizing the results into question.

Video games can be especially appealing to people with ASD because they offer a structured, clear, and predictable environment, provide practically unlimited opportunities for satisfying specific and repetitive interests, do not set high social demands, and are based on a limited set of rules. Various audiovisual effects can have a reinforcing effect on people with autism (Mazurek & Engelhardt, 2013b), which is especially pronounced in situations where the reward system has been changed. There is neurobiological evidence that individuals with autism and comorbid GD have reduced connectivity in cortical, subcortical, and limbic areas responsible for reward processing, and in cortical areas associated with executive control (Kuriki et al., 2020). ADHD in people with autism also increases the risk of GD (Murray et al., 2021; Normand et al., 2021). Due to their impulsivity, difficulty in inhibiting responses, and easy loss of control, people with ASD have high addictive potential (Coutelle et al., 2021; Craig et al., 2021). On the other hand, some games have been designed to create a strong desire to continue gaming. This particularly refers to massively multiplayer online role-playing games (e.g., World of Warcraft). Role-playing games usually require more time to reach a goal compared to shooter games or real-time strategy games. In addition, rewards and punishments are significant structural components of these games, so they easily cause addiction in predisposed individuals (Kaye et al., 2021; Normand et al., 2021).

In a systematic review of studies on GD in people with ASD, Craig et al. (2021) point out that the game genre is one of the possible GD predictors. Other most commonly mentioned predictors are average daily time and the amount of free time spent on gaming, higher cognitive abilities, insufficient parental control and guidance, attention deficits, and oppositional behavior. Alienation from other people and low cognitive reappraisal are significant GD predictors in adults with ASD (Murray et al., 2022). People with autism are more prone to solitary gaming than TD participants who prefer multiplayer mode (Paulus et al., 2020), which could also increase the risk of GD. Although studies indicating possible gender differences are scarce, it seems that males with ASD are more prone to GD than females, which corresponds to research findings in the typical population (Craig et al., 2021).

10.3 Cyberbullying

Cyberbullying is most often defined as a form of aggressive behavior exhibited intentionally and repeatedly through electronic contacts with people who cannot easily defend themselves (Kowalski et al., 2014). The mentioned and other similar definitions clearly attempt to associate cyberbullying with traditional bullying by listing three main characteristics of this aggressive behavior: intentionality, repetitiveness, and power imbalance between perpetrators and their victims. While intentionality is evident, the remaining two criteria are not always easily applied in cyberbullying. Regardless of their severity, single acts of aggressive behavior toward different people in different circumstances do not fit the definition of traditional bullying. However, only one malicious act in cyberspace, such as posting inappropriate photographs or videos online or distributing them to multiple users, may lead to long-term humiliation of the victim due to the possibility to share and reproduce such content indefinitely (Dooley et al., 2009). It is also difficult to determine the power imbalance in online interactions. The feeling of not being able to control aggressive attacks in online space is enough to put an individual in the position of a victim (Dooley et al., 2009), regardless of the actual or apparent superiority of a potential perpetrator. A cyberbully is often anonymous. Also, people who do not have significant social power in the actual environment can be perpetrators of cyberbullying. Unlike traditional bullying that involves a specific location or time, cyberbullying can occur anywhere and anytime. Although in many ways similar, traditional and cyberbullying cannot be assessed by the same criteria (Law et al., 2012).

Some authors distinguish between cyber-teasing, which does not meet any of the mentioned criteria; cyber-arguing, which involves only the intention to hurt others; and cyberbullying, which should satisfy all three criteria (Vandebosch & Van Cleemput, 2008). Cyberbullying is sometimes referred to as electronic, online, or Internet violence with unclear boundaries in the scope and content of these terms.

Cyberbullying perpetrators can use email, social media, chat rooms, instant messaging, websites, online games, blogs, etc. (Eldrige et al., 2021; Hu et al., 2019; Kowalski et al., 2014). There are many different forms of cyberbullying. They include flaming, bashing, or cyberharrasing (expressing hostility through insults, swearing, and other forms of abusive language, from name-calling to death threats), cyberstalking, social exclusion, masquerading (the perpetrator pretends to be someone else and sends messages as that other person to harm the victim), and outing and trickery (the perpetrator tricks the victim into revealing personal information and then shares it; sending humiliating photographs, messages, or videos; distributing embarrassing photographs and videos of the victim; trolling; identity theft etc.) (Bauman, 2010; Eldrige et al., 2021; Hwang et al., 2018; Moor et al., 2010; Wright, 2018). Although cyberbullying is by nature psychological, indirect violence, there are cases where traditional physical violence and cyberbullying are combined through the happy slapping phenomenon, which involves recording and sharing aggressive or sexual attacks on a victim (Wright, 2018).

Cyberbullying can have numerous negative consequences, especially in adolescence, such as anxiety, depression, adjustment disorders, substance abuse, and somatic problems. Cyberbullying victims are also more prone to self-harm (e.g., self-cutting and self-burning), which involves deliberately hurting oneself without suicide attempts but with the increased risk of suicidal behavior (Dorol & Mishara, 2021). In a research study on large samples of adolescents from Israel, Lithuania, and Luxembourg, 6.5% of the participants 15 years of age were victims of cyberbullying. Boys were at a twice greater risk than girls. In all three countries, cyberbullying victims were significantly more likely to have suicidal ideas and plan and attempt suicide than their peers who did not have such experience (Zaborskis et al., 2019).

As a stressful life event, bullying cannot fully account for these psychopathological manifestations. There are biologically and cognitively vulnerable individuals in whom the negative effects of bullying are much more pronounced (Swearer & Hymel, 2015). Although the effects of bullying have usually been examined in a typical population, some studies show that people with disability are at greater risk and have more severe consequences of traditional and cyberbullying than their TD peers (Dorol & Mishara, 2021; Eldrige et al., 2021; Wright & Wachs, 2019).

10.3.1 Cyberbullying in People with Autism

Adolescents with ASD are at greater risk of victimization than their TD peers (Chan et al., 2018; Wright, 2018). It is not uncommon for them to be the victims of traditional and cyberbullying at the same time and suffer the consequences of different types of bullying—physical, verbal, and relational (Holfeld et al., 2019; Kloosterman et al., 2013; Kowalski & Fedina, 2011). Hellström (2019) points out the danger of polyvictimization that involves being exposed to different forms of victimization in different contexts, which, apart from bullying, also include conventional crimes, maltreatment, and indirect victimization when the victim is a witness of maltreatment. When an individual is targeted as a victim because of autism, it is a hate crime that can have various forms: verbal abuse, harassment, intimidation, cyberbullying, property destruction, physical violence, etc. It is believed that people with severe forms of autism get the support they need more easily because their difficulties are more noticeable. However, specific support needs of people with HFA can be neglected in this field, making them even more exposed to hate crime (Chaplin & Mukhopadhyay, 2018).

Hellström (2019) believes that the existing research underestimates the severity of cyber victimization in people with autism and that it is difficult to determine its actual extent due to different methodological designs. Different data can be obtained depending on whether the assessment is based on parent or self-reports of people with ASD. Thus, on a sample of adolescents with ADHD and Asperger syndrome, Kowalski and Fedina (2011) determined significant differences in the assessment of time spent online (the adolescents admitted that they spent more time online than their parents thought) and perceived safety (the adolescents considered the Internet a safer place compared to their parents). Almost every fifth participant stated that they had never discussed cyberspace safety with their parents, while 24% said to have done it very rarely. On the other hand, the parents usually believed that they had often discussed that topic with their children. Research shows that the participation rates of adolescents with HFA in cyberbullying, both as victims and perpetrators, are significantly higher when the assessment is based on self-reports rather than on parent reports (Hu et al., 2019). Kloosterman et al. (2013) found no such differences.

Just as parents may not have a clear insight into their children's online activities, including cyberbullying, adolescents with autism may also lack the capacity to recognize the situations in which they are either perpetrators or victims of cyberbullying. Thus, Hwang et al. (2018) created vignettes that described possible situations of traditional and cyberbullying, aiming to examine whether participants with autism could recognize them. The research was conducted on a sample of 89 adolescents with HFA and 490 TD peers. After a short explanation of what was meant by bullying and cyberbullying, the participants were presented with the vignettes. The results showed that the adolescents with HFA somewhat better understood cyberbullying situations than the control group. Their mistakes mainly involved false-positive findings on the vignettes describing some forms of cyber violence that were not cyberbullying.

The main clinical characteristics of autism are considered significant risk factors for cyber victimization. This primarily refers to difficulties in social communication, theory of mind deficit, inadequate understanding of social signals, motor mannerisms, and other unusual behaviors and rituals (Hu et al., 2019; Matthias et al., 2021). Difficulties in understanding and producing paralinguistic communication elements (according to Đorđević et al., 2016) and problems in understanding sarcasm and irony can result in inappropriate reactions in a specific communication context (Holfeld et al., 2019). Some people with ASD may exhibit fear in social contact with strangers. Socially anxious individuals sometimes look for a way out in the online world. However, the more time they spend online, the greater the chances of victimization are. Cyber victimization further increases social anxiety in people with ASD, thus closing the vicious circle (Liu et al., 2021). Repeated victimization and peer rejection reduce the coping strategies of adolescents with autism, leading them to anxiety and depression. Peer rejection has proved to moderate a positive relation between cyber victimization and depression (Wright & Wachs, 2019).

Research on cyberbullying in people with ASD is scarce. One of the first studies included a sample of children with ADHD and/or Asperger syndrome 10–20 years of age. It was shown that the participants were often the victims of traditional (57%) and cyberbullying (21%), while 5.8% were the perpetrators of cyberbullying (Kowalski & Fedina, 2011). Since the results refer to the sample as a whole, it is not possible to precisely determine whether there are differences between the children with ADHD and HFA. Information about ADHD, either as a separate or co-occurring condition, is very significant since ADHD is a possible risk factor for the participation of people with autism in cyberbullying, both as victims and as perpetrators (Kloosterman et al., 2013).

A study conducted in Canada showed that adolescents with HFA were more likely to be the victims of cyberbullying (12.5%) by using computers and sending emails compared to their peers with other disabilities (4.5%) and TD participants (4.2%). They were also the perpetrators more frequently than the other two groups (Kloosterman et al., 2013). A more recent Canadian study was conducted on a sample of 23 participants with autism 10–17 years of age. It showed that 73.9% of the participants were the victims, while 17.4% were the perpetrators of cyberbullying. Two-thirds of the participants did not know why they were being attacked in the online environment, while disability and physical appearance were reported as reasons by 11% of the participants, respectively. Researchers from different parts of the world have concluded that adolescents with ASD are much more often the victims than the perpetrators of cyberbullying. Research conducted in Taiwan shows that the ratio is 13.7%:8.2% (Liu et al., 2021), in Spain 51.6%:9.7% (Iglesias et al., 2019), and in Canada 12.5%:8.5% (Kloosterman et al., 2013).

Victimization in cyberspace is associated with mental health problems of adolescents with autism, primarily anxiety, depression, and suicidal behavior (Holfeld et al., 2019; Hu et al., 2019; Wright & Wachs, 2019). On a sample of adolescents with HFA 11–18 years of age, Hu et al. (2019) found that older participants were more likely to participate in cyberbullying both as perpetrators and victims, possibly because they spent more time online. Adolescents with numerous symptoms of oppositional defiant disorder also had both roles more frequently. Their irritability and aggression directed them to aggressively attack others, while they were also targeted as potential victims. When the influence of sociodemographic factors was controlled, the role of cyberbullying perpetrators in people with autism was not related to increased anxiety, depression, and suicidal behavior.

Unfortunately, at this point, studies on people with ASD as perpetrators of cyberbullying are scarce, while the roles of cyberbully victims and bystanders have not been researched. Almost all existing research is aimed at people with HFA as cyberbully victims, and individuals with lower cognitive abilities may also be at certain risk. In addition, researchers often start from the fact that young people most frequently use modern technology. Thus, the focus is on adolescents with ASD.

One of the scarce studies on cyberbullying in adults with ASD included 78 participants 18–59 years of age, mainly from European countries. Data on their victimization experience while using social media was collected. Much more participants had the role of victims (31%) than perpetrators (2.7%) of cyberbullying. Six (8%) participants were in the category of cyberbully victims. Almost a quarter of the victims (24%) experienced social exclusion since they were ignored by other users of social networking sites or Internet chat rooms. The feeling of belonging to the online community positively correlated with the self-esteem of adults with autism, while the experience of being ignored and rejected was associated with low self-esteem. Somewhat fewer participants reported that other social media users had spoken ill of them in the online space (23%) or had sent them unpleasant messages (22%) (Triantafyllopoulou et al., 2021).

Based on the obtained data, it is clear that preventive and intervention programs related to cyberbullying in people with ASD should be aimed at individuals with autism, their family members, and school. The starting point for all participants would be education about possible forms of cyberbullying and their consequences. In order to reduce the vulnerability of people with ASD, we should work on the development of their coping skills, communication, theory of mind, social skills, and digital citizenship (according to Liu et al., 2021). The role of parents as mediators (e.g., setting the rules for using digital technologies, limiting the availability of specific content and time spent online, discussing appropriate online behavior) and their support may alleviate the negative psychological effects of cyber victimization (Wright, 2018). There are indications that students with autism who attend special schools are at a lower risk of bullying than those attending regular schools (Chan et al., 2018; Eldridge et al., 2021). School connectedness is a significant protective factor (Dorol & Mishara, 2021), and peer acceptance mitigates the negative effects of cyber victimization (Wright & Wachs, 2019). Thus, one strategy to prevent cyberbullying and its consequences would be to improve the overall school climate. To our knowledge, there are no evaluated prevention and intervention programs related to cyberbullying in people with ASD.

10.4 Cybercrime

Cybercrime is an umbrella term for various illegal activities carried out using a computer and the Internet (Ledingham & Mills, 2015). These activities can roughly be divided into two groups: cyber-enabled crimes and cyber-dependent crimes. Some criminal activities, such as fraud, have existed for centuries, and the Internet has only increased their effect. Such activities are cyber-enabled crimes. On the other hand, hacking, deliberate virus spreading, denial of service, and many other forms of cybercrime can only be carried out using digital technologies, which is why they are called cyber-dependent crimes. Virtually all devices providing online access (desktop and laptop computers, game consoles, smart TVs, and phones) can be attack targets (Brosnan, 2021).

Due to the need to harmonize national cybercrime legislation and foster international cooperation in implementing crime prevention and legal measures, the

Council of Europe adopted the European Convention on Cybercrime in 2001, also known as the Budapest Convention (Council of Europe, 2001). The Convention lists the following criminal activities:

- Offences against confidentiality, integrity, and availability of computer data and systems (illegal access, illegal interception, data interference, system interference, misuse of devices).
- Computer-related offences (forgeries and frauds committed on computers).
- Content-related offences (e.g., child pornography).
- Offences related to copyright infringement.

Hacking is one of the most well-known forms of cybercrime that can have various forms, from identity theft to industrial and military espionage. There are also ethical or white hat hackers that do not belong to the criminal milieu but use their skills to pursue a career in cyber security. Sending fake emails to collect personal information is relatively common. Denial of access involves attacks on specific computer systems in order to disable them. It is usually performed by overloading the selected system with content to block its operation. Cybercrime also includes downloading other people's files without permission, downloading screenshots of someone's computer screen, recording what is typed on the keyboard, etc. (Brosnan, 2021; Ledingham & Mills, 2015; NCA, 2017).

Cybercrime motives are various: financial gain, revenge, curiosity, desire for recognition, accepting a challenge to defeat the security system, etc. Hacktivism is a form of hacking motivated by political, ideological, or religious reasons. The existing research usually takes a broader perspective and rarely deals with specific forms of cybercrime (Edwards et al., 2022). Cybercrime perpetrators are usually younger, educated men (Edwards et al., 2022; NCA, 2017).

Some researchers are trying to determine the factors that may predispose some people to participate in cybercrime. Harvey et al. (2016) compared a group of students, ethical hackers, with their colleagues who were not computer experts. The results showed that ethical hackers paid more attention to detail and showed a greater tendency toward systematization than the comparison group. Systematization is a tendency to analyze and construct systems, i.e., find the rules according to which certain systems, including computer systems, function. In addition to noticing details, people with ASD have a relatively preserved, sometimes even superior, ability to systematize (Baron-Cohen, 2009). Thus, the question arises as to whether people with autism are at higher risk of participating in cybercrime than the general population.

10.4.1 Cybercrime in People with Autism

Despite the fact that people with autism may not always understand social signals and rules of behavior and have great difficulties in adapting to change, research shows that they do not commit crimes more frequently than people in the general population (King & Murphy, 2014; Yu et al., 2021). With regard to the type of crime, people with autism are most commonly charged with crimes against person, crimes against property, and offences against public order, which also does not distinguish them from non-autistic perpetrators (Yu et al., 2021). Some research studies show that comorbid conditions, such as ADHD or psychotic disorders, can play a significant role in the occurrence of criminal behavior in people with ASD (Blackmore et al., 2022). The mentioned studies mainly focus on different types of "traditional" criminal activities. Therefore, the question remains whether these people are more susceptible to specific types of crime, such as cybercrime.

Developed technical skills are certainly a prerequisite for a criminal career in cyberspace. Baron-Cohen (2012) speculates that there are many people with autism among Silicon Valley employees. He also points out that fathers of autistic children more frequently have technology careers than fathers of other children with developmental disorders or TD ones. Although these attitudes have been widely criticized over the past decade, a recent study in Denmark indicates a relation between fathers' occupations based on superior systematization skills and their children's autism. Children whose both parents had extremely developed systematization skills had 35% greater chances of being diagnosed with autism compared to children whose parents had equally developed systematization and empathy skills (Daysal et al., 2021). In a sample of over 450,000 participants from the UK, Ruzich et al. (2015) showed that the mean values of the Autism-Spectrum Quotient (AQ) in individuals with occupations in science, technology, engineering, and math (STEM) were significantly higher than in the participants with non-STEM jobs. AQ is a well-known self-administered instrument used to determine whether and to what extent individuals have autistic traits (Baron-Cohen et al., 2001). Of course, not all people with autism or autistic traits have superior computer skills, nor are those with advanced knowledge in digital technologies more prone to cybercrime.

Ledingham and Mills (2015) published the results of a preliminary study indicating a possible relation between autism and cybercrime. The research was based on collecting data through a questionnaire distributed to six national cybercrime units and two fraud and cybercrime units from eight different countries. The obtained data only detected that the participants had experience with people with ASD who committed a cybercrime, but the results could not be generalized.

Another study was published in the same year, examining the relation between autistic traits and cyberdeviancy in a sample of 296 university students (Seigfried-Spellar et al., 2015). This research observed cyberdeviancy as a broad concept that included different forms of cybercrime and cyberbullying. The results showed that very few cybercrime perpetrators (0.01%) had clinically significant AQ scores. There was no difference between hackers and non-hackers in the mean value of AQ. However, virus writers and identity thieves had significantly higher AQ scores than the students not included in the mentioned cyber-dependent crimes.

Payne et al. (2019) conducted a research study on the relation between cyber-dependent crimes and autism. Apart from TD participants, their sample also included participants diagnosed with autism. The sample consisted of computer science students and alumni assumed to be well versed in digital technologies. These authors found that autistic traits increased the risk of participating in cybercrime in the general population, with advanced digital skills contributing to about 40% of the relation between autistic traits and cyber-dependent crimes. On the other hand, the diagnosis of autism was not a particular risk factor for cybercrime.

A methodologically advanced study (Lim et al., 2021) did not determine a significant relation between autistic traits and cybercrime. If criminal activities are evaluated by an instrument measuring only cyber-dependent crimes, the autism diagnosis does not increase the risk of participating in criminal activity. However, if a specific instrument evaluates both cyber-enabled and cyber-dependent crimes, people with autism are almost three times more likely to participate in criminal activity. Neither advanced digital skills nor theory of mind deficits contributed to the relation between autism and cybercrime. Compared to the general population participants, people with autism were more likely to download other people's computer screenshots; they tried to crack passwords to access other people's data, used wireless without permission, and harassed other people through emails and social media. Unlike previously mentioned studies that used the AQ version with 50 items (Baron-Cohen et al., 2001), Lim et al. (2021) used a short version of the scale with only 12 items (Lundqvist & Lindner, 2017) which, according to the authors, measures the unidimensional construct of autistic traits better. In addition, various instruments were used to evaluate a broader scope of cybercrime. Unlike Payne et al. (2019), whose sample included digital technology experts, this research did not specify any particular inclusion criteria. To ensure the reliability of the obtained data, the authors excluded all participants who used automatic question-answering methods. Furthermore, a bogus question was included in the digital skills assessment questionnaire. The participants were asked to mark on a 5-point scale to what extent they were familiar with GFTI snooping video software, which actually does not exist. All participants who did not choose the answer "not at all true" in this question were also excluded from the sample.

It seems that future research on cybercrime in people with autism will have to consider numerous methodological questions: whether all forms of cybercrime are covered by the existing assessment instruments; to what extent we can rely on self-report surveys as reliable information sources; whether all participants, especially those with autism, understand what cybercrime is; whether the possibility that perpetrators of the most serious Internet crimes unwillingly report on their activities affects sample selection even when the research is anonymous; etc.

Most studies in this field rely on data collection through online surveys with anonymous participants. One of the scarce studies involving people with autism in forensic secure care settings aimed to examine specific autism characteristics that could be related to criminal activities on the Internet (Higham et al., 2021). They identified 23 Internet offenders with autism. The most common form of cybercrime was related to producing, using, and distributing child pornography, while email and social media harassment and terrorist activities were significantly rarer. Internet offenders with autism in secure units usually had some comorbid conditions (e.g., paranoid schizophrenia, delusional disorder, unspecified psychosis, bipolar disorder, depression, etc.), violent behavior, and traumatic experiences in the past.

In order to understand the true nature of cybercrime, especially its most severe forms, it is necessary to expand research and include security units, taking into account specific deficits of people with autism, comorbid conditions, and previous life experiences. There are still no evidence-based interventions that can be used to prevent and treat cybercrime in people with ASD.

References

American Psychiatric Association (Ed.). (2013). *Diagnostic and statistical manual of mental disorders* (5th ed.). American Psychiatric Association.

Baron-Cohen, S. (2009). Autism: The empathizing–systemizing (E-S) theory. *Annals of the New York Academy of Sciences, 1156*(1), 68–80. https://doi.org/10.1111/j.1749-6632.2009.04467.x

Baron-Cohen, S. (2012). Autism and the technical mind. *Scientific American, 307*(5), 72–75.

Baron-Cohen, S., Wheelwright, S., Skinner, R., Martin, J., & Clubley, E. (2001). The autism-spectrum quotient (AQ): Evidence from Asperger syndrome/high-functioning autism, males and females, scientists and mathematicians. *Journal of Autism and Developmental Disorders, 31*(1), 5–17. https://doi.org/10.1023/A:1005653411471

Bauman, S. (2010). Cyberbullying in a rural intermediate school: An exploratory study. *The Journal of Early Adolescence, 30*(6), 803–833. https://doi.org/10.1177/0272431609350927

Blackmore, C. E., Woodhouse, E. L., Gillan, N., Wilson, E., Ashwood, K. L., Stoencheva, V., Nolan, A., McAlonan, G. M., Robertson, D. M., Whitwell, S., Deeley, Q., Craig, M. C., Zinkstok, J., Wichers, R., Spain, D., Roberts, G., Murphy, D. G. M., Murphy, C. M., & Daly, E. (2022). Adults with autism spectrum disorder and the criminal justice system: An investigation of prevalence of contact with the criminal justice system, risk factors and sex differences in a specialist assessment service. *Autism*, 13623613221081343. https://doi.org/10.1177/13623613221081343

Brand, M., Young, K. S., Laier, C., Wölfling, K., & Potenza, M. N. (2016). Integrating psychological and neurobiological considerations regarding the development and maintenance of specific Internet-use disorders: An Interaction of Person-Affect-Cognition-Execution (I-PACE) model. *Neuroscience & Biobehavioral Reviews, 71*, 252–266. https://doi.org/10.1016/j.neubiorev.2016.08.033

Brosnan, M. (2021). Cyber-dependent crime, autism, and autistic-like traits. In F. R. Volkmar, R. Loftin, A. Westphal, & M. Woodbury-Smith (Eds.), *Handbook of autism spectrum disorder and the law* (pp. 219–231). Springer. https://doi.org/10.1007/978-3-030-70913-6_10

Chan, K. L., Lo, C. K., & Ip, P. (2018). Associating disabilities, school environments, and child victimization. *Child Abuse & Neglect, 83*, 21–30. https://doi.org/10.1016/j.chiabu.2018.07.001

Chaplin, E., & Mukhopadhyay, S. (2018). Autism spectrum disorder and hate crime. *Advances in Autism, 4*(1), 30–36. https://doi.org/10.1108/AIA-08-2017-0015

Coskun, M., Hajdini, A., Alnak, A., & Karayagmurlu, A. (2020). Internet use habits, parental control and psychiatric comorbidity in young subjects with Asperger syndrome. *Journal of Autism and Developmental Disorders, 50*(1), 171–179. https://doi.org/10.1007/s10803-019-04243-2

Council of Europe. (2001). *Convention on cybercrime*. Available at https://www.coe.int/en/web/cybercrime/the-budapest-convention

Coutelle, R., Weiner, L., Paasche, C., Pottelette, J., Bertschy, G., Schröder, C. M., & Lalanne, L. (2021). Autism spectrum disorder and video games: Restricted interests or addiction? *International Journal of Mental Health and Addiction, 19*, 1–22. https://doi.org/10.1007/s11469-021-00511-4

Craig, F., Tenuta, F., De Giacomo, A., Trabacca, A., & Costabile, A. (2021). A systematic review of problematic video-game use in people with Autism Spectrum Disorders. *Research in Autism Spectrum Disorders, 82*, 101726. https://doi.org/10.1016/j.rasd.2021.101726

Daysal, N. M., Elder, T. E., Hellerstein, J. K., Imberman, S. A., & Orsini, C. (2021). *Parental skills, assortative mating, and the incidence of autism spectrum disorder* (No. w28652). National Bureau of Economic Research. https://doi.org/10.3386/w28652

Dooley, J. J., Pyżalski, J., & Cross, D. (2009). Cyberbullying versus face-to-face bullying: A theoretical and conceptual review. *Zeitschrift für Psychologie/Journal of Psychology, 217*(4), 182–188. https://doi.org/10.1027/0044-3409.217.4.182

Đorđević, M., Glumbić, N., & Brojčin, B. (2016). Paralinguistic abilities of adults with intellectual disability. *Research in Developmental Disabilities, 48*, 211–219. https://doi.org/10.1016/j.ridd.2015.11.001

Dorol, O., & Mishara, B. L. (2021). Systematic review of risk and protective factors for suicidal and self-harm behaviors among children and adolescents involved with cyberbullying. *Preventive Medicine, 152*, 106684. https://doi.org/10.1016/j.ypmed.2021.106684

Edwards, M., Williams, E., Peersman, C., & Rashid, A. (2022). Characterising cybercriminals: A review. *ArXiv preprint arXiv:2202.07419.*

Eldridge, M. A., Demaray, M. L. K., Emmons, J. D., & Riffle, L. N. (2021). Cyberbullying and cybervictimization among youth with disabilities. In *Child and Adolescent Online Risk Exposure* (pp. 255–281). Academic Press. https://doi.org/10.1016/B978-0-12-817499-9.00013-2

Engelhardt, C. R., Mazurek, M. O., & Hilgard, J. (2017). Pathological game use in adults with and without Autism Spectrum Disorder. *PeerJ, 5*, e3393. https://doi.org/10.7717/peerj.3393

Harvey, I., Bolgan, S., Mosca, D., McLean, C., & Rusconi, E. (2016). Systemizers are better code-breakers: Self-reported systemizing predicts code-breaking performance in expert hackers and naïve participants. *Frontiers in Human Neuroscience, 10*, 229. https://doi.org/10.3389/fnhum.2016.00229

Hellström, L. (2019). A systematic review of polyvictimization among children with attention deficit hyperactivity or autism spectrum disorder. *International Journal of Environmental Research and Public Health, 16*(13), 2280. https://doi.org/10.3390/ijerph16132280

Higham, L., Girardi, A., & Edwards, H. V. (2021). Clinical and criminal profile of internet offenders with ASD. *Journal of Intellectual Disabilities and Offending Behaviour, 12*(2), 61–74. https://doi.org/10.1108/JIDOB-09-2020-0016

Hirota, T., McElroy, E., & So, R. (2021). Network analysis of internet addiction symptoms among a clinical sample of Japanese adolescents with autism spectrum disorder. *Journal of Autism and Developmental Disorders, 51*(8), 2764–2772. https://doi.org/10.1007/s10803-020-04714-x

Holfeld, B., Stoesz, B., & Montgomery, J. (2019). Traditional and cyber bullying and victimization among youth with autism spectrum disorder: An investigation of the frequency, characteristics, and psychosocial correlates. *Journal on Developmental Disabilities, 24*(2), 61–76.

Hu, H. F., Liu, T. L., Hsiao, R. C., Ni, H. C., Liang, S. H. Y., Lin, C. F., Chan, H. L., Hsieh, Y. H., Wang, L. J., Lee, M. J., Chou, W. J., & Yen, C. F. (2019). Cyberbullying victimization and perpetration in adolescents with high-functioning autism spectrum disorder: Correlations with depression, anxiety, and suicidality. *Journal of Autism and Developmental Disorders, 49*(10), 4170–4180. https://doi.org/10.1007/s10803-019-04060-7

Hwang, Y. S., Dillon-Wallace, J., Campbell, M., Ashburner, J., Saggers, B., Carrington, S., & Hand, K. (2018). How students with autism spectrum conditions understand traditional bullying and cyberbullying. *International Journal of Inclusive Education, 22*(4), 391–408. https://doi.org/10.1080/13603116.2017.1370736

Iglesias, O. B., Sánchez, L. E. G., & Rodríguez, M. Á. A. (2019). Do young people with Asperger syndrome or intellectual disability use social media and are they cyberbullied or cyberbullies in the same way as their peers? *Psicothema, 31*(1), 30–37. https://doi.org/10.7334/psicothema2018.243

Kawabe, K., Horiuchi, F., Miyama, T., Jogamoto, T., Aibara, K., Ishii, E., & Ueno, S. I. (2019). Internet addiction and attention-deficit/hyperactivity disorder symptoms in adolescents with autism spectrum disorder. *Research in Developmental Disabilities, 89*, 22–28. https://doi.org/10.1016/j.ridd.2019.03.002

Kaye, L. K., Kuss, D. J., & Rumpf, H. J. (2021). Conceptual and methodological considerations of gaming disorder and internet gaming disorder. In N. el-Guebaly, G. Carrà, M. Galanter, & A. M. Baldacchino (Eds.), *Textbook of addiction treatment* (pp. 967–977). Springer. https://doi.org/10.1007/978-3-030-36391-8_68

Kim, H. S., Son, G., Roh, E. B., Ahn, W. Y., Kim, J., Shin, S. H., Chey, J., & Choi, K. H. (2022). Prevalence of gaming disorder: A meta-analysis. *Addictive Behaviors, 126*, 107183. https://doi.org/10.1016/j.addbeh.2021.107183

King, C., & Murphy, G. H. (2014). A systematic review of people with autism spectrum disorder and the criminal justice system. *Journal of Autism and Developmental Disorders, 44*(11), 2717–2733. https://doi.org/10.1007/s10803-014-2046-5

Király, O., & Demetrovics, Z. (2021). Problematic internet use. In N. el-Guebaly, G. Carrà, M. Galanter, & A. M. Baldacchino (Eds.), *Textbook of addiction treatment* (pp. 955–965). Springer. https://doi.org/10.1007/978-3-030-36391-8_67

Kloosterman, P. H., Kelley, E. A., Craig, W. M., Parker, J. D., & Javier, C. (2013). Types and experiences of bullying in adolescents with an autism spectrum disorder. *Research in Autism Spectrum Disorders, 7*(7), 824–832. https://doi.org/10.1016/j.rasd.2013.02.013

Kowalski, M. R., & Fedina, C. (2011). Cyberbullying in ADHD and Asperger syndrome populations. *Research in Autism Spectrum Disorders, 5*(3), 1201–1208. https://doi.org/10.1016/j.rasd.2011.01.007

Kowalski, R. M., Giumetti, G. W., Schroeder, A. N., & Lattanner, M. R. (2014). Bullying in the digital age: A critical review and meta-analysis of cyberbullying research among youth. *Psychological Bulletin, 140*(4), 1073–1137. https://doi.org/10.1037/a0035618

Kuriki, S., Higuchi, S., Nakayama, H., Mihara, S., Okazaki, Y., Ono, Y., & Kobayashi, H. (2020). Neurobiological influence of comorbid conditions in young patients diagnosed with gaming disorder: A whole-brain functional connectivity study based on a data driven method. *PLoS One, 15*(5), e0233780. https://doi.org/10.1371/journal.pone.0233780

Kuss, D. J., & Griffiths, M. D. (2017). Social networking sites and addiction: Ten lessons learned. *International Journal of Environmental Research and Public Health, 14*(3), 311. https://doi.org/10.3390/ijerph14030311

Law, D. M., Shapka, J. D., Hymel, S., Olson, B. F., & Waterhouse, T. (2012). The changing face of bullying: An empirical comparison between traditional and internet bullying and victimization. *Computers in Human Behavior, 28*(1), 226–232. https://doi.org/10.1016/j.chb.2011.09.004

Leader, G., Hogan, A., Chen, J. L., Maher, L., Naughton, K., O'Rourke, N., Casburn, M., & Mannion, A. (2022). Age of autism spectrum disorder diagnosis and comorbidity in children and adolescents with autism spectrum disorder. *Developmental Neurorehabilitation, 25*(1), 29–37. https://doi.org/10.1080/17518423.2021.1917717

Ledingham, R., & Mills, R. (2015). A preliminary study of autism and cybercrime in the context of international law enforcement. *Advances in Autism, 1*(1), 2–11. https://doi.org/10.1108/AIA-05-2015-0003

Lim, A., Brewer, N., & Young, R. L. (2021). Revisiting the relationship between cybercrime, autistic traits, and autism. *Journal of Autism and Developmental Disorders, 51*, 1–12. https://doi.org/10.1007/s10803-021-05207-1

Liu, T. L., Hsiao, R. C., Chou, W. J., & Yen, C. F. (2021). Social anxiety in victimization and perpetration of cyberbullying and traditional bullying in adolescents with autism spectrum disorder and attention-deficit/hyperactivity disorder. *International Journal of Environmental Research and Public Health, 18*(11), 5728. https://doi.org/10.3390/ijerph18115728

Liu, S., Xu, B., Zhang, D., Tian, Y., & Wu, X. (2022). Core symptoms and symptom relationships of problematic internet use across early, middle, and late adolescence: A network analysis. *Computers in Human Behavior, 128*, 107090.

Lundqvist, L. O., & Lindner, H. (2017). Is the autism-spectrum quotient a valid measure of traits associated with the autism spectrum? A Rasch validation in adults with and without autism spectrum disorders. *Journal of Autism and Developmental Disorders, 47*(7), 2080–2091. https://doi.org/10.1007/s10803-017-3128-y

MacMullin, J. A., Lunsky, Y., & Weiss, J. A. (2016). Plugged in: Electronics use in youth and young adults with Autism Spectrum Disorder. *Autism, 20*(1), 45–54. https://doi.org/10.1177/1362361314566047

Matthias, C., LaVelle, J. M., Johnson, D. R., Wu, Y. C., & Thurlow, M. L. (2021). Exploring predictors of bullying and victimization of students with autism spectrum disorder (ASD): Findings from NLTS 2012. *Journal of Autism and Developmental Disorders, 51*(12), 4632–4643. https://doi.org/10.1007/s10803-021-04907-y

Mazurek, M. O., & Engelhardt, C. R. (2013a). Video game use and problem behaviors in boys with autism spectrum disorders. *Research in Autism Spectrum Disorders, 7*(2), 316–324. https://doi.org/10.1016/j.rasd.2012.09.008

Mazurek, M. O., & Engelhardt, C. R. (2013b). Video game use in boys with autism spectrum disorder, ADHD, or typical development. *Pediatrics, 132*(2), 260–266. https://doi.org/10.1542/peds.2012-3956

Mazurek, M. O., & Wenstrup, C. (2013). Television, video game and social media use among children with ASD and typically developing siblings. *Journal of Autism and Developmental Disorders, 43*(6), 1258–1271. https://doi.org/10.1007/s10803-012-1659-9

Moor, P. J., Heuvelman, A., & Verleur, R. (2010). Flaming on YouTube. *Computers in Human Behavior, 26*(6), 1536–1546. https://doi.org/10.1016/j.chb.2010.05.023

Moreno, M., Riddle, K., Jenkins, M. C., Singh, A. P., Zhao, Q., & Eickhoff, J. (2022). Measuring problematic internet use, internet gaming disorder, and social media addiction in young adults: Cross-sectional survey study. *JMIR Public Health and Surveillance, 8*(1), e27719.

Murray, A., Koronczai, B., Király, O., Griffiths, M. D., Mannion, A., Leader, G., & Demetrovics, Z. (2021). Autism, problematic internet use and gaming disorder: A systematic review. *Review Journal of Autism and Developmental Disorders, 9*, 120–140. https://doi.org/10.1007/s40489-021-00243-0

Murray, A., Mannion, A., Chen, J. L., & Leader, G. (2022). Gaming disorder in adults with autism spectrum disorder. *Journal of Autism and Developmental Disorders, 52*(6), 2762–2769.

NCA. (2017). *Pathways into cyber crime*. Available at https://www.nationalcrimeagency.gov.uk/who-we-are/publications/6-pathways-into-cyber-crime-1/file

Normand, C. L., Fisher, M. H., Simonato, I., Fecteau, S. M., & Poulin, M. H. (2021). A systematic review of problematic internet use in children, adolescents, and adults with autism spectrum disorder. *Review Journal of Autism and Developmental Disorders, 8*, 1–14. https://doi.org/10.1007/s40489-021-00270-x

Paulus, F. W., Sander, C. S., Nitze, M., Kramatschek-Pfahler, A. R., Voran, A., & von Gontard, A. (2020). Gaming disorder and computer-mediated communication in children and adolescents with autism spectrum disorder. *Zeitschrift für Kinder-und Jugendpsychiatrie und Psychotherapie, 48*(2), 113–122. https://doi.org/10.1024/1422-4917/a000674

Payne, K. L., Russell, A., Mills, R., Maras, K., Rai, D., & Brosnan, M. (2019). Is there a relationship between cyber-dependent crime, autistic-like traits and autism? *Journal of Autism and Developmental Disorders, 49*(10), 4159–4169. https://doi.org/10.1007/s10803-019-04119-5

Ruzich, E., Allison, C., Chakrabarti, B., Smith, P., Musto, H., Ring, H., & Baron-Cohen, S. (2015). Sex and STEM occupation predict autism-spectrum quotient (AQ) scores in half a million people. *PLoS One, 10*(10), e0141229. https://doi.org/10.1371/journal.pone.0141229

Seigfried-Spellar, K. C., O'Quinn, C. L., & Treadway, K. N. (2015). Assessing the relationship between autistic traits and cyberdeviancy in a sample of college students. *Behaviour & Information Technology, 34*(5), 533–542. https://doi.org/10.1080/0144929X.2014.978377

Shane-Simpson, C., Brooks, P. J., Obeid, R., Denton, E. G., & Gillespie-Lynch, K. (2016). Associations between compulsive internet use and the autism spectrum. *Research in Autism Spectrum Disorders, 23*, 152–165. https://doi.org/10.1016/j.rasd.2015.12.005

So, R., Makino, K., Fujiwara, M., Hirota, T., Ohcho, K., Ikeda, S., Tsubouchi, S., & Inagaki, M. (2017). The prevalence of internet addiction among a Japanese adolescent psychiatric clinic sample with autism spectrum disorder and/or attention-deficit hyperactivity disorder: A cross-sectional study. *Journal of Autism and Developmental Disorders, 47*(7), 2217–2224. https://doi.org/10.1007/s10803-017-3148-7

So, R., Makino, K., Hirota, T., Fujiwara, M., Ocho, K., Ikeda, S., Tsubouchi, S., & Inagakip, M. (2019). The 2-year course of internet addiction among a Japanese adolescent psychiatric clinic sample with autism spectrum disorder and/or attention-deficit hyperactivity disorder. *Journal of Autism and Developmental Disorders, 49*(11), 4515–4522. https://doi.org/10.1007/s10803-019-04169-9

Swearer, S. M., & Hymel, S. (2015). Understanding the psychology of bullying: Moving toward a social-ecological diathesis–stress model. *American Psychologist, 70*(4), 344–353. https://doi.org/10.1037/a0038929

Triantafyllopoulou, P., Clark-Hughes, C., & Langdon, P. E. (2021). Social media and cyberbullying in autistic adults. *Journal of Autism and Developmental Disorders, 51*, 1–9. https://doi.org/10.1007/s10803-021-05361-6

Umeda, M., Shimoda, H., Miyamoto, K., Ishikawa, H., Tachimori, H., Takeshima, T., & Kawakami, N. (2021). Comorbidity and sociodemographic characteristics of adult autism spectrum disorder and attention deficit hyperactivity disorder: Epidemiological investigation in the World Mental Health Japan 2nd Survey. *International Journal of Developmental Disabilities, 67*(1), 58–66. https://doi.org/10.1080/20473869.2019.1576409

Vandebosch, H., & Van Cleemput, K. (2008). Defining cyberbullying: A qualitative research into the perceptions of youngsters. *Cyberpsychology & Behavior, 11*(4), 499–503. https://doi.org/10.1089/cpb.2007.0042

World Health Organization. (2022). *ICD-11 for mortality and morbidity statistics*. Retrieved April 20, 2022, from https://icd.who.int/browse11/l-m/en#/http://id.who.int/icd/entity/1448597234

Wright, M. F. (2018). Cyber victimization and depression among adolescents with autism spectrum disorder: The buffering effects of parental mediation and social support. *Journal of Child & Adolescent Trauma, 11*(1), 17–25. https://doi.org/10.1007/s40653-017-0169-5

Wright, M. F., & Wachs, S. (2019). Does peer rejection moderate the associations among cyberbullying victimization, depression, and anxiety among adolescents with autism spectrum disorder? *Children (Basel), 6*(3), 41. https://doi.org/10.3390/children6030041

Young, K. S. (1996). Psychology of computer use: XL. Addictive use of the Internet: A case that breaks the stereotype. *Psychological Reports, 79*(3), 899–902.

Young, K. S. (1998). *Caught in the net: How to recognize the signs of internet addiction and a winning strategy for recovery*. Wiley.

Yu, Y., Bradley, C. C., Boan, A. D., Charles, J. M., & Carpenter, L. A. (2021). Young adults with autism spectrum disorder and the criminal justice system. *Journal of Autism and Developmental Disorders, 51*(10), 3624–3636. https://doi.org/10.1007/s10803-020-04805-9

Zaborskis, A., Ilionsky, G., Tesler, R., & Heinz, A. (2019). The association between cyberbullying, school bullying, and suicidality among adolescents. *Crisis, 40*(2), 100–114. https://doi.org/10.1027/0227-5910/a000536

Chapter 11
Self-Advocacy

11.1 Self-Advocacy: Defining the Concept

Self-advocacy is a civil rights movement developed in the 1960s and 1970s in the USA and the UK and then spread to other parts of the world. Although there is no universal definition of self-advocacy, we could understand this concept as the possibility for a person with disability to speak up for what they want or need (individual self-advocacy), or for individuals to form groups and fight together for their rights and common goals (group or collective self-advocacy) (Dowse, 2001; Ryan & Griffiths, 2015). Self-advocacy is very closely related to the concept of self-determination, which implies that each person should make decisions about and manage their lives (Ryan & Griffiths, 2015; Sebag, 2010; Wehmeyer et al., 2000).

Self-advocacy activities often go beyond "speaking up" and include many other daily activities such as reading, writing, traveling, scheduling and holding meetings, preparing for performances, doing administrative work, etc. (Petri et al., 2020). According to Test et al. (2005), self-advocacy involves four basic components—knowledge of self, knowledge of rights, communication, and leadership. This means that self-advocates should be familiar with their rights and responsibilities, be provided with opportunities to stand up for them, fight for the right to make decisions that concern them through speeches and activities, and encourage others to take control over their lives (Pennell, 2001). Self-advocacy skills are learned. By analyzing and reviewing the literature, Roberts et al. (2014) identified the following opportunities and ways to teach these skills—including self-advocacy in the curricula and vocational training, practicing these skills with peers, writing strategies, transition planning involvement, direct instruction, college-based transition programs, a weeklong program, and supporting students to lead their Individualized Education Plan (IEP) meetings. Teaching self-advocacy skills is associated with an increased perception of social support in the environment, a higher level of academic self-efficacy (Gillespie-Lynch et al., 2017), improved skills for requesting

N. Glumbić et al., *Digital Inclusion of Individuals with Autism Spectrum Disorder*, Autism and Child Psychopathology Series,
https://doi.org/10.1007/978-3-031-12037-4_11

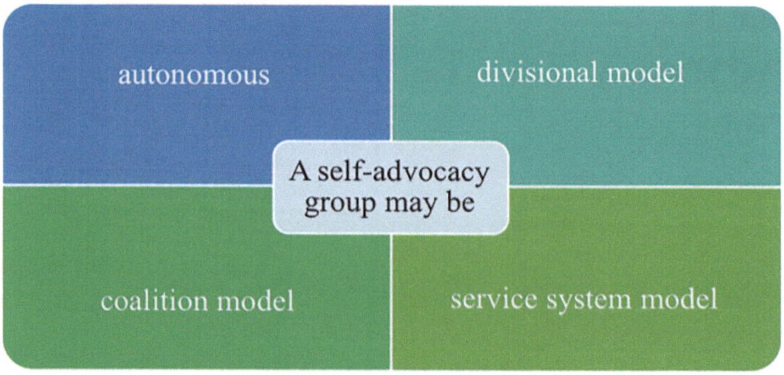

Fig. 11.1 Different types of organization of self-advocacy groups

accommodations (White et al., 2014), improved health self-advocacy skills (Feldman et al., 2012), and greater likelihood of continuing education after high school, finding a job, and living independently (Zhang et al., 2019).

Self-advocacy groups may have different organizational structures (Fig. 11.1). Some may function independently of external factors, others may be a part of a greater organizational structure or coalition with other groups that include people with different disabilities, or they can be linked to organizations that provide support and a wider range of services (Crawley 1988, according to Ryan & Griffiths, 2015). Self-advocates agree that different forms of self-advocacy should not be mistaken for representative advocacy, within which people without disabilities speak on behalf of children or adults with disabilities (Waltz et al., 2015).

11.2 Self-Advocacy and Autism

Until the 1990s, parents or relatives of people with autism, or professionals who worked with them, usually advocated for their rights. After that, the first groups of autistic self-advocates appeared. Since then, there have been constant debates, disagreements, and sometimes even open conflicts between advocates for autism and autistic self-advocates about which group truly articulates the interests of the population it represents (McCoy et al., 2020).

Petri et al. (2020) state that autistic self-advocates fight for the rights of people with autism, inform and educate people about what autism is and is not, support other autistic people, initiate and sign petitions related to topics important for this population, acquire new skills, etc. At the same time, autistic self-advocates fight for different ways of neurocognitive functioning to be respected, i.e., for neurodiversity. Advocating for the rights of people different from neurotypical also involves insisting on specific terminology, i.e., on referring to people from the autistic spectrum as autistic persons or autistics, sometimes even with an initial capital letter ("identity-first" language) (Hughes, 2016; Lei et al., 2021).

Also, autistic self-advocates insist that autistic persons should have the opportunities to develop their sexual identity (Rosqvist, 2013). Advocating for continuing education is another important topic on the list of self-advocacy priorities. With the aim to support autistic people in college in self-advocacy, Autistic Self Advocacy Network (ASAN, 2011) published a handbook with all the necessary information, personal experiences of autistic people, and suggested ideas and guidelines.

Leadbitter et al. (2021) indicate that autistic self-advocates are also for redefining the concept of (early) interventions' effectiveness, abandoning the instruments that assess the degree of symptoms manifestation, and partnership with autistic people in creating research design. Some autistic activists are academics, and their self-advocacy, among other things, also includes publishing articles in journals, at conferences and seminars (Grant & Kara, 2021; Woods et al., 2018); memberships in various scientific organizations such as *Participatory Autism Research Collective*, *International Society for Autism Research (INSAR)*, and *Autistic Researchers Committee*; and using #AutisticsinAcademia on social media (Dwyer et al., 2021). Autistic academics advocate that different research teams include autistic researchers believing that this can contribute to quality and productivity (Dwyer et al., 2021; Grant & Kara, 2021), that autistic researchers are the ones who define the field of research, that it inevitably relies on the social model of disability, and that its results are aimed at improving the lives of people with autism (Chown et al., 2017). In addition, autistic researchers point out numerous barriers that prevent the employment of autistic academics at universities and advocate for overcoming them (Martin, 2020).

Autistic people also state that they would like more self-advocacy related to the lack of support services in situations of late diagnosis, unpleasant and painful experiences with the system, feeling rejected and excluded, and communication barriers (Townson et al., 2007). With regard to this, autistic self-advocates insist on prioritizing the mental health of autistic people in healthcare research, i.e., traumatic experiences these people have had during their lifetime, and on examining all potential adverse effects of medications and interventions they received as children (Benevides et al., 2020).

Although autistic self-advocates are often criticized for fighting only for the rights of high-functioning persons, the representatives of these movements insist that their advocacy includes the rights of people with intellectual disability, entirely dependent persons, those living in institutions, and those who cannot communicate conventionally but use augmentative and alternative communication devices (Ne'eman & Bascom, 2020).

Self-advocacy is not an easy process, and autistic people can face many obstacles such as the lack of financial resources, the lack of time for performing these activities, personal burnout due to overload, doubts the rest of the community may have related to the diagnoses of self-advocates, ideas they promote, conflicts and disagreements with advocacy groups or other formal bodies and organizations, etc. (Waltz et al., 2015).

11.3 Digital Technology and Self-Advocacy

Petri et al. (2021) indicate that new forms of self-advocacy have recently emerged in the population of autistic people through online space, which do not rely on formal organizations but on individual self-advocates. Furthermore, by researching self-advocacy, Petri et al. (2020) point out that autistic self-advocates create websites, record videos, blog, vlog, and share information through social media.

Virtual space can be considered suitable for activism of autistic people (e.g., by posting on forums—writing texts, posting photographs, creating and sharing videos; participating in chat rooms; playing games; sharing experiences; etc.) because the usual distractors from daily face-to-face interactions are reduced to a minimum and because each autistic individual can easily articulate or interpret the messages of neurodiversity (Belek, 2017). According to Rosqvist et al. (2015), members of global online self-advocacy communities are people who function at different neurocognitive levels and those who differ in their verbal abilities.

Online platforms can also be a tool that allows autistic people to be heard. In relation to this, Hughes (2016) points out that, for example, organizers of various gatherings or conferences where these people are discussed should provide different ways in which they can participate—e.g., typing a message, instead of saying it, on *Twitter*, email, or group discussions in virtual space (e.g., *Google*).

According to Autistic Minority International (2019), the Internet contributed to the visibility of autism and enabled the creation of a global self-advocacy movement. However, 44% of the world population still has no access to this network. Thus, in order to increase the availability and accessibility of the Internet to autistic people, this organization advocates for the availability of online education, recognition of written electronic communication as universal design, special training for sellers of technological devices in working with autistic customers, deinstitutionalization of autistic people, and accessibility of information and communication technology (ICT) to people who live in institutions.

Furthermore, autistic people can take different online courses or may use available online resources (articles, books, videos, etc.) to learn about self-advocacy, ways in which they can advocate for themselves, and the possibilities offered by *Facebook*, *Twitter*, *Pinterest*, *Instagram*, video blogs, etc. These courses and resources are free and usually available on the websites of organizations that bring together autistic people and people from their environment, such as ASAN, Asperger/Autism Network (ANNE), Autism After 21, etc. Also, autistic self-advocates can participate in creating online courses on various topics for people with autism (Gillespie-Lynch et al., 2021; Rothman et al., 2022), developing safe online platforms for autistic people to socialize (Zhu et al., 2022), and designing games and applications that can be useful for autistic people (Libbi, 2021; Murphy, 2015).

The analysis of research literature on self-advocacy and technology shows that there are at least three paths that stand out—activities of online self-advocacy communities through text messages, videos, and augmentative and alternative communication (AAC) devices.

11.3.1 Online Discussion Groups: Autistic Space, Forums, and Blogs

The Internet can be the space where significant discussions of people with autism take place, through which experts and other people can learn about autism in a positive light, i.e., go beyond the boundaries of traditional ways of thinking about people with autism. Brownlow and O'Dell (2006) followed the work of an online community of 39 autistic people for 4 months and analyzed all the messages they exchanged. Then, they singled out two important topics through a qualitative discourse analysis: "expert" knowledge of autism and self-identity with group labels. Within the first topic, autistic people discussed who real experts in autism were, whether professional or experiential insights were more important, and who should make the diagnosis—professionals or people with autism themselves. The second topic included questions about how to refer to people with and without autism, how neurotypical persons were different from autistic persons, positive aspects of autism, and whether neurotypicality could be observed in a negative context.

Bertilsdotter Rosqvist et al. (2013) analyzed the content of four online discussion groups of autistic adults over 4 months, or 998 exchanged messages. According to the results, autistic people believe that groups on the Internet are a great way to meet other people and communicate with them and an excellent opportunity to meet like-minded people. Furthermore, this analysis indicates that many autistic people consider real-life spaces to be hostile environments completely adapted to neurotypical people, while the Internet communities support "autistic identity" and enable the creation of online autistic spaces with rules set by autistic people.

By analyzing the interactions between the members of *Aspies Central*, *Wrong Planet*, *Aspies For Freedom*, and *Spectrumville* online communities, Parsloe (2015) used a netnographic approach to analyze online posts and interviews of ten members of these groups. The results show that autistic people in online communities distinguish between naming and labeling, pointing out that labeling is an imposed medical diagnosis while naming means that a person feels autistic and thus identifies with a group with similar experiences. Also, participating in online communities allows autistic people to contact people like them from all over the world and not feel lonely but as a part of a larger group, culture, and community.

Giles (2014) followed the reactions to the announced changes in the DSM-5 classification of the American Psychiatric Association (APA, 2013) with regard to removing the Asperger syndrome category by analyzing 19 threads on over 100 posts in the online communities such as *Wrong Planet, Aspies For Freedom, Aspergers and ASD UK Online Forum, and German Aspies* in the period from 2010 to 2012. The results showed that autistic people in these forums had six main reactions—acceptance, fear, rejection, defiance, reassurance, and suspicion. Some participants felt that any kind of elitism was unacceptable and that fitting Asperger syndrome into the whole spectrum contributed to the sense of belonging. On the other hand, others feared that removing this category might deprive some people of their benefits or that families of people with severe forms of autism would be offended if they were all seen as members of the same group. Some people rejected this idea stating that APA was a nonscientific association that could not be trusted, or they expressed hostility and anger because they were not invited or consulted when the manual was written. Spillers et al. (2014) conducted a similar study examining the reactions to the DSM-5 classification (APA, 2013) in the *Wrong Planet* community by analyzing posts from 2009 to 2012. The participants in this research feared for their identity and the services they were provided with until then and were appalled by how a culture created in the previous decades was being annulled.

Sarrett (2016) examined how self-advocates in the *Wrong Planet* community considered self-diagnosis. The basis of this research was provided by a forum participant who asked why people generally hated those who self-diagnosed. Sarrett (2016) classified all the answers and obtained three main topics—*I accept and support self-diagnosis*, *I reject self-diagnosis*, and *my attitude is halfway*. Forum participants who were against self-diagnosis believed that the diagnosis process was very complex, thus requiring extensive professional training, and that it should be free of bias. Some participants believed that a person could not claim to have autism without a professional diagnosis, i.e., that such claims may be considered speculation. On the other hand, self-advocates who supported self-diagnosis pointed out that too much power and knowledge were attributed to professionals, that non-autistic people could never have the insights and knowledge about autism as autistic people did, and that formal diagnoses were very changeable and often speculative. This group of self-advocates also stated that the formal diagnosis process focused too much on a child's age and that some adults may encounter various obstacles in their environment when trying to reach a professional who would diagnose them with autism in adulthood, which they believed was another argument in favor of self-diagnosis. Also, some people may consider formal diagnosis to be a source of discrimination.

Ringland (2019) analyzed *Autcraft*, an online community for people with autism with over 7000 members, created around the *Minecraft* server. According to this author, this community is a safe place for all persons on the spectrum or those who feel as if they belong to the spectrum. This space provides support to all members and space for nurturing and expressing their identities, but it also shows understanding for all unpleasant experiences of autistic people. In memory of all the violence experienced, one self-advocate built a virtual memorial center with bright glass walls (Fig. 11.2). Within the center, there are about 420 names of the people the creator knows had unpleasant experiences from 1980 to 2016. This place sends a message to the people on the spectrum that they are neither alone nor forgotten.

Nicolaidis et al. (2011) described one way of online collaboration between the autistic and academic community in the field of community-based participatory research. They presented the practice applied within the *Academic Autism Spectrum*

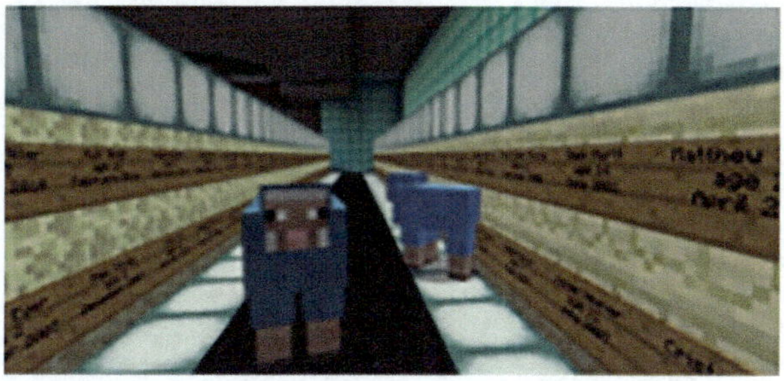

Fig. 11.2 Colorful sheep wander through the rows of names in a memorial to those with disabilities as victims of filicide. (Reproduced from Ringland, 2019)

Partnership in Research and Education (AASPIRE) team consisting of autistic self-advocates from the USA and Germany and non-autistic representatives of the academic community. All members of the AASPIRE team are equal. The team meets online and communicates between meetings by emails, text-based chat, or telephone, especially those participants who feel there was not enough time for a real-time discussion. Written communication uses the text message format with three necessary categories—the purpose of the message, proposed actions, and time to react. Each meeting has a moderator, who takes care of the agenda, the content of the messages participants type during the discussion, and that there are 30–60 s after the last comment and before moving on to a new topic. The AASPIRE team has its own way of voting when making important decisions—the five-finger method for making decisions or reaching consensus. This method allows all participants to vote and understand what is being decided. One finger means that the participant fully agrees and approves the decision; two fingers mean that the participant is not very enthusiastic about the decision but still agrees; three fingers mean that they are not sure how to vote and need more information; four fingers mean they do not like and will not approve it, but can vote for the opposite decision; five fingers mean they dislike it so much that they cannot bear to have their name associated with such decision. A discussion precedes each voting, after which the participants are invited to vote through the five-finger method. The votes are then counted. If everyone has voted with one or two fingers, the decision is made. However, if there are votes with three, four, or five fingers, a new discussion starts with special emphasis on additional explanations and new solutions. After that, the participants are invited to vote with their fingers again, and the votes are counted. The team has the rule to close the discussions after reaching consensus to save time. They can be reopened with reasonable arguments to do so.

Autistic self-advocates sometimes use public online spaces like *Twitter*, *YouTube*, and *Facebook* to influence public policies. Hughes (2016), for example, mentions an event from 2014 when ASAN members made Congress amend the Combating Autism Act by using the *#StopCombatingMe* on most social media and online spaces. This campaign resulted in renaming and modifying the proposed legislation.

Many autistic people participate in blogs, i.e., they write some kind of online personal diaries or messages for the general public to raise awareness about autism

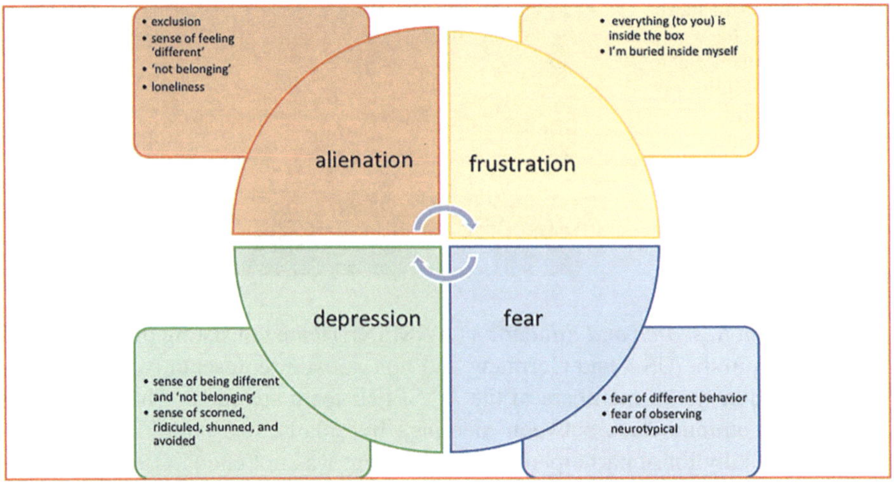

Fig. 11.3 The range of different emotions that people with autism expressed in blogs on the Internet

or share their opinions on various topics related to the spectrum. Jones et al. (2001) analyzed the content of emotional experiences in five first-hand accounts in blogs written by autistic people. The results indicate four basic emotions—a sense of alienation, a sense of frustration, depression, and a pervasive sense of fear or apprehension (Fig. 11.3)

In a similar study, Jones et al. (2003) analyzed five public blogs run by people with autism to learn more about how autistic people experienced sensations from the environment and how they dealt with their sensory experiences. By reviewing the textual content, the authors grouped all topics into four categories—turbulent sensory perceptual experiences, coping mechanisms, enjoyable sensory perceptual experiences, and awareness of being different. From personal stories in the blogs, it could be concluded that autistic people very often had atypical reactions and altered experiences to common daily auditory, visual, tactile, and other sensations and that these altered experiences could be unpleasant for some but pleasure for others.

To understand the autistic burnout construct, Mantzalas et al. (2021) analyzed the discussions of 683 autistic people over the age of 18 on *Twitter* and *Wrong Planet* from 2005 to 2019. They concluded on the participants' autistic status based on the use of the *#ActuallyAutistic*. The results show that burnout in autistic adults can result from chronic stress or a chronic condition. Autistic people pointed out that burnout was the final point they reached when the demands exceeded the possibilities to overcome them. Burnout can occur at all stages of life, and transitions and stressful life events can pose increased risks for its occurrence. Although almost all participants pointed out the adverse effects of burnout on overall life functioning, some stated that burnout was a catalyst for their diagnosis in adulthood and thus offered new perspectives on their own lives.

Seidmann (2018) did a research study on 17 autistic bloggers, analyzed the content of their blogs, and conducted in-depth interviews to examine the process of creating an autistic identity. The results showed that bloggers believed blogging enabled them to self-present and create a personal identity through questioning their autistic experience, the act of diagnosis, and understanding the normalcy and agency concepts. Seidmann (2018) concluded that autistic identity on blogs developed by rejecting normality assumptions, perceiving autism as a difference, and self-accepting autism as an integral part of "me."

11.3.2 Vlogs and Self-Advocacy

Unlike text messages and discussions on various websites, a vlog is a weblog that includes video content where people comment on specific topics, express personal opinions, etc. Apart from verbal messages, these videos can also show certain nonverbal characteristics of speakers—extralinguistic and paralinguistic. By analyzing the vlogs of autistic persons, professionals and other people from the environment can learn a lot about autism and attitudes, beliefs, and feelings of people on the spectrum and then consequently change their attitudes toward them. Another advantage of vlogs and uploading them to *YouTube* is that people do not need special skills or equipment for this activity (Brownlow et al., 2013).

Angulo-Jiménez and DeThorne (2019) analyzed 39 videos from different vlogs uploaded to *YouTube* from 2007 to 2015. The videos lasted between 2 and 39 minutes. Almost all vloggers were from the USA and spoke in English. With regard to gender, there were 26 men and 13 women. The results showed that about 62% of vloggers used language in accordance with the neurodiversity paradigm, i.e., that they narrated about strengths and differences of people on the spectrum, and that 51% of vloggers insisted on presenting positive dimensions of autism. It is interesting that other videos included attitudes related to the medical model of disability and that videos advocating neurodiversity also occasionally mixed social and medical models of disability.

Angulo et al. (2019) selected 36 vlogs to examine how autistics understood neurotypicality. The analysis determined three perspectives—neurotypicality as an achievement, masquerade, and curse. Some autistic people believe that neurotypicality is a tendency to conventional achievements, i.e., fitting into the world of "normal" and "neurotypical." The path to achievement is a process that requires overcoming many barriers, fighting against disability, and striving to alleviate the manifestations of the autistic disorder. With such content, autistic vloggers show other followers that they can achieve a lot despite their difficulties, flaws, and imperfections and that neurotypicality can be achievable. For another group of vloggers, neurotypicality is a masquerade, a game played every day, pretending and camouflaging, i.e., consciously putting effort, energy, and time into making their behavior resemble the behavior of other people in the environment. The third group of vloggers think that neurotypicality is a curse because the appearance of an autistic person corresponds to the appearance of neurotypical people, i.e., an autistic person looks "normal" but is actually not. They point out that the demands of the environment are set too high for the people on the spectrum and that not meeting these demands causes pain and suffering in these people.

Reading (2018) analyzed *YouTube* videos made by autistic people or their parents and campaign videos and films aimed at translating nonverbal behavior of autistic people. She aimed to determine the extent to which these digital products contributed to strengthening the idea of neurodiversity and neuroqueer approach. The analysis singled out the videos considered to help neurotypical persons reconsider their usual sensory perception and better understand different reactions of autistic people (e.g., "Too Much Information"), understand that autism also occurs in females and that they can be creative and imaginative (e.g., Rosie King films), and think about what communication means to them and whether verbal messages are overrated (e.g., Amanda Baggs videos). In addition, Reading (2018) pointed out that, by analyzing videos, she came across those that could have adverse effects on autistic people, i.e., videos that could embarrass or belittle them. These were most frequently documentaries made by parents filming their autistic children when they were injured and had meltdowns and seizures. Although the author was aware that these recordings were published so that the parents could show other neurotypical people that living with an autistic child could sometimes be very challenging, and advocate for specific services or rights in the community, she pointed to an important ethical issue related to the consent of the children being filmed.

11.3.3 Self-Advocacy with the Help of Augmentative and Alternative Communication Devices

IEP meetings are the place for students to put their self-advocacy skills into practice. The question arises as to what happens at IEP meetings with students on the spectrum who have complex support needs or are nonverbal. In her research, Krishnan (2021) included two students with complex support needs around 15 years of age, one of whom had autism and visual impairment. In order to encourage student engagement in class and their performance at IEP meetings, the research used a multiliteracies approach. This means that the students, together with their teachers, created the multimodal book (with personal photographs, videos, and pictures) and their identity charts on the Book Creator tablet application. The results showed that both students were significantly more active at IEP meetings; that they used the created presentations, changed slides and options with their fingers, and expressed satisfaction when showing the videos and photographs they made; and that the autistic student started applauding himself after completing the presentation to encourage others to do the same.

Also, the transition period after high school is a time when young autistic people enter the world of adults and get many opportunities in the environment to talk about themselves, their interests, preferences, or barriers they face. Digital transition portfolios such as This is Me (TiME) may be a potential solution for self-advocacy in people with more pronounced communication difficulties. This application enables young autistic people to share their stories, accompanied by pictures and videos, with other people in their environment with the help of iPhones and iPads. The stories are created by taking into account the receptive and expressive speech of the users, and their pragmatic abilities and executive functions. Each story must include the "About me" section containing important information about the users, such as what they like or dislike, whether they have any health problems, etc. (Müller & Evans, 2022).

Although there are various technological devices nonverbal autistic people can use to speak for themselves during their education, ASAN (2016) points out that it happens that schools do not provide AAC devices to autistic students, i.e., that these students turn to ASAN to draw attention to such behavior of school administrators. ASAN emphasizes that some schools are very rigid and use outdated approaches insisting on verbal communication, although the legislation states that schools are obliged to provide effective ways of communication to all students (e.g., sign-language interpreter, sound amplification, CART technology, materials in Braille and AAC—such as iPad apps, speech-generating devices, letter boards, and symbol systems). Schools sometimes limit the communication of autistic students by giving them only a specific number of pictures to express themselves, so if the student's needs exceed the provided images, they are deprived of the opportunity to express their ideas.

Zisk and Dalton (2019) go one step further and point out that AAC is useful and necessary to many verbal autistic adults for their more adequate self-advocacy, for example, to people who have intermittent, unreliable, and/or insufficient speech. However, these people often face obstacles in using AAC—some of them are not familiar with the existing options; others think that this type of technology is only for those who cannot speak at all; for some insurance does not cover the cost of the equipment because it is believed they have developed speech and do not need this type of aid. Also, some parents do not support AAC, believing it will slow down the improvement of speech production.

Donaldson et al. (2021) state that autistic people were often forced to speak during childhood, although some other forms of communication may have suited them better. They were forced by their parents and therapists, which was exhausting for them. Sometimes AAC devices were taken from them without their consent. Many autistic adults believe that their communication autonomy is reflected in the fact that they can choose how to communicate, with whom, and in what circumstances. Thus, they also believe that they have an indisputable right to AAC. The barriers related to AAC they recognize in adulthood are mainly related to the fact that other people in the environment show impatience while waiting for them to type the answer and usually hurry them. Autistic adults in this research think that professionals should not make assumptions about who needs or requires AAC but that it should be available to everyone from the earliest age.

It can be concluded that, with the help of digital technologies, autistic people can share their attitudes, ideas, and opinions on all topics related to their lives. Digital self-advocacy activities are useful on several levels—they enable autistic people to connect and share their views but also fight for common goals; they provide opportunities for autistic persons and neurotypical representatives of the academic community to work together on different projects, research studies, or services that are in line with the priorities of autistic people; they provide an opportunity for all people in the world to learn more about autism "first hand" and accept the theory of neurodiversity.

References

American Psychiatric Association. (2013). *Diagnostic and statistical manual of mental disorders (DSM-5)* (5th ed.). American Psychiatric Publishing.

Angulo, H., Chan, M., & DeThorne, L. (2019). Life is a stage: Autistic perspectives on neurotypicality. *Autism in Adulthood, 1*(4), 276–285. https://doi.org/10.1089/aut.2019.0024

Angulo-Jiménez, H., & DeThorne, L. (2019). Narratives about autism: An analysis of YouTube videos by individuals who self-identify as autistic. *American Journal of Speech-Language Pathology, 28*(2), 569–590. https://doi.org/10.1044/2018_AJSLP-18-0045

ASAN. (2016, May 19). *A voice for all: Why I'm fighting to help Autistic students access the form of communication that works best for them*. https://autisticadvocacy.org/2016/05/a-voice-for-all-why-im-fighting-to-help-autistic-students-access-the-form-of-communication-that-works-best-for-them/

Autistic Minority International. (2019, June 11). *ICT accessibility for autistic persons and self-advocacy online and off*. https://www.itu.int/en/ITU-T/jca/ahf/Pages/201906-docs.aspx

Autistic Self-Advocacy Network. (2011). *Navigating College: A Handbook on self advocacy written for autistic students from autistic adults*. Available at: http://www.navigatingcollege.org/download.php

Belek, B. (2017). I feel, therefore I matter: Emotional rhetoric and autism self-advocacy. *Anthropology Now, 9*(2), 57–69. https://doi.org/10.1080/19428200.2017.1337967

Benevides, T. W., Shore, S. M., Palmer, K., Duncan, P., Plank, A., Andresen, M. L., Caplan, R., Cook, B., Gassner, D., Hector, B. L., Morgan, L., Nebeker, L., Purkis, Y., Rankowski, B., Witting, K., & Coughlin, S. S. (2020). Listening to the autistic voice: Mental health priorities to guide research and practice in autism from a stakeholder-driven project. *Autism, 24*(4), 822–833. https://doi.org/10.1177/1362361320908410

Bertilsdotter Rosqvist, H., Brownlow, C., & O'Dell, L. (2013). Mapping the social geographies of autism–online and off-line narratives of neuro-shared and separate spaces. *Disability & Society, 28*(3), 367–379. https://doi.org/10.1080/09687599.2012.714257

Brownlow, C., & O'Dell, L. (2006). Constructing an autistic identity: AS voices online. *Mental Retardation, 44*(5), 315–321. https://doi.org/10.1352/0047-6765(2006)44[315:caaiav]2.0.co

Brownlow, C., O'Dell, L., & Rosqvist, H. B. (2013). Commentary: Challenging representations of autism-exploring possibilities for broadcasting the self on YouTube. *Journal on Developmental Disabilities, 19*(1), 90–95.

Chown, N., Robinson, J., Beardon, L., Downing, J., Hughes, L., Leatherland, J., Fox, K., Hickman, L., & MacGregor, D. (2017). Improving research about us, with us: A draft framework for inclusive autism research. *Disability & Society, 32*(5), 720–734. https://doi.org/10.1080/09687599.2017.1320273

Donaldson, A. L., Corbin, E., & McCoy, J. (2021). "Everyone deserves AAC": Preliminary study of the experiences of speaking autistic adults who use augmentative and alternative communication. *Perspectives of the ASHA Special Interest Groups, 6*(2), 315–326. https://doi.org/10.1044/2021_PERSP-20-00220

Dowse, L. (2001). Contesting practices, challenging codes: Self advocacy, disability politics and the social model. *Disability & Society, 16*(1), 123–141. https://doi.org/10.1080/713662036

Dwyer, P., Acevedo, S. M., Brown, H. M., Grapel, J., Jones, S. C., Nachman, B. R., Raymaker, D., & Williams, Z. J. (2021). An expert roundtable discussion on experiences of autistic autism researchers. *Autism in Adulthood, 3*(3), 209–220. https://doi.org/10.1089/aut.2021.29019.rtb

Feldman, M. A., Owen, F., Andrews, A., Hamelin, J., Barber, R., & Griffiths, D. (2012). Health self-advocacy training for persons with intellectual disabilities. *Journal of Intellectual Disability Research, 56*(11), 1110–1121. https://doi.org/10.1111/j.1365-2788.2012.01626.x

Giles, D. C. (2014). 'DSM-V is taking away our identity': The reaction of the online community to the proposed changes in the diagnosis of Asperger's disorder. *Health, 18*(2), 179–195. https://doi.org/10.1177/1363459313488006

Gillespie-Lynch, K., Bublitz, D., Donachie, A., Wong, V., Brooks, P. J., & D'Onofrio, J. (2017). "For a long time our voices have been hushed": Using student perspectives to develop supports for neurodiverse college students. *Frontiers in Psychology, 8*, 1–14. https://doi.org/10.3389/fpsyg.2017.00544

Gillespie-Lynch, K., Bisson, J. B., Saade, S., Obeid, R., Kofner, B., Harrison, A. J., Daou, N., Tricarico, N., Delos Santos, J., Pinkawa, J., & Jordan, A. (2021). If you want to develop an effective autism training, ask autistic students to help you. *Autism*, 1–13. https://doi.org/10.1177/13623613211041006

Grant, A., & Kara, H. (2021). Considering the autistic advantage in qualitative research: The strengths of autistic researchers. *Contemporary Social Science, 16*(5), 589–603. https://doi.org/10.1080/21582041.2021.1998589

Hughes, J. M. (2016). *Increasing neurodiversity in disability and social justice advocacy groups*. Autistic Self Advocacy Network.

Jones, R. S. P., Zahl, A., & Huws, J. C. (2001). First-hand accounts of emotional experiences in autism: A qualitative analysis. *Disability & Society, 16*(3), 393–401. https://doi.org/10.1080/09687590120045950

Jones, R. S. P., Quigney, C., & Huws, J. C. (2003). First-hand accounts of sensory perceptual experiences in autism: A qualitative analysis. *Journal of Intellectual & Developmental Disability, 28*(2), 112–121. https://doi.org/10.1080/1366825031000147058

Krishnan, S. (2021). The role of multiliteracies in changing learning spaces and promoting self-advocacy for students with complex support needs. *Research and Practice for Persons with Severe Disabilities, 46*(2), 108–124. https://doi.org/10.1177/15407969211010307

Leadbitter, K., Buckle, K. L., Ellis, C., & Dekker, M. (2021). Autistic self-advocacy and the neurodiversity movement: Implications for autism early intervention research and practice. *Frontiers in Psychology, 12*. https://doi.org/10.3389/fpsyg.2021.635690

Lei, J., Jones, L., & Brosnan, M. (2021). Exploring an e-learning community's response to the language and terminology use in autism from two massive open online courses on autism education and technology use. *Autism*, 1362361320987963. https://doi.org/10.1177/1362361320987963

Libbi, C. A. (2021). *When life gives you lemons: designing a game with and for autistic girls* [Master's thesis, University of Twente] http://essay.utwente.nl/88356/

Mantzalas, J., Richdale, A. L., Adikari, A., Lowe, J., & Dissanayake, C. (2021). *What is autistic burnout? A thematic analysis of posts on two online platforms*. Autism in Adulthood. https://doi.org/10.1089/aut.2021.0021

Martin, N. (2020). Perspectives on UK university employment from autistic researchers and lecturers. *Disability & Society*, 1–21. https://doi.org/10.1080/09687599.2020.1802

McCoy, M. S., Liu, E. Y., Lutz, A. S., & Sisti, D. (2020). Ethical advocacy across the autism spectrum: Beyond partial representation. *The American Journal of Bioethics, 20*(4), 13–24. https://doi.org/10.1080/15265161.2020.1730482

Müller, E., & Evans, D. P. (2022, January 1). *This Is Me: Using a personalized, electronic transition tool to support self-advocacy in transition-aged young adults*. https://autismspectrumnews.

org/this-is-me-using-a-personalized-electronic-transition-tool-to-support-self-advocacy-in-transition-aged-young-adults/

Murphy J. (2015, August 6). Having a meltdown? Use the emergency chat app for help. *Geek club books: Autism storytelling*. https://geekclubbooks.com/2015/08/meltdown-emergency-chat-app-help

Ne'eman, A., & Bascom, J. (2020). Autistic self advocacy in the developmental disability movement. *The American Journal of Bioethics, 20*(4), 25–27. https://doi.org/10.1080/15265161.2020.1730

Nicolaidis, C., Raymaker, D., McDonald, K., Dern, S., Ashkenazy, E., Boisclair, C., Robertson, S., & Baggs, A. (2011). Collaboration strategies in nontraditional community-based participatory research partnerships: Lessons from an academic–community partnership with autistic self-advocates. *Progress in Community Health Partnerships, 5*(2), 143–150. https://doi.org/10.1353/cpr.2011.0022

Parsloe, S. M. (2015). Discourses of disability, narratives of community: Reclaiming an autistic identity online. *Journal of Applied Communication Research, 43*(3), 336–356. https://doi.org/10.1080/00909882.2015.1052

Pennell, R. L. (2001). Self determination and self-advocacy: Shifting the power. *Journal of Disability Policy Studies, 11*(4), 223–227. https://doi.org/10.1177/104420730101100404

Petri, G., Beadle-Brown, J., & Bradshaw, J. (2020). Redefining self-advocacy: A practice theory-based approach. *Journal of Policy and Practice in Intellectual Disabilities, 17*(3), 207–218. https://doi.org/10.1111/jppi.12343

Petri, G., Beadle-Brown, J., & Bradshaw, J. (2021). 'Even a self-advocate needs to buy milk' – Economic barriers to self-advocacy in the autism and intellectual disability movement. *Scandinavian Journal of Disability Research, 23*(1), 180–191. https://doi.org/10.16993/sjdr.738

Reading, A. (2018). Neurodiversity and communication ethics: How images of autism trouble communication ethics in the globital age. *Cultural Studies Review, 24*(2), 113–129. https://doi.org/10.5130/csr.v24i2.6040

Ringland, K. E. (2019). "Autsome": Fostering an autistic identity in an online Minecraft community for youth with autism. *Lecture Notes in Computer Science*, 132–143. https://doi.org/10.1007/978-3-030-15742-5_12

Roberts, E. L., Ju, S., & Zhang, D. (2014). Review of practices that promote self-advocacy for students with disabilities. *Journal of Disability Policy Studies, 26*(4), 209–220. https://doi.org/10.1177/1044207314540213

Rosqvist, H. B. (2013). Becoming an "autistic couple": Narratives of sexuality and couplehood within the Swedish autistic self-advocacy movement. *Sexuality and Disability, 32*(3), 351–363. https://doi.org/10.1007/s11195-013-9336-2

Rosqvist, H. B., Brownlow, C., & O'Dell, L. (2015). 'An association for all' – Notions of the meaning of autistic self-advocacy politics within a parent-dominated autistic movement. *Journal of Community & Applied Social Psychology, 25*, 219–231. https://doi.org/10.1002/casp.2210

Rothman, E. F., Graham Holmes, L., Caplan, R., Chiang, M., Haberer, B., Gallop, N., Kadel, R., Person, M., Sanchez, A., Quinn, A., & Wharmby, P. (2022). Healthy Relationships on the Autism Spectrum (HEARTS): A feasibility test of an online class co-designed and co-taught with autistic people. *Autism*, 13623613211069421. https://doi.org/10.1177/13623613211069421

Ryan, T. G., & Griffiths, S. (2015). Self-advocacy and its impacts for adults with developmental disabilities. *Australian Journal of Adult Learning, 55*(1), 31–53.

Sarrett, J. C. (2016). Biocertification and neurodiversity: The role and implications of self-diagnosis in autistic communities. *Neuroethics, 9*(1), 23–36. https://doi.org/10.1007/s12152-016-9247-x

Sebag, R. (2010). Behavior management through self-advocacy: A strategy for secondary students with learning disabilities. *Teaching Exceptional Children, 42*(6), 22–29. https://doi.org/10.1177/004005991004200603

Seidmann, V. (2018). *Voice and identity in the autistic space of the blogosphere*. Doctoral thesis, Nanyang Technological University, Singapore. https://doi.org/10.32657/10356/73378

Spillers, J. L. H., Sensui, L. M., & Linton, K. F. (2014). Concerns about identity and services among people with autism and Asperger's regarding DSM–5 changes. *Journal of Social Work in Disability & Rehabilitation, 13*(3), 247–260. https://doi.org/10.1080/1536710x.2014.9121

Test, D. W., Fowler, C. H., Wood, W. M., Brewer, D. M., & Eddy, S. (2005). A conceptual framework of self-advocacy for students with disabilities. *Remedial and Special Education, 26*(1), 43–54. https://doi.org/10.1177/07419325050260010601

Townson, L., Macauley, S., Harkness, E., Docherty, A., Dias, J., Eardley, M., & Chapman, R. (2007). Research project on advocacy and autism. *Disability & Society, 22*(5), 523–536. https://doi.org/10.1080/09687590701427669

Waltz, M., van den Bosch, K., Ebben, H., Van Hal, L., & Schippers, A. (2015). Autism self-advocacy in the Netherlands: Past, present and future. *Disability & Society, 30*(8), 1174–1191. https://doi.org/10.1080/09687599.2015.1090954

Wehmeyer, M. L., Palmer, S. B., Agran, M., Mithaug, D. E., & Martin, J. E. (2000). Promoting causal agency: The self-determination learning model of instruction. *Exceptional Children, 66*, 439–453. https://doi.org/10.1177/001440290006600401

White, G. W., Summers, J. A., Zhang, E., & Renault, V. (2014). Evaluating the effects of a self-advocacy training program for undergraduates with disabilities. *Journal of Postsecondary Education and Disability, 27*(3), 229–244.

Woods, R., Milton, D., Arnold, L., & Graby, S. (2018). Redefining critical autism studies: A more inclusive interpretation. *Disability and Society, 33*(6), 974–979. https://doi.org/10.1080/09687599.2018.1454380

Zhang, D., Roberts, E., Landmark, L., & Ju, S. (2019). Effect of self-advocacy training on students with disabilities: Adult outcomes and advocacy involvement after participation. *Journal of Vocational Rehabilitation, 50*(2), 207–218. https://doi.org/10.3233/JVR-181001

Zhu, R., Hardy, D., & Myers, T. (2022). Community led co-design of a social networking platform with adolescents with autism spectrum disorder. *Journal of Autism and Developmental Disorders, 52*(1), 38–51. https://doi.org/10.1007/s10803-021-04918-9

Zisk, A. H., & Dalton, E. (2019). Augmentative and alternative communication for speaking autistic adults: Overview and recommendations. *Autism in Adulthood, 1*(2), 93–100. https://doi.org/10.1089/aut.2018.0007

Index

N. Glumbić et al., *Digital Inclusion of Individuals with Autism Spectrum Disorder*, Autism and Child Psychopathology Series,
https://doi.org/10.1007/978-3-031-12037-4

Printed by Printforce, the Netherlands